Medical Tests
SOURCEBOOK

Sixth Edition

Health Reference Series

Sixth Edition

Medical Tests
SOURCEBOOK

Basic Consumer Health Information about Preventive Care Guidelines, Routine Health Screenings, Home-Use Tests, Blood, Stool, and Urine Tests, Genetic Testing, Biopsies, Endoscopic Exams, and Imaging Tests, Such as X-Ray, Ultrasound, Computed Tomography (CT), and Nuclear and Magnetic Resonance Imaging (MRI) Exams

Along with Facts about Diagnostic Tests for Allergies, Cancer, Diabetes, Heart and Lung Disease, Infertility, Osteoporosis, Sleep Problems, and Other Specific Conditions, a Glossary of Related Terms, and Directories of Additional Resources

OMNIGRAPHICS

615 Griswold, Ste. 901, Detroit, MI 48226

Bibliographic Note
Because this page cannot legibly accommodate all the copyright notices, the Bibliographic Note portion of the Preface constitutes an extension of the copyright notice.

* * *

OMNIGRAPHICS
Angela L. Williams, *Managing Editor*
***

Copyright © 2018 Omnigraphics
ISBN 978-0-7808-1640-4
E-ISBN 978-0-7808-1641-1

Library of Congress Cataloging-in-Publication Data

Names: Omnigraphics, Inc., issuing body.

Title: Medical tests sourcebook: basic consumer health information about preventive care guidelines, routine health screenings, home-use tests, blood, stool, and urine tests, genetic testing, biopsies, endoscopic exams, and imaging tests, such as X-ray, ultrasound, computed tomography (CT), and nuclear and magnetic resonance imaging (MRI) exams; along with facts about diagnostic tests for allergies, cancer, diabetes, heart and lung disease, infertility, osteoporosis, sleep problems, and other specific conditions, a glossary of related terms, and directories of additional resources.

Description: Sixth edition. | Detroit, MI: Omnigraphics, [2018] | Series: Health reference series | Includes bibliographical references and index.

Identifiers: LCCN 2018024599 (print) | LCCN 2018025555 (ebook) | ISBN 9780780816411 (eBook) | ISBN 9780780816404 (hardcover: alk. paper)

Subjects: LCSH: Diagnosis--Popular works. | Diagnosis, Laboratory--Popular works. | Medicine, Popular.

Classification: LCC RC71.3 (ebook) | LCC RC71.3.M45 2018 (print) | DDC 616.07/5--dc23

LC record available at https://lccn.loc.gov/2018024599

Table of Contents

Part IV: Catheterization, Endoscopic, and Electrical Tests and Assessments

Part V: Screening and Assessments for Specific Conditions and Diseases

Part VI: Home and Self-Ordered Tests

Part VII: Additional Help and Information

Preface

About This Book

Regular medical tests can help find problems before they start. They also can help find problems early, when one's chances for treatment and cure are better. Screening tests identify risk factors for specific disorders, while diagnostic tests find markers of disease or dysfunction. Medical tests assist in diagnosing the causes of symptoms, making treatment decisions, and assessing treatment effectiveness. When faced with decisions about health, consumers need to understand the benefits and limitations of medical tests and how test results guide treatment and lifestyle choices.

Medical Tests Sourcebook, Sixth Edition provides updated information about exams, tests, and other screening, diagnostic, and disease monitoring procedures. It discusses preventive care guidelines and the screening tests used for such specific conditions as allergies, cancer, celiac disease, cardiovascular disorders, diabetes, kidney and thyroid dysfunction, and others. Details about laboratory blood tests, biopsies, throat cultures, toxicology screens, urinalysis, and genetic tests are also presented. Imaging tests, such as X-ray, ultrasound, computed tomography, and magnetic resonance, nuclear, and thermal imaging are described, and facts are offered about electrical, endoscopic, and home-use tests. The book concludes with a glossary of related terms, a list of online health screening tools, and directories of breast and cervical cancer early detection programs and other resources for more information.

How to Use This Book

This book is divided into parts and chapters. Parts focus on broad areas of interest. Chapters are devoted to single topics within a part.

Part I: Screening and Preventive Care Tests are used to identify individuals with specific risk factors for which the timely provision of medical care or other interventions can help avoid or reduce health consequences. These include high blood pressure, high cholesterol, and certain genetic characteristics. Information is included about regular health exams, newborn screening tests, and preventive screening recommendations for all ages.

Part II: Laboratory Tests begins with an overview of lab tests. It identifies the features that distinguish quality services and provides help for understanding lab reports. Information about commonly used diagnostic and preventive care tests is provided along with details about tests of body fluids, such as those that analyze blood, urine, and bone marrow. Specific biopsies and cultures are also explained.

Part III: Imaging Tests describes the many types of imaging available and the accompanying risks associated with exposure to radiation emissions. Imaging tests include radiography (X-rays), contrast studies, ultrasound exams, computed tomography (CT) scans, magnetic resonance imaging (MRI), nuclear imaging, and optical imaging. Mammograms, neurological imaging, and new imaging techniques are also discussed.

Part IV: Catheterization, Endoscopic, and Electrical Tests and Assessments describes tests that use scopes, cameras, and electrical assessments. Cardiac catheterization, endoscopy, and laparoscopy enable physicians to see the structure of the heart, colon, and other areas inside the body. Electrical tests provide data about the functioning of the cardiovascular, brain, and nervous systems.

Part V: Screening and Assessments for Specific Conditions and Diseases explains tests used to identify and monitor conditions such as allergy, cancer, celiac disease, cystic fibrosis, diabetes, heart disease, infectious disease, kidney disease, lung disease, sleep disorders, and thyroid disorders. Information is also provided about hearing assessments, vision tests, and prenatal and infertility tests.

Part VI: Home and Self-Ordered Tests discusses products that offer consumers a private option for the initial screening of fecal occult blood, drug abuse, human immunodeficiency virus (HIV), and other health concerns. The pros and cons of each test are given, and consumers are cautioned to use only tests approved by the U.S. Food and

Drug Administration (FDA). All questions about home or self-ordered test results should be discussed with a healthcare provider.

Part VII: Additional Help and Information provides a glossary of terms related to medical tests and a list of online health screening tools. Directories of early detection programs for breast and cervical cancer and other resources for people undergoing medical tests are also included.

Bibliographic Note

This volume contains documents and excerpts from publications issued by the following government agencies: Agency for Healthcare Research and Quality (AHRQ); Centers for Disease Control and Prevention (CDC); *Eunice Kennedy Shriver* National Institute of Child Health and Human Development (NICHD); Genetics Home Reference (GHR); National Cancer Institute (NCI); National Eye Institute (NEI); National Heart, Lung, and Blood Institute (NHLBI); National Institute of Diabetes and Digestive and Kidney Diseases (NIDDK); National Institute of Environmental Health Sciences (NIEHS); National Institute of Biomedical Imaging and Bioengineering (NIBIB); National Institutes of Health (NIH); National Institute on Deafness and Other Communication Disorders (NIDCD); Office of Disease Prevention and Health Promotion (ODPHP); Office on Women's Health (OWH); U.S. Department of Health and Human Services (HHS); U.S. Department of Veterans Affairs (VA); and U.S. Food and Drug Administration (FDA).

It may also contain original material produced by Omnigraphics and reviewed by medical consultants.

About the Health Reference Series

The *Health Reference Series* is designed to provide basic medical information for patients, families, caregivers, and the general public. Each volume takes a particular topic and provides comprehensive coverage. This is especially important for people who may be dealing with a newly diagnosed disease or a chronic disorder in themselves or in a family member. People looking for preventive guidance, information about disease warning signs, medical statistics, and risk factors for health problems will also find answers to their questions in the *Health Reference Series*. The *Series*, however, is not intended to serve as a tool for diagnosing illness, in prescribing treatments, or as a substitute for the physician/patient relationship. All people concerned about medical symptoms or the possibility of disease are encouraged to seek professional care from an appropriate healthcare provider.

A Note about Spelling and Style

Health Reference Series editors use *Stedman's Medical Dictionary* as an authority for questions related to the spelling of medical terms and the *Chicago Manual of Style* for questions related to grammatical structures, punctuation, and other editorial concerns. Consistent adherence is not always possible, however, because the individual volumes within the *Series* include many documents from a wide variety of different producers, and the editor's primary goal is to present material from each source as accurately as is possible. This sometimes means that information in different chapters or sections may follow other guidelines and alternate spelling authorities. For example, occasionally a copyright holder may require that eponymous terms be shown in possessive forms (Crohn's disease vs. Crohn disease) or that British spelling norms be retained (leukaemia vs. leukemia).

Medical Review

Omnigraphics contracts with a team of qualified, senior medical professionals who serve as medical consultants for the *Health Reference Series*. As necessary, medical consultants review reprinted and originally written material for currency and accuracy. Citations including the phrase "Reviewed (month, year)" indicate material reviewed by this team. Medical consultation services are provided to the *Health Reference Series* editors by:

Dr. Vijayalakshmi, MBBS, DGO, MD
Dr. Senthil Selvan, MBBS, DCH, MD
Dr. K. Sivanandham, MBBS, DCH, MS (Research), PhD

Our Advisory Board

We would like to thank the following board members for providing initial guidance on the development of this series:

- Dr. Lynda Baker, Associate Professor of Library and Information Science, Wayne State University, Detroit, MI

- Nancy Bulgarelli, William Beaumont Hospital Library, Royal Oak, MI

- Karen Imarisio, Bloomfield Township Public Library, Bloomfield Township, MI

- Karen Morgan, Mardigian Library, University of Michigan-Dearborn, Dearborn, MI

- Rosemary Orlando, St. Clair Shores Public Library, St. Clair Shores, MI

Health Reference Series *Update Policy*

The inaugural book in the *Health Reference Series* was the first edition of *Cancer Sourcebook* published in 1989. Since then, the *Series* has been enthusiastically received by librarians and in the medical community. In order to maintain the standard of providing high-quality health information for the layperson the editorial staff at Omnigraphics felt it was necessary to implement a policy of updating volumes when warranted.

Medical researchers have been making tremendous strides, and it is the purpose of the *Health Reference Series* to stay current with the most recent advances. Each decision to update a volume is made on an individual basis. Some of the considerations include how much new information is available and the feedback we receive from people who use the books. If there is a topic you would like to see added to the update list, or an area of medical concern you feel has not been adequately addressed, please write to:

Managing Editor
Health Reference Series
Omnigraphics
615 Griswold, Ste. 901
Detroit, MI 48226

Part One

Screening and
Preventive Care Tests

Chapter 1

Regular Health Exams Are Important

Chapter Contents

Section 1.1

Why Regular Health Exams Are Important

This section contains text excerpted from the following sources: Text beginning with the heading "Why Are Check-Ups Important?" is excerpted from "Health Equity—Regular Check-Ups Are Important," Centers for Disease Control and Prevention (CDC), August 2, 2017; Text beginning with the heading "When Getting Medical Tests" is excerpted from "When Getting Medical Tests," Agency for Healthcare Research and Quality (AHRQ), U.S. Department of Health and Human Services (HHS), September 2012. Reviewed July 2018.

Why Are Check-Ups Important?

Regular health exams and tests can help find problems before they start. They also can help find problems early, when your chances for treatment and cure are better. By getting the right health services, screenings, and treatments, you are taking steps that help your chances for living a longer, healthier life. Your age, health and family history, lifestyle choices (i.e., what you eat, how active you are, whether you smoke), and other important factors impact what and how often you need healthcare.

Where Can I Go for Health Services?

The best place to go for health services is your regular healthcare provider. However, if you do not have one, the links below provide other options.

What Health Services Are Recommended?

The health services are listed below:

- Breast and cervical cancer early detection
- Cholesterol
- Colorectal cancer screening
- High blood pressure
- Immunization schedules
- Oral health for adults
- Prostate cancer screening

4

- Skin cancer: basic information
- Human immunodeficiency virus (HIV)/acquired immunodeficiency virus (AIDS)
- Viral hepatitis

How Can I Prepare for My Appointment?

- Check-Up Checklist: Things to Do Before Your Next Check-Up
- Family History: Tools and Resources
- Women's Preventive Services: Required Health Plan Coverage Guidelines

Check-Up Checklist: Things to Do before Your Next Check-Up

Getting check-ups is one of many things you can do to help stay healthy and prevent disease and disability. You've made the appointment to see your healthcare provider. You've reviewed the instructions on how to prepare for certain tests. You've done the usual paperwork. Done, right? Not quite. Before your next check-up, make sure you do these four things.

Review Your Family Health History

Are there any new conditions or diseases that have occurred in your close relatives since your last visit? If so, let your healthcare provider know. Family history might influence your risk of developing heart disease, stroke, diabetes, or cancer. Your provider will assess your risk of disease based on your family history and other factors. Your provider may also recommend things you can do to help prevent disease, such as exercising more, changing your diet, or using screening tests to help detect disease early.

Find out If You Are Due for Any General Screenings or Vaccinations

Have you had the recommended screening tests based on your age, general health, family history, and lifestyle? Check with your healthcare provider to see if its time for any vaccinations, follow-up exams, or tests. For example, it might be time for you to get a Papanicolaou test (Pap) test, mammogram, prostate cancer screening, colon cancer screening, sexually transmitted disease (STD) screening, blood pressure check, tetanus shot, eye check, or other screening.

Write down a List of Issues and Questions to Take with You

Review any existing health problems and note any changes.

- Have you noticed any body changes, including lumps or skin changes?
- Are you having pain, dizziness, fatigue, problems with urine or stool, or menstrual cycle changes?
- Have your eating habits changed?
- Are you experiencing depression, anxiety, trauma, distress, or sleeping problems?

If so, note when the change began, how it's different from before, and any other observation that you think might be helpful.

Be honest with your provider. If you haven't been taking your medication as directed, exercising as much, or anything else, say so. You may be at risk for certain diseases and conditions because of how you live, work, and play. Your provider develops a plan based partly on what you say you do. Help ensure that you get the best guidance by providing the most up-to-date and accurate information about you.

Be sure to write your questions down beforehand. Once you're in the office or exam room, it can be hard to remember everything you want to know. Leave room between questions to write down your provider's answers.

Consider Your Future

Are there specific health issues that need addressing concerning your future? Are you thinking about having infertility treatment, losing weight, taking a hazardous job, or quitting smoking? Discuss any issues with your provider so that you can make better decisions regarding your health and safety.

When Getting Medical Tests

Doctors order blood tests, X-rays, and other tests to help diagnose medical problems. Perhaps you do not know why you need a particular test or you don't understand how it will help you. Here are some questions to ask:

- How is the test done?
- What kind of information will the test provide?
- Is this test the only way to find out that information?
- What are the benefits and risks of having this test?
- How accurate is the test?
- What do I need to do to prepare for the test? (What you do or don't do may affect the accuracy of the test results.)
- Will the test be uncomfortable?
- How long will it take to get the results, and how will I get them?
- What's the next step after the test?

What Can You Do?

- For tests your doctor sends to a lab, ask which lab he or she uses, and why. You may want to know that the doctor chooses a certain lab because he or she has business ties to it. Or, the health plan may require that the tests go there.
- Check to see that the lab is accredited by a group such as the College of American Pathologists (CAP) (800-323-4040) or the Joint Commission on Accreditation of Healthcare Organizations (JCAHO) (telephone: 630-792-5800; website: jointcommission.org).
- If you need a mammogram, make sure the facility is approved by the U.S. Food and Drug Administration (FDA). You can find out by checking the certificate in the facility. Or, call 800-4-CANCER (800-422-6237) 9:00 a.m. to 4:30 p.m. EST to find out the names and locations of certified facilities near you.

What about the Test Results?

- Do not assume that no news is good news. If you do not hear from your doctor, call to get your test results.
- If you and your doctor think the test results may not be right, have the test done again. Remember, quality matters, especially when it comes to your health.

Section 1.2

Women: Stay Healthy at Any Age

This section includes text excerpted from "Women:
Stay Healthy at Any Age," Agency for Healthcare Research and
Quality (AHRQ), U.S. Department of Health and Human
Services (HHS), May 2014. Reviewed July 2018.

Get the Screenings You Need

Screenings are tests that look for diseases before you have symptoms. Blood pressure checks and mammograms are examples of screenings. You can get some screenings, such as blood pressure readings, in your doctor's office. Others, such as mammograms, need special equipment, so you may need to go to a different office. After a screening test, ask when you will see the results and who to talk to about them.

Breast cancer. Talk with your healthcare team about whether you need a mammogram.

BRCA1 and BRCA2 genes. If you have a family member with breast, ovarian, or peritoneal cancer, talk with your doctor or nurse about your family history. Women with a strong family history of certain cancers may benefit from genetic counseling and *BRCA* genetic testing.

Cervical cancer. Starting at age 21, get a Papanicolaou (Pap) test (Pap smear) every 3 years until you are 65 years old. Women 30 years of age or older can choose to switch to a combination Pap smear and human papillomavirus (HPV) test every 5 years until the age of 65. If you are older than 65 or have had a hysterectomy, talk with your doctor or nurse about whether you still need to be screened.

Colon cancer. Between the ages of 50 and 75, get a screening test for colorectal cancer. Several tests—for example, a stool test or a colonoscopy—can detect this cancer. Your healthcare team can help you decide which is best for you. If you are between the ages of 76 and 85, talk with your doctor or nurse about whether you should continue to be screened.

Depression. Your emotional health is as important as your physical health. Talk to your healthcare team about being screened for depression, especially if during the last 2 weeks:

- You have felt down, sad, or hopeless

- You have felt little interest or pleasure in doing things

Diabetes. Get screened for diabetes (high blood sugar) if you have high blood pressure or if you take medication for high blood pressure. Diabetes can cause problems with your heart, brain, eyes, feet, kidneys, nerves, and other body parts.

Hepatitis C virus (HCV). Get screened one time for HCV infection if:

- You were born between 1945 and 1965
- You have ever injected drugs
- You received a blood transfusion before 1992

If you currently are an injection drug user, you should be screened regularly.

High blood cholesterol. Have your blood cholesterol checked regularly with a blood test if:

- You use tobacco
- You are overweight or obese
- You have a personal history of heart disease or blocked arteries
- A male relative in your family had a heart attack before age 50 or a female relative, before age 60

High blood pressure. Have your blood pressure checked at least every 2 years. High blood pressure can cause strokes, heart attacks, kidney and eye problems, and heart failure.

Human immunodeficiency virus (HIV). If you are 65 or younger, get screened for HIV. If you are older than 65, talk to your doctor or nurse about whether you should be screened.

Lung cancer. Talk to your doctor or nurse about getting screened for lung cancer if you are between the ages of 55 and 80, have a 30 pack-year smoking history, and smoke now or have quit within the past 15 years. (Your pack-year history is the number of packs of cigarettes smoked per day times the number of years you have smoked.) Know that quitting smoking is the best thing you can do for your health.

Overweight and obesity. The best way to learn if you are overweight or obese is to find your body mass index (BMI). You can find your BMI by entering your height and weight into a BMI calculator.

A BMI between 18.5 and 25 indicates a normal weight. Persons with a BMI of 30 or higher may be obese. If you are obese, talk to your doctor or nurse about getting intensive counseling and help with changing your behaviors to lose weight. Overweight and obesity can lead to diabetes and cardiovascular disease.

Osteoporosis (Bone thinning). Have a screening test at age 65 to make sure your bones are strong. The most common test is a dual-energy X-ray absorptiometry (DEXA) scan—a low-dose X-ray of the spine and hip. If you are younger than 65 and at high risk for bone fractures, you should also be screened. Talk with your healthcare team about your risk for bone fractures.

Sexually transmitted infections (STIs). STIs can make it hard to get pregnant, may affect your baby, and can cause other health problems.

- Get screened for chlamydia and gonorrhea infections if you are 24 years or younger and sexually active. If you are older than 24 years, talk to your doctor or nurse about whether you should be screened.

- Ask your doctor or nurse whether you should be screened for other STI.

Get Preventive Medicines If You Need Them

Aspirin. If you are 55 or older, ask your healthcare team if you should take aspirin to prevent strokes. Your healthcare team can help you decide whether taking aspirin to prevent stroke is right for you.

Breast cancer drugs. Talk to your doctor about your risks for breast cancer and whether you should take medicines that may reduce those risks. Medications to reduce breast cancer have some potentially serious harms, so think through both the potential benefits and harms.

Folic acid. If you of an age at which you can get pregnant, you should take a daily supplement containing 0.4–0.8 mg of folic acid.

Vitamin D to avoid falls. If you are 65 or older and have a history of falls, mobility problems, or other risks for falling, ask your doctor about taking a vitamin D supplement to help reduce your chances of falling. Exercise and physical therapy may also help.

Immunizations:

- Get a flu shot every year

- Get shots for tetanus, diphtheria, and whooping cough. Get tetanus booster if it has been more than 10 years since your last shot.

- If you are 60 or older, get a shot to prevent shingles

- If you are 65 or older, get a pneumonia shot

- Talk with your healthcare team about whether you need other vaccinations

Take Steps to Good Health

- Be physically active and make healthy food choices

- Get to a healthy weight and stay there. Balance the calories you take in from food and drink with the calories you burn off by your activities.

- Be tobacco free. For tips on how to quit, go to www.smokefree. gov. To talk to someone about how to quit, call the National Quitline: 800-QUIT-NOW (800-784-8669).

- If you drink alcohol, have no more than one drink per day. A standard drink is one 12-ounce bottle of beer or wine cooler, one 5-ounce glass of wine, or 1.5 ounces of 80-proof distilled spirits.

Section 1.3

Men: Take Charge of Your Health

This section includes text excerpted from "Men: Take
Charge of Your Health," Office of Disease Prevention and Health
Promotion (ODPHP), U.S. Department of Health and
Human Services (HHS), May 15, 2018.

Most men need to pay more attention to their health. Compared to women, men are more likely to:

- Smoke

- Drink alcohol

- Make unhealthy or risky choices

- Put off regular checkups and medical care

The good news is that you can start taking better care of your health today

How Can I Take Charge of My Health?

See a doctor for regular checkups even if you feel fine. This is important because some diseases and health conditions don't have symptoms at first. Plus, seeing a doctor will give you a chance to learn more about your health.

You can also take care of your health by:

- Getting screening tests that are right for you

- Making sure you are up-to-date on important shots

- Watching out for signs of health problems like diabetes or depression

- Eating healthy and being active

It's Not Too Late to Start Healthier Habits

Make eating healthy and being active part of your daily routine. A healthy diet and regular physical activity can help lower your:

- Blood pressure

- Blood sugar

- Cholesterol

- Weight

By keeping these numbers down, you can lower your risk of serious health problems like type 2 diabetes and heart disease.

You can also help prevent health problems by:

- Drinking alcohol only in moderation

- Quitting smoking

Take Action!

Use these tips to take charge of your health.

Talk about It

Don't be embarrassed to talk about your health. Start by talking to family members to find out which diseases run in your family.

Get Preventive Care to Stay Healthy

Many people think of the doctor as someone to see when they are sick. But doctors also provide services—like shots and screening tests—that help keep you from getting sick in the first place.

Get Screening Tests to Find Problems Early

Screenings are medical tests that doctors use to check for diseases and health conditions before there are any signs or symptoms. Screenings help find problems early, when they may be easier to treat.

- Get your blood pressure checked regularly starting at age 18. Find out how often you need to get your blood pressure checked.

- Talk to your doctor about getting your cholesterol checked. You could have high cholesterol and not know it.

- If you are age 50–75, get tested regularly for colorectal cancer. Ask your doctor what type of colorectal cancer screening test is right for you.

- If you are a man age 65–75 and have ever smoked, talk with your doctor about your risk for abdominal aortic aneurysm (AAA).

- Ask your doctor to screen you for depression. Most people with depression feel better when they get treatment.

13

Make Small Changes Every Day

Small changes can add up to big results—like lowering your risk of type 2 diabetes or heart disease.

- Take a walk instead of having a cigarette
- Try a green salad instead of fries
- Drink water instead of soda or juice

Ask Your Doctor about Taking Aspirin Every Day

If you are age 50–59, taking aspirin every day can lower your risk of heart attack and colorectal cancer. Talk with your doctor about whether daily aspirin is right for you.

What about Cost?

Depending on your insurance plan, you may be able to get screenings and shots at no cost to you.

The Affordable Care Act (ACA), the healthcare reform law passed in 2010, requires most insurance plans to cover many screening tests. This means you may be able to get screening tests at no cost to you. Check with your insurance provider to find out what's included in your plan.

- Find out which services are covered under the ACA.
- Find out which services are covered by Medicare.

Even if you don't have insurance, you can still get healthcare. Find a health center near you and make an appointment.

Section 1.4

Five Minutes (Or Less) for Health

This section includes text excerpted from "Health Equity—Five Minutes (Or Less) for Health," Centers for Disease Control and Prevention (CDC), December 23, 2015.

Take five for your health! Being healthy and safe takes commitment, but it doesn't have to be time-consuming. Most things are so simple and take so little time, that you'll wonder why you've been avoiding them. Taking just a few of the 1440 minutes in a day is worth having a safer and healthier life for you and your family. Below are some steps you can take to help protect your health and safety in five minutes or less.

Test Smoke Alarms

Every month, check your smoke alarms to ensure they work properly. Check or replace the battery to your smoke alarm and carbon monoxide detector when you change the time on your clocks each spring and fall. If the alarm or detector sounds, leave your home immediately, and call 911.

Do a Skin and Body Check

Check your skin and body regularly for lumps, rashes, sores, discolorations, limitations, and other changes. Do checks during and after bathing. Take note of other changes such as those related to urine or bowel habits, thirst, hunger, fatigue, discharge, vision, and weight. If you find or experience anything suspicious, see your healthcare provider.

Make an Appointment

One of the best and easiest ways for adults to keep themselves healthy is to make sure they get recommended exams, screenings and immunizations. Screenings are designed to help detect some diseases in their early, most treatable stages. Make the appointment now.

Know Your Numbers

Keep track of your numbers for blood pressure, blood sugar, cholesterol, body mass index (BMI), and others. These numbers can provide a glimpse of your health status and risk for certain diseases and conditions, including heart disease, diabetes, obesity, and more. Be sure to ask your healthcare provider what tests you need and how often. If your numbers are too high or too low, he/she can make recommendations to help you get them to a healthier range.

Make Sure You Are Up-to-Date on Your Vaccinations

Keep track of your and your family's vaccinations, and make sure they stay up-to-date. Children, young adults, and older adults all need vaccinations. Vaccinations help protect people from diseases and save lives.

Eat Healthy

Take the extra time to make better food choices. Eat more fruits and vegetables as a meal, less saturated fat, and healthy grab-and-go snacks. There are many quick and easy ways to add healthier choices to your day.

Wash Children's Hands and Toys Regularly

Hands and toys can become contaminated from household dust or exterior soil, both of which are sources of harmful lead.

Know Important Asthma Triggers

An asthma attack can occur when you are exposed to things in the environment, such as house dust mites and tobacco smoke. These are called asthma triggers. Your personal triggers can be very different from those of another person.

Learn the Signs for Developmental Problems

Check to see if your children can do the things associated with their age. From birth to 5 years, your children should reach milestones in how they play, learn, speak, and act. A delay in any of these areas could be a sign of a developmental problem.

Know the Signs and Symptoms for Heart Attack and Stroke

If you or someone you know is having a heart attack or stroke, call 911 immediately. With timely treatment, a person's chance of surviving a heart attack is increased, and the risk of death and disability from stroke can be lowered.

Encourage Health through Play

Encourage kids to adopt safe and healthy habits with these fun pages and activity book. Children and adolescents should do 60 minutes (1 hour) or more of physical activity each day.

Take a Break

If you think you're getting sick, feel yourself losing control, or are dealing with stress, take a break. Just taking a few minutes can give you the opportunity to clear your head so you can make better decisions about your and your family's health and safety.

Take Care of Your Teeth and Gums

Drink fluoridated water and use a fluoride toothpaste. Fluoride's protection against tooth decay works at all ages. Brush and floss your teeth thoroughly to reduce dental plaque and help prevent gingivitis (a form of gum disease).

Keep Foods Safe

Refrigerate leftovers promptly. Bacteria can grow quickly at room temperature, so refrigerate leftover foods if they are not going to be eaten within 4 hours. Wash hands, utensils, and cutting boards after they have been in contact with raw meat or poultry and before they touch another food. Wash produce. Cook meat, poultry, and eggs thoroughly. Report suspected foodborne illnesses to your local health department.

Ask Questions

Before seeing your healthcare provider, write down all of your questions and bring the list with you to your appointment. Write down the answers during your discussion. Make sure all of your questions are answered before you leave and you know exactly what the next steps are. Don't risk injury or other problems because you are not clear on what to do.

If instructions are confusing, get help. Talk to your healthcare provider. Call or visit the website of the pharmacy, clinic, equipment manufacturer, or business for information. Make sure you use credible sources and websites and ask your healthcare provider if the information you found applies to you. With more knowledge, you can make better decisions about your health.

Listen to a Health Podcast

Podcasts on a variety of health and safety topics are available online. Most are one to five minutes long, and some are longer.

Disinfect Surfaces to Keep Germs Away

Cleaning removes germs from surfaces, and disinfecting destroys germs from surfaces. Disinfecting after cleaning gives an extra level of protection from germs. Areas with the largest amounts of germs and frequently used areas—such as the kitchen and bathroom—should be disinfected with a bleach solution or another disinfectant as often as possible to avoid the spread of germs.

If You Have Diabetes, Check for Sores and Vision Changes

If you have diabetes, check your feet every day for cuts, blisters, red spots, and swelling. Call your doctor immediately if you have sores that will not heal. Also, tell your doctor if you notice any changes in your eyesight.

Get a Radon Test for Your Home

Radon is a cancer-causing natural radioactive gas that you can't see, smell or taste. Its presence in your home can pose a danger to your family's health. Radon is the second leading cause of lung cancer in America and claims about 20,000 lives annually. Nearly 1 out of every 15 homes in the United States is estimated to have elevated radon levels. Testing is inexpensive and easy.

Go Green

Lower greenhouse gases in the environment, reuse products, and recycle items that can no longer be used.

Learn Healthy Contact Lens Wear and Care

You only have one pair of eyes, so take care of them! Healthy Habits = Healthy Eyes. Enjoy the comfort and benefits of contact lenses while lowering your chance of complications. Failure to wear, clean, and store your lenses as directed by your eye doctor raises the risk of developing serious infections. Your habits, supplies, and eye doctor are all essential to keeping your eyes healthy.

Chapter 2

Questions about
Medical Tests

A registered nurse in her mid-40s, Nancy Keelan was concerned that her heavy, irregular bleeding could be something more serious than the start of menopause. But her doctor did not agree and told her on several occasions not to worry.

Three years later, at age 46, Keelan discovered she had advanced endometrial and ovarian cancer.

At present, she speaks to women's groups and advises them not to wait to see their doctors if they develop new, unusual symptoms, according to a recent Cable News Network (CNN) news report. Keelan also urges women who are worried about new symptoms to ask their doctors if they should be tested to diagnose or rule out a disease or illness.

If a nurse like Keelan—who is familiar with medical tests and terms—didn't insist that her doctor perform a test when she experienced symptoms, I wouldn't be surprised if you were also reluctant to ask for a test. That's why her story and her advice are so important. Asking questions about medical tests—which ones you need, which ones you don't, and what the results tell you—can help you stay healthy and alert your doctor to the signs of a medical problem.

This chapter includes text excerpted from "Asking Questions about Medical Tests," Agency for Healthcare Research and Quality (AHRQ), U.S. Department of Health and Human Services (HHS), October 2014. Reviewed July 2018.

A wide array of medical tests are available today that can detect disease or illness at an early stage, when many conditions can be treated effectively. Your physician shouldn't prescribe tests that you don't need, but you should get the tests that are right for your age, gender, and medical history.

Ask your doctor:

- How is the test done?

- What kind of information will the test provide?

- Is this test the only way to find out that information?

- What are the risks and benefits of having this test?

- How accurate is the test?

- What do I need to do to prepare for the test?

- Will the test be uncomfortable?

- How long will it take to get the results, and how will I get them?

- What's the next step after the test?

Your doctor should be able to tell you when the results of your medical test will be ready. Do not assume that everything is fine if you don't hear from your doctor. Tests results can get lost, or people can think someone else gave you the results. No news is not necessarily good news.

In fact, a study conducted at Harvard Medical School (HMS) found that up to 33 percent of doctors did not always notify patients about abnormal test results. If you don't hear from your doctor, call to get your results.

It is also possible that your test results are incorrect. If you or your doctor think the test results may not be right, retake the test. A second test can confirm or rule out a diagnosis.

It's also a good idea to get information on the lab your doctor uses to analyze test results. For example, you may want to know if your doctor uses a lab because he or she has a business arrangement with them or if a health insurance company requires your doctor to use a certain lab.

You can find out if a lab is accredited by or has a seal of approval from groups such as the College of American Pathologists (CAP) or the Joint Commission. Both groups require labs to meet certain standards, which are linked to better-quality services.

If you need a mammogram, which is a test to detect breast cancer, make sure the test is performed at a facility that is approved by the U.S. Food and Drug Administration (FDA). You can ask this when you make your appointment, or you can call 800-4-CANCER (800-422-6237) to find out the names and locations of approved facilities in your area. By asking your doctor questions about medical tests and your test results, you will have the information that you need to make smart decisions about your healthcare.

Chapter 3

Newborn Screening Tests

Newborn screening programs across the United States screen 4 million infants each year. This public health program detects treatable disorders in newborns, allowing treatment to begin often before symptoms or permanent problems occur. Newborn screening not only saves lives, but can also improve the health and quality of life for children and their families.

Within the first 24–48 hours after birth, babies undergo a simple heel stick and a few drops of blood are collected on a special paper card. Healthcare providers then test those blood spots for a number of congenital disorders (conditions that are present at birth). Infants are also screened for hearing disorders and for other serious heart problems using methods other than dried blood spots.

When a screen is positive for any condition, the newborn's parents are informed that their infant has an "out-of-range" test result for one of the conditions. But a positive screening test does not mean the infant has a disorder. Additional testing is needed to confirm and diagnose the condition.

Only about one out of 300 newborns is later diagnosed with a treatable condition. Once the condition is confirmed, the infant is referred to an appropriate specialist so that treatment can begin as early as possible.

This chapter contains text excerpted from the following sources: Text in this section begins with excerpts from "About Newborn Screening," *Eunice Kennedy Shriver* National Institute of Child Health and Human Development (NICHD), September 1, 2017; Text beginning with the heading "Screening Costs" is excerpted from "Talk with Your Doctor about Newborn Screening," U.S. Department of Health and Human Services (HHS), June 26, 2018.

What Is the Purpose of Newborn Screening?

The purpose of newborn screening is to detect potentially fatal or disabling conditions in newborns as early as possible, often before the infant displays any signs or symptoms of a disease or condition. Such early detection allows treatment to begin immediately, which reduces or even eliminates the effects of the condition. Many of the conditions detectable in newborn screening, if left untreated, have serious symptoms and effects, such as lifelong nervous system damage; intellectual, developmental, and physical disabilities; and even death.

The Advisory Committee on Heritable Disorders in Newborns and Children (ACHDNC), formerly the Discretionary Advisory Committee on Heritable Disorders in Newborns and Children (DACHDNC), is the federal government committee charged with reducing morbidity and mortality in newborns and children who have or are at risk for heritable disorders such as sickle cell anemia, cystic fibrosis, and hearing impairment.

The committee issues a Recommended Uniform Screening Panel (RUSP) that identifies a number of core conditions—those that states are highly recommended to screen for—and secondary conditions, for which screening is optional. The committee's recommendations are based on the *Newborn Screening: Towards a Uniform Screening Panel and System* and on current research evidence, which means that the number of core and secondary conditions may change. As of November 2016, the RUSP included 34 core conditions and 26 secondary conditions.

The committee also advises the U.S. Department of Health and Human Services (HHS) Secretary on the most appropriate application of universal newborn screening tests, technologies, policies, guidelines, and standards. Specifically, the committee provides to the Secretary the following:

- advice and recommendations concerning grants and projects authorized under the Heritable Disorders Program administered by the Health Resources and Services Administration (HRSA);

- technical information to develop Heritable Disorders Program policies and priorities that will enhance the ability of the state and local health agencies to provide screening, counseling, and healthcare services for newborns and children who have or are at risk for heritable disorders; and

- recommendations, advice, and information to enhance, expand, or improve the ability of the Secretary to reduce mortality and morbidity from heritable disorders in newborns and children.

What Disorders Are Newborns Screened for in the United States?

The ACHDNC issues a RUSP that identifies a number of core conditions—those for which screening is highly recommended—and secondary conditions, for which screening is optional. As of November 2016, the RUSP included 34 core conditions and 26 secondary conditions.

The committee's recommendations are based on the *Newborn Screening:* **Towards a Uniform Screening Panel and System** and on research evidence, which means that the number of core and secondary conditions may change.

What Are Some Examples of Newborn Screening Successes?

Many conditions included in U.S. newborn screening programs no longer cause serious disability or illness because they are detected early and treated immediately—but they once did. The three examples that follow are conditions that cause serious developmental and intellectual disabilities, or death, if they are not detected and treated early. Successful newborn screening for these conditions and follow-up treatment means that babies who might have died or needed specialized long-term care, can now grow into healthy adulthood.

Severe Combined Immunodeficiency (SCID)

One of the additions added to the RUSP is an inherited condition, called severe combined immunodeficiency (SCID), that makes a child's body unable to fight off even mild infections. The condition, also known as "bubble boy syndrome," causes parts of the immune system to not work properly. If untreated, infants with SCID are unlikely to live past the age of 2 years. However, when SCID is detected and treated early, children can live longer, healthier lives.

SCID is rare, with between 40–100 infants diagnosed each year in the United States. Because SCID is a newcomer to the RUSP, not all states screen for it yet, meaning infants with the condition might be getting sick without being diagnosed.

Infants should be evaluated for SCID and other types of immune system problems if they have:

- a high number of infections

- infections that do not improve with antibiotic treatment for 2 or more months

- diarrhea

- poor weight gain or growth (called "failure to thrive")

- fungal infections in the mouth (called "thrush") that will not go away

An infant with any of these warning signs should be tested for SCID as soon as possible.

Phenylketonuria (PKU)

Phenylketonuria (PKU) is a metabolic disorder that is detected by newborn screening. In PKU, the body cannot digest or process one of the building blocks of proteins, an amino acid called phenylalanine, or Phe. Phe is found naturally in many foods, especially high-protein foods.

PKU was the first condition for which a screening test was developed, and the first condition for which widespread newborn testing was implemented in the 1960s.

If PKU is left untreated, the Phe builds up in the body and brain. By 3–6 months of age, infants with untreated PKU begin to show symptoms of intellectual and developmental disability. These disabilities can become severe if Phe remains at high levels.

Fortunately, PKU is treatable. The treatment consists of a diet containing little or no Phe and higher levels of other amino acids. If children with the condition are placed on this diet at birth, they grow normally and usually show no symptoms or health problems. The *Eunice Kennedy Shriver* National Institute of Child Health and Human Development (NICHD)-sponsored research has shown that people with PKU should stay on the restricted diet as they enter adulthood and, in fact, throughout their lives. This is especially important for women of childbearing age who wish to or who might become pregnant.

Before newborn screening programs could detect PKU in the first few hours after birth, PKU was one of the leading causes of intellectual and developmental disabilities (IDD) in the United States. Today, as a result of newborn screening programs that allow for almost immediate treatment of the condition, PKU has been virtually eliminated as a cause of IDD in this country.

Galactosemia

Another metabolic disorder included in newborn screening is galactosemia, which means being unable to use galactose. Galactose is one of two simple sugars that make up lactose, the sugar in milk. People with galactosemia cannot have any milk or milk products.

If someone with galactosemia consumes milk or milk products (human or animal), the galactose builds up in their blood and causes serious damage to their liver, brain, kidneys, and eyes. Infants with untreated galactosemia can die of a serious blood infection or of liver failure. Those that may survive usually have IDD and other damage to the brain and nervous system. Even milder forms of galactosemia still require treatment to prevent early cataracts, an unsteady gait, and delays in learning, talking, and growth.

The treatment for galactosemia is not to consume any milk or milk products and to avoid other foods that contain this sugar. If this disease is diagnosed very early and the infant is placed on a strict galactose-free diet, she or he is likely to live a relatively normal life, although mild IDD may still develop. If not placed on a galactose-free diet immediately, an infant will develop symptoms in the first few days after birth.

Before it could be detected either before birth or through a newborn screening program, galactosemia was a frequent cause of IDD and early death. Oregon began screening newborns for galactosemia 50 years ago, and all states now screen for this condition. Screening has identified more than 2,500 infants with the condition, many of whom would have died without the screening.

How Many Newborns Are Screened in the United States?

At present, all 50 states, the District of Columbia (DC), and the Commonwealth of Puerto Rico have newborn screening programs. This means that nearly every child born in the United States or Puerto Rico is screened shortly after birth.

- All states require newborn screening for at least 29 health conditions. Each state's public health department decides both the number and types of conditions on its testing panel. Most states allow parents to opt out for religious or other reasons. Many states also offer supplemental screening programs that screen for disorders beyond those required by the state; costs for these supplemental tests are usually covered by insurance.

- About 4 million infants are born each year in the United States, and most of them are screened.

- Most states report participation of 99.9 percent or higher.

- The Centers for Disease Control and Prevention (CDC) data show that about 12,500 newborns each year are diagnosed with one of the core conditions detected through newborn screening. This means that almost 1 out of every 300 newborns screened is eventually diagnosed.

- Early diagnosis and treatment in many cases can significantly improve the chances of healthy development and positive outcomes and nearly eliminates death from the conditions.

Who Pays for Newborn Screening?

Although most states collect a fee for newborn screening, all U.S. infants go through newborn screening regardless of whether their family can pay for it.

The specific cost of screening varies from state to state in part because the states test for different conditions and pay for their programs in different ways. Birthing centers and hospitals sometimes bill directly for newborn screening or include the fee in charges for maternity care. Many private and public health insurance programs pay the fees for newborn screening. For example, the State Children's Health Insurance Program (CHIP) or Medicaid can pay the fees for newborn screening for eligible families.

The National Newborn Screening and Genetics Resource Center (NNSGRC) (genes-r-us.uthscsa.edu/resources/consumer/statemap. htm) provides information about the cost of newborn screening in each state and the DC.

How Is Newborn Screening Done?

Newborn screening usually starts with a blood test, followed by a hearing test and possibly other tests.

First, hospital staff fill out a newborn screening card with the infant's vital information—name, sex, weight, and date and time of birth—and the date and time of the blood collection. Part of the card consists of special absorbent paper used to collect the blood sample.

After warming and careful sterilizing of the infant's heel, medical staff do a "heel stick," in which they make a small puncture in the baby's heel and squeeze out a few drops of blood. They put the absorbent part of the card in contact with the blood drop. They continue until all the printed circles on the card contain a blood sample. The card is then sent to a laboratory, where the blood is tested for the various conditions as part of the newborn screening panel.

Hearing Test

Hospital staff typically use one of two methods for the hearing test. Both are quick (5–10 minutes) and safe.

- **Otoacoustic emissions (OAE).** This test determines if certain parts of the infant's ear respond to sound. A miniature earphone and microphone are placed in the ear, and sounds are played. If the infant has normal hearing, the microphone picks up an echo reflected back into the ear canal. Failure to detect an echo means there may be a loss of hearing.

- **Auditory brain stem response (ABR).** This test evaluates the auditory brain stem—the part of the auditory nerve that carries sound from the ear to the brain—and the brain's response to sound. Miniature earphones are placed in the ear, and sounds are played. Electrodes (small, sticky electric conductors) are placed on the infant's head to detect the brain's response to the sounds. If the infant's brain does not respond consistently to the sounds, there may be a hearing problem.

Pulse Oximetry

In some cases, hospital staff will perform pulse oximetry to measure how much oxygen is in the infant's blood. Pulse oximetry is usually performed at least 24 hours after birth. Hospital staff place a sensor on the infant's skin for a couple of minutes, and the sensor measures the level of oxygen in the blood through the skin.

Low blood oxygen can indicate that a newborn has heart problems. Pulse oximetry can help identify infants with a condition called critical congenital heart disease (CCHD). According to the CDC, 25 percent of babies with congenital heart disease (one that is present at birth) have a CCHD. There is evidence that medical care is allowing more infants with CCHD to survive.

Other Blood Tests

Some states require a second blood test that repeats the initial set of screenings.

- The first screening is performed 24–48 hours after the infant is born, ideally before the infant leaves the hospital. For some conditions, the screening is not valid if the blood is taken within 24 hours of birth.

31

• The second screening is performed when the infant is 10 days to 2 weeks old to ensure that the healthcare provider has the most accurate results possible.

How Are My Newborn's Screening Results Used?

In most cases, parents don't hear anything at all about the results of their baby's newborn screening tests. This usually means that the tests did not detect any of the conditions screened for—or, as the child's healthcare provider might say, the results were "negative" or "in-range." Parents with concerns should talk with their healthcare provider and ask about the results. Most states notify parents only when the results are "positive" or "out of range" for a particular condition(s).

Out of Range Results

If the screening detects one or more conditions, the result is "positive" or, more accurately, "out of range." The child's healthcare provider or someone from the state health department will notify the parents, usually within 2–3 weeks, if the results are out of range.

This result does not mean the child definitely has the condition detected. Sometimes, the tests produce a "false positive," meaning that even though the test result was positive, the infant does not actually have the disease.

If the test result is positive, it is very important for the infant to undergo additional testing right away to confirm and diagnose any specific condition(s). Screening tests and diagnostic tests are not the same. If a baby is diagnosed with a condition, his or her healthcare provider and other providers will recommend a course of treatment.

The Importance of Following Up

Newborn screening is used to detect serious medical conditions. If not treated, some of these conditions can cause lifelong health problems; others can cause death.

If your child's healthcare provider or the state health department calls you about your infant's newborn screening results, it is important to follow up quickly. Follow their instructions to get care for your baby. Newborn screening makes early diagnosis possible so that treatment can begin immediately—before serious problems can occur or become permanent. This approach helps to ensure the best possible outcomes for babies.

Screening Costs

Some newborn screening tests are covered under the Affordable Care Act, the healthcare reform law passed in 2010. Depending on your insurance plan, you may be able to get your baby screened at no cost to you.

Check with your insurance provider to find out what's included in your plan.

If you don't have insurance, you can still get medical care for yourself and your baby. Call one of the toll-free phone numbers below to connect with the health department in your area. Be sure to ask about free care.

For information in English, call 800-311-BABY (800-311-2229).

For information in Spanish, call 800-504-7081.

Schedule Checkups

A well-baby checkup is a full checkup from your baby's doctor that you schedule ahead of time. This is different from other visits for sickness or injury. Most babies have their first well-baby checkup 2 to 3 days after coming home from the hospital.

Maintaining Child Health Records

Keep track of your baby's test results and shots. Put medical information in a safe place—you will need it for child care, school, and other activities.

Your family's health history is another important part of your baby's health record. Use this family health history tool to keep track of your family's health. Keep a copy with your baby's other health information.

Chapter 4

Preventive Care Screening Tests for Children and Adolescents

Chapter Contents

Section 4.1

Recommended Screening Tests for Children and Adolescents

This section includes text excerpted from "Section 3.
Recommendations for Children and Adolescents,"
Agency for Healthcare Research and Quality (AHRQ),
June 2014. Reviewed July 2018.

The U.S. Preventive Services Task Force (USPSTF) is an independent panel of nonfederal experts in prevention and evidence-based medicine and is composed of primary care providers (such as internists, pediatricians, family physicians, gynecologists/obstetricians, nurses, and health behavior specialists). The USPSTF conducts scientific evidence reviews of a broad range of clinical preventive healthcare services (such as screening, counseling, and preventive medications) and develops recommendations for primary care clinicians and health systems. The USPSTF assigns one of five letter grades to each of its recommendations (A, B, C, D, or I).

- **A:** The USPSTF recommends the service. There is high certainty that the net benefit is substantial.

- **B:** The USPSTF recommends the service. There is high certainty that the net benefit is moderate or there is moderate certainty that the net benefit is moderate to substantial.

- **C:** The USPSTF recommends against routinely providing the service. There may be considerations that support providing the service in an individual patient. There is at least moderate certainty that the net benefit is small.

- **D:** The USPSTF recommends against the service. There is moderate or high certainty that the service has no net benefit or that the harms outweigh the benefits.

- **I:** The USPSTF concludes that the available evidence is insufficient to assess the balance of benefits and harms of the service. Evidence is lacking, of poor quality, or conflicting, and the balance of benefits and harms cannot be determined.

Following are recommendations made by the USPSTF for children and adolescents.

Screening for Congenital Hypothyroidism

The USPSTF recommends screening for congenital hypothyroidism (CH) in newborns.

Grade: A recommendation. This recommendation applies to all infants born in the United States. Premature, very low birth weight, and ill infants may benefit from additional screening because these conditions are associated with decreased sensitivity and specificity of screening tests. Screening for CH is mandated in all 50 states and the District of Columbia (DC), though methods of screening vary. There are two main methods used in the United States:

1. Primary thyroid-stimulating hormone (TSH) with backup (thyroxine) T4; and

2. Primary T4 with backup TSH.

A few states use both tests in initial screening. Families should be provided with appropriate information about newborn screening tests, including the benefits and harms of screening. They should be aware of the potential of a false-positive test, and the process required for definitive testing. Nationally, only one in 25 positive screening tests are confirmed to be CH. Normal newborn screening results for CH should not preclude appropriate evaluation of infants presenting with clinical signs and symptoms suggestive of hypothyroidism. Infants should be tested between 2–4 days of age. Infants discharged from hospitals before 48 hours of life should be tested immediately before discharge. Specimens obtained in the first 24–48 hours of age may be falsely elevated for TSH regardless of the screening method used. Primary care clinicians should ensure that infants with abnormal screens receive confirmatory testing and begin appropriate treatment with thyroid hormone replacement within two weeks after birth. Children with positive confirmatory testing in whom no permanent cause of CH is found (such as lack of thyroid tissue on thyroid ultrasound or thyroid scan), should, at some time point after the age of three years, undergo a 30-day trial of reduced or discontinued thyroid hormone replacement therapy to determine if the hypothyroidism is permanent or transient.

Screening for Phenylketonuria

The USPSTF recommends screening for phenylketonuria (PKU) in newborns.

Grade: A recommendation. This recommendation applies to newborns. Screening for PKU is mandated in all 50 states, though methods of screening vary. There are three principal methods used for PKU screening in the United States:

1. The Guthrie Bacterial Inhibition Assay (BIA),

2. Automated fluorometric assay, and

3. Tandem mass spectrometry.

Screening tests are most accurate if performed after 24 hours of life but before the infant is seven days old. It is essential that phenylalanine restrictions be instituted shortly after birth to prevent the neurodevelopmental effects of PKU. Infants who are tested within the first 24 hours after birth should receive a repeat screening test by two weeks of age. Premature infants and those with illnesses should be tested at or near seven days of age, but in all cases before newborn nursery discharge.

Screening for Sickle Cell Disease (SCD) in Newborns

The USPSTF recommends screening for sickle cell disease in newborns.

Grade: A recommendation. Screening for sickle cell disease in newborns is mandated in all 50 states and the DC. Most states use either thin-layer isoelectric focusing (IEF) or high-performance liquid chromatography (HPLC) as the initial screening test. Both methods have extremely high sensitivity and specificity for sickle cell anemia. Specimens must be drawn prior to any blood transfusion due to the potential for a false negative result as a result of the transfusion. Extremely premature infants may have false-positive results when adult hemoglobin is undetectable. All newborns should undergo testing regardless of birth setting. In general, birth attendants should make arrangements for samples to be obtained, and the first physician to see the child at an office visit should verify screening results. Confirmatory testing should occur no later than two months of age.

Universal Screening for Hearing Loss in Newborns

The USPSTF recommends screening for hearing loss in all newborn infants.

Grade: B recommendation. The patient population considered here includes all newborn infants. Screening programs should be conducted by using a 1- or 2-step validated protocol. A frequently used protocol requires a 2-step screening process, which includes otoacoustic emissions (OAEs) followed by auditory brainstem response (ABR) in those who failed the first test.

Equipment should be well maintained, staff should be thoroughly trained, and quality-control programs should be in place to reduce avoidable false-positive test results. Programs should develop protocols to ensure that infants with positive screening test results receive appropriate audiologic evaluation and follow up after discharge. Newborns delivered at home, birthing centers, or hospitals without hearing screening facilities should have some mechanism for referral for newborn hearing screening, including tracking of follow-up. All infants should have hearing screening before one month of age. Those infants who do not pass the newborn screening should undergo audiologic and medical evaluation before three months of age for confirmatory testing. Because of the elevated risk of hearing loss in infants with risk indicators, an expert panel made a recommendation in 2000 that these children should undergo periodic monitoring for three years.

Screening for Visual Impairment in Children Younger than Age Five Years

The USPSTF recommends screening to detect amblyopia, strabismus, and defects in visual acuity in children age 3–5 years.

Grade: B recommendation. Various screening tests are used in primary care to identify visual impairment in children, including: Visual acuity test, stereo-acuity test, cover-uncover test, Hirschberg light reflex test, autorefraction, and photo screening. Various tests are used widely in the United States to identify visual defects in children, and the choice of tests is influenced by the child's age. During the first year of life, strabismus can be assessed by the cover test and the Hirschberg light reflex test. Screening children younger than age three years for visual acuity is more challenging than screening older children and typically requires testing by specially trained personnel. Newer automated techniques can be used to test these children.

Screening and Treatment for Major Depressive Disorder (MDD) in Children and Adolescents

The U.S. Preventive Services Task Force (USPSTF) recommends screening of adolescents (12–18 years of age) for major depressive disorder (MDD) when systems are in place to ensure accurate diagnosis, psychotherapy (cognitive/behavioral or interpersonal), and follow-up.

Grade: B recommendation. This USPSTF recommendation addresses screening for MDD in adolescents (12–18 years of age) and children (7–11 years of age) in the general population. There is a spectrum of depressive disorders. Instruments developed for primary care (Patient Health Questionnaire for Adolescents (PHQ-A) and the Beck Depression Inventory-Primary Care Version (BDI-PC)) have been used successfully in adolescents. There are limited data describing the accuracy of using MDD screening instruments in younger children (7–11 years of age).

Screening for Obesity in Children and Adolescents

The USPSTF recommends that clinicians screen children aged six years and older for obesity and offer them or refer them to comprehensive, intensive behavioral interventions to promote improvement in weight status.

Grade: B recommendation. This recommendation statement applies to children and adolescents aged 6–18 years.

The USPSTF is using the following terms to define categories of increased body mass index (BMI):

- overweight is defined as an age- and gender-specific BMI between the 85th to 95th percentiles, and

- obesity is defined as an age- and gender-specific BMI at greater than or equal to the 95th percentile.

The USPSTF did not find sufficient evidence for screening children younger than six years. The USPSTF found adequate evidence that body mass index (BMI) was an acceptable measure for identifying children and adolescents with excess weight. BMI is calculated from the measured weight and height of an individual. No evidence was found regarding appropriate intervals for screening. Height and weight, from which BMI is calculated, are routinely measured during health maintenance visits.

Section 4.2

Body Mass Index Screening for Weight Problems

Text under the heading "What Is Obesity?" is excerpted from "Obesity," National Institute of Environmental Health Sciences (NIEHS), July 16, 2018; Text beginning with the heading "What Is Body Mass Index (BMI)?" is excerpted from "Healthy Weight—about Child and Teen BMI," Centers for Disease Control and Prevention (CDC), May 15, 2015.

What Is Obesity?

Childhood obesity is a serious problem in the United States. Obesity means having too much body fat. Obesity occurs over time when a person eats more calories than they can use.

Being obese puts people at risk for many health problems. The more body fat a person has and the more they weigh, the more likely they are to develop diseases such as diabetes, heart disease, stroke, arthritis, breathing problems, and some cancers.

The good news is that even modest weight loss can improve or prevent many of the health problems associated with obesity. Dietary changes, increased physical activity and behavior changes are all things that can help person lose weight.

What Is Body Mass Index (BMI)?

Body mass index (BMI) is a person's weight in kilograms divided by the square of height in meters. For children and teens, BMI is age- and sex-specific and is often referred to as BMI-for-age. In children, a high amount of body fat can lead to weight-related diseases and other health issues and being underweight can also put one at risk for health issues.

A high BMI can be an indicator of high body fatness. BMI does not measure body fat directly, but research has shown that BMI is correlated with more direct measures of body fat, such as skinfold thickness measurements, bioelectrical impedance, densitometry (underwater weighing), dual-energy X-ray absorptiometry (DXA) and other methods. BMI can be considered an alternative to direct measures of body fat. In general, BMI is an inexpensive and easy-to-perform method of screening for weight categories that may lead to health problems.

41

How Is BMI Calculated for Children and Teens?

Calculating BMI using the BMI Percentile Calculator involves the following steps:

1. Measure height and weight

2. Use the child and teen BMI calculator to calculate BMI. The BMI number is calculated using standard formulas.

What Is a BMI Percentile and How Is It Interpreted?

After BMI is calculated for children and teens, it is expressed as a percentile which can be obtained from either a graph or a percentile calculator. These percentiles express a child's BMI relative to children in the United States who participated in national surveys that were conducted from 1963–65 to 1988–94. Because weight and height change during growth and development, as does their relation to body fatness, a child's BMI must be interpreted relative to other children of the same sex and age.

The BMI-for-age percentile growth charts are the most commonly used indicator to measure the size and growth patterns of children and teens in the United States. BMI-for-age weight status categories and the corresponding percentiles were based on expert committee recommendations and are shown in the following table.

Table 4.1. Body Mass Index (BMI) Table

Weight Status Category	Percentile Range
Underweight	Less than the 5th percentile
Normal or healthy weight	5th percentile to less than the 85th percentile
Overweight	85th to less than the 95th percentile
Obese	Equal to or greater than the 95th percentile

How Is BMI Used with Children and Teens?

For children and teens, BMI is not a diagnostic tool and is used to screen for potential weight and health-related issues. For example, a child may have a high BMI for their age and sex, but to determine if excess fat is a problem, a healthcare provider would need to perform further assessments. These assessments might include skinfold thickness measurements, evaluations of diet, physical activity, family history, and other appropriate health screenings. The American Academy of Pediatrics (AAP) recommends the use of BMI to screen for overweight and obesity in children beginning at 2 years old. For children under the age of 2 years old, consult the World Health Organization (WHO) standards.

Is BMI Interpreted the Same Way for Children and Teens as It Is for Adults?

BMI is interpreted differently for children and teens even though it is calculated as weight ÷ height². Because there are changes in weight and height with age, as well as their relation to body fatness, BMI levels among children and teens need to be expressed relative to other children of the same sex and age. These percentiles are calculated from the Centers for Disease Control and Prevention (CDC) growth charts, which were based on national survey data.

Obesity is defined as a BMI at or above the 95th percentile for children and teens of the same age and sex. For example, a 10-year-old boy of average height (56 inches) who weighs 102 pounds would have a BMI of 22.9 kg/m². This would place the boy in the 95th percentile for BMI, and he would be considered to have obesity. This means that the child's BMI is greater than the BMI of 95 percent of 10-year-old boys in the reference population.

Why Can't Healthy Weight Ranges Be Provided for Children and Teens?

Normal or healthy weight, weight status is based on BMI between the 5th–85th percentile on the CDC growth chart. It is difficult to provide healthy weight ranges for children and teens because the interpretation of BMI depends on weight, height, age, and sex.

What Are the BMI Trends for Children and Teens in the United States?

The prevalence of children and teens who measure in the 95th percentile or greater on the CDC growth charts has greatly increased over the past 40 years. However, this trend has leveled off and has even declined in certain age groups.

How Can You Tell If Your Child Is Overweight or Obese?

CDC and the AAP recommend the use of BMI to screen for overweight and obesity in children and teens age 2 through 19 years. For children under the age of 2 years old, consult the WHO standards. Although BMI is used to screen for overweight and obesity in children and teens, BMI is not a diagnostic tool. To determine whether the child has excess fat, further assessment by a trained health professional would be needed.

Can You Determine If Your Child or Teen Is Obese by Using an Adult BMI Calculator?

In general, it's not possible to do this. The adult calculator provides only the BMI value (weight/height^2) and not the BMI percentile that is needed to interpret BMI among children and teens. It is not appropriate to use the BMI categories for adults to interpret the BMI of children and teens.

However, if a child or teen has a BMI of $\geq$ 30 kg/m^2, the child is almost certainly obese. A BMI of 30 kg/m^2 is approximately the 95th percentile among 17-year-old girls and 18-year-old boys.

Your Two Children Have the Same BMI Values, but One Is Considered Obese and the Other Is Not. Why Is That?

The interpretation of BMI varies by age and sex. So if the children are not the same age and the same sex, the interpretation of BMI has different meanings. For children of different age and sex, the same BMI could represent different BMI percentiles and possibly different weight status categories.

What Are the Health Consequences of Obesity during Childhood?

Health Risks Now

- Childhood obesity can have a harmful effect on the body in a variety of ways:

  - High blood pressure and high cholesterol, which are risk factors for cardiovascular disease (CVD). In one study, 70 percent of obese children had at least one CVD risk factor, and 39 percent had two or more.

- Increased risk of impaired glucose tolerance, insulin resistance and type 2 diabetes

- Breathing problems, such as sleep apnea, and asthma

- Joint problems and musculoskeletal discomfort

- Fatty liver disease, gallstones, and gastroesophageal reflux (i.e., heartburn)

- Psychological stress such as depression, behavioral problems, and issues in school

- Low self-esteem and low self-reported quality of life

- Impaired social, physical, and emotional functioning

Health Risks Later

- Obese children are more likely to become obese adults. Adult obesity is associated with a number of serious health conditions including heart disease, diabetes, and some cancers.

- If children are overweight, obesity in adulthood is likely to be more severe.

Section 4.3

Screening Test for Child's Vision

This section includes text excerpted from "Get Your Child's Vision Checked," Office of Disease Prevention and Health Promotion (ODPHP), U.S. Department of Health and Human Services (HHS), September 22, 2017.

It's important for all children to have their vision checked at least once between ages 3–5. Even if children don't show signs of eye problems, they still need their vision checked. Finding and treating eye problems early on can save a child's sight. Healthy eyes and vision are very important to a child's development. Growing children constantly use their eyes, both at play and in the classroom.

What Are Common Eye Problems in Children?

These common eye problems can be treated if they are found early enough:

- Lazy eye (amblyopia)
- Crossed eyes (strabismus)

Other conditions—like being nearsighted or farsighted—can be corrected with glasses or contact lenses. Conditions like these are called refractive errors.

Is Your Child at Risk for Vision Problems?

If your family has a history of childhood vision problems, your child may be more likely to have eye problems. Talk to the doctor about eye problems in your family.

Eye Exams Are Part of Regular Checkups

The doctor will check your child's eyes during each checkup, beginning with your child's first well-baby visit. Around age 3 or 4, the doctor will give your child a more complete eye exam to make sure her vision is developing normally. If there are any problems, the doctor may send your child to an eye doctor.

Take Action!

Follow these steps to protect your child's vision.

Talk to Your Child's Doctor

Ask the doctor or nurse if there are any problems with your child's vision.

If the doctor recommends a visit to an eye care professional:

- Ask your child's doctor for the name of an eye doctor who is good with kids. You can also use these tips to find an eye doctor.
- Write down any information about your child's vision problem.
- Plan your child's visit to the eye.

What about Cost?

Under the Affordable Care Act (ACA), the healthcare reform law passed in 2010, health insurance plans must cover vision screening for kids.

- If you have private insurance, your child may be able to get screened at no cost to you. Check with your insurance provider.

- Medicaid and the children's health insurance program (CHIP) also cover vision care for kids.

Look Out for Problems

Schedule an eye exam for your child if you see signs of an eye problem, like if your child's eyes:

- Look crossed

- Turn outwards

- Don't focus together

- Are red, crusted, or swollen around the eyelids

Protect Your Child's Eyes

- Don't let your child play with toys that have sharp edges or points

- Keep sharp or pointed objects, like knives and scissors, away from your child

- Protect your child's eyes from the sun. Look for kids' sunglasses that block 100 percent of ultraviolet (UV) i.e., ultraviolet A (UVA) and ultraviolet B (UVB) rays.

- Keep chemicals and sprays (like cleaners and bug spray) where kids can't reach them

- Make sure your child wears the right eye protection for sports

Help Develop Your Child's Vision

It takes skill to match up what we see with what we want to do— like when we want to bounce a ball or read a book.

Here are ways to help your child develop vision skills:

- Read to your child and let your child see what you are reading.

- Play with your child using a chalkboard, finger paints, or blocks.

- Take your child to the playground to climb the jungle gym and walk on the balance beam.

- Play catch with your child.

Section 4.4

Get Your Teen Screened for Depression

This section includes text excerpted from "Get Your Teen Screened for Depression," Office of Disease Prevention and Health Promotion (ODPHP), U.S. Department of Health and Human Services (HHS), July 25, 2017.

If your child is between ages 12–18, ask the doctor about screening (checking) for depression—even if you don't see signs of a problem.

Why Do You Need to Get Your Teen Screened for Depression?

More than 1 in 10 teens show some signs of depression. Depression can be serious, and most teens with depression don't get the help they need. The good news is that depression can be treated with counseling or medicine. When you ask the doctor about screening for depression, find out what services are available (like therapy or counseling) in case your teen needs follow-up care.

What Is Depression?

Teen depression can be a serious mental health problem. If your child is depressed, she may:

- Feel sad or irritable (easily upset) most of the time

- Lose interest in favorite activities

- Have aches and pains for no reason

- Sleep too much or be unable to sleep

- Eat too much or have trouble eating

- Use drugs or alcohol

- Think about death or suicide

It's normal for teens to have mood swings, and it can be hard to tell if your child is just feeling down or if she's depressed. That's why it's so important for all teens to be screened for depression.

What Causes Depression?

Depression can happen to anyone. It's not your fault or your teen's fault. Some experiences may make it more likely that a teen will develop depression, like:

- Dealing with a big loss, like a death or divorce in the family

- Living with someone who is depressed

- Having another mental health problem, like anxiety or an eating disorder

- Feeling stressed at school or at home

- Having a family history of depression

Teen girls are more likely to get depressed than teen boys.

What Happens during a Depression Screening?

The doctor will ask your teen questions about his feelings and behaviors. This may include asking how often your teen:

- feels hopeless or sad

- has low energy or feels tired during the day

- has trouble paying attention at school

- eats too much or has trouble eating

Screening for depression usually takes about 5 minutes. It can be done as part of your teen's yearly checkup.

What If the Doctor Finds Signs of Depression?

If your child is showing signs of depression, the doctor will:

- refer your teen to a therapist or doctor with special training in helping young people with emotional or behavioral problems

- talk about medicines or other treatments that could help your teen with depression

- order tests to check for other health problems

Make sure to include your teen when you make any decisions about treatment.

Take Action!

Take steps to protect your teen's mental health.

Talk to Your Teen's Doctor about Depression Screening

Ask the doctor to screen your child for depression. If you are worried about your teen, be sure to let the doctor know. Find out what services are available in case your teen needs treatment.

What about Cost?

Screening for depression is covered under the Affordable Care Act (ACA), the healthcare reform law passed in 2010. Depending on your insurance plan, your teen may be able to get screened at no cost to you. Check with your insurance provider.

If you don't have health insurance, use this treatment locator to find mental health services near you. Some programs offer free or low-cost treatment for depression.

Write Down Any Concerns You Have

Keep track of your teen's actions and words that make you think she might be depressed. If you see a change in your child's behavior, make a note about the change and when it happened. Include details like:

- How long the behavior has been going on

- How often the behavior happens

- How serious you think it is

Share these notes with your teen's doctor. You can also use them to start a conversation with your teen.

Watch for Signs That Your Teen May Be Thinking about Suicide

Most people who are depressed don't attempt suicide, but depression can increase the risk of suicide and suicide attempts. Suicide is the second leading cause of death for people ages 15–24.

These behaviors may be signs your teen is thinking about suicide:

- Talking about wanting to kill or hurt himself
- Taking dangerous risks, like driving recklessly
- Spending less and less time with friends and family
- Talking about not being around in the future or "going away"
- Giving away prized possessions
- Increasing the use of alcohol or drugs
- Talking about feeling hopeless, or very angry

If your child is showing some or all of these warning signs, get help right away. Visit the National Suicide Prevention or call 800-273-TALK (800-273-8255) to learn how to help. If you think your child may be in immediate danger, call 911 or take him to the emergency room.

Find Resources for Your Teen

If your child isn't ready to talk to you about her feelings, there are still things you can do. Help your teen find resources online and in the community.

Let her know that, in a crisis, she can get support anonymously (without giving her name) by:

- Texting the Crisis Text
- Chatting online with someone from the National Suicide Prevention
- Calling the National Suicide Prevention Hotline at 800-273-TALK (800-273-8255)

Make a list with your teen of other people she can go to with problems or questions—like a teacher, guidance counselor, or adult friend. Remind your teen that you are always there if she wants to talk.

51

Chapter 5

Preventive Care and Screening Tests for Adults

Chapter Contents

Section 5.1

Women's Health Screening Recommendations

This section includes text excerpted from "Get Recommended Screening Tests and Immunizations for Women," U.S. Department of Veterans Affairs (VA), June 6, 2018.

The Veterans Health Administration (VHA) aims to help you stay healthy. The images below list the preventive health services (screening tests, medications, health counseling, and vaccines) that VHA recommends. Screening tests are used to look for health conditions before there are symptoms. These recommendations apply only to adult women of average risk. You are a woman of average risk if you have no personal or family history or symptoms of the conditions listed below. If you are having symptoms of a condition, please talk with your provider.

HEALTH CONDITION	18–29 years	30–39 years	40–49 years	50–59 years	60–69 years	70–79 years	80 years and older
Abdominal Aortic Aneurysm (AAA)	Not recommended (age 18–64)					Talk with your provider (age 65–75)	Not recommended (age 76 and older)
Breast Cancer	Not recommended (age 18–39)		Recommended annually (45-54) Recommend biennial (55 and older or have opportunity to continue annually) Have opportunity to begin annual screening (40-44)				Recommended for some women — talk with your provider (age 75+)
Cervical Cancer	Every 3 years (age 21–29)	Recommended. Every 3 or 5 years, depending on tests chosen (age 30–65)			Not recommended (age 66 and older)		
Colon Cancer	Not recommended (age 18–49)			Recommended. Frequency varies by test chosen (age 50–75)		Talk with your provider (age 76–85)	NR (age 86 and older)
Depression	Recommended every year						
Hepatitis B Infection	Recommended for some women – talk with your provider (age 18 and older)						
Hepatitis C Infection	Recommended for some women – talk with your provider (age 18 and older)						
High Blood Pressure	Recommended every 2 years (age 18 and older)						
High Cholesterol	Talk with your provider (age 20 and older)						
HIV Infection	Recommended once (age 18 and older)						
Osteoporosis	Recommended for some women – talk with your provider (age 18–64)				Recommended once (age 65 and older)		
Overweight & Obesity	Recommended every year (age 18 and older)						
Sexually Transmitted Infections	Recommended. Test for gonorrhea and chlamydia every year (age 18–24). Talk with your provider about syphilis testing.	Talk with your provider about testing for gonorrhea, chlamydia, and syphilis (age 25 and older)					

Figure 5.1. *Screening Tests for Women*

HEALTH CONDITION	18–29 years	30–39 years	40–49 years	50–59 years	60–69 years	70–79 years	80 years and older
Folic Acid for Pregnancy Planning	Recommended. Daily folic acid supplement for any woman who may become pregnant			Not recommended after child-bearing age			
Aspirin to Prevent Stroke	Not recommended (age 18–54)				Talk with your provider (age 55–79)		NR (age 80 and older)

Figure 5.2. *Medications for Women*

HEALTH CONDITION	18–29 years	30–39 years	40–49 years	50–59 years	60–69 years	70–79 years	80 years and older
Tobacco Use	Recommended every visit (if using tobacco) (age 18 and older)						
Alcohol Use	Talk with your provider about healthy alcohol use (age 18 and older)						
Healthy Diet and Physical Activity	Talk with your provider about a healthy diet and physical activity (age 18 and older)						

Figure 5.3. *Health Counseling for Women*

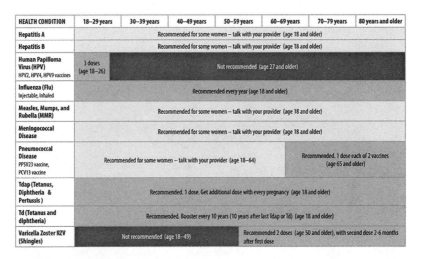

HEALTH CONDITION	18–29 years	30–39 years	40–49 years	50–59 years	60–69 years	70–79 years	80 years and older
Hepatitis A	Recommended for some women – talk with your provider (age 18 and older)						
Hepatitis B	Recommended for some women – talk with your provider (age 18 and older)						
Human Papilloma Virus (HPV) HPV2, HPV4, HPV9 vaccines	3 doses (age 18–26)	Not recommended (age 27 and older)					
Influenza (Flu) Injectable, Inhaled	Recommended every year (age 18 and older)						
Measles, Mumps, and Rubella (MMR)	Recommended for some women – talk with your provider (age 18 and older)						
Meningococcal Disease	Recommended for some women – talk with your provider (age 18 and older)						
Pneumococcal Disease PPSV23 vaccine, PCV13 vaccine	Recommended for some women – talk with your provider (age 18–64)				Recommended. 1 dose each of 2 vaccines (age 65 and older)		
Tdap (Tetanus, Diphtheria & Pertussis)	Recommended. 1 dose. Get additional dose with every pregnancy (age 18 and older)						
Td (Tetanus and diphtheria)	Recommended. Booster every 10 years (10 years after last Tdap or Td) (age 18 and older)						
Varicella Zoster RZV (Shingles)	Not recommended (age 18–49)			Recommended 2 doses (age 50 and older), with second dose 2-6 months after first dose			

Figure 5.4. *Vaccines for Women*

Medium Gray: *Recommended*
Light Gray: *Recommended for some Women—talk with your provider*
Dark Gray: *Not recommended (NR)*

Section 5.2

Men's Health Screening Recommendations

This section includes text excerpted from "Get
Recommended Screening Tests and Immunizations for Men,"
U.S. Department of Veterans Affairs (VA), June 6, 2018.

The Veterans Health Administration (VHA) aims to help you
stay healthy. The images below list the preventive health services

(screening tests, medications, health counseling, and vaccines) that VHA recommends. Screening tests are used to look for health conditions before there are symptoms. These recommendations apply only to adult men of average risk. You are a man of average risk if you have no personal or family history or symptoms of the conditions listed below. If you are having symptoms of a condition, please talk with your provider.

HEALTH CONDITION	18–29 years	30–39 years	40–49 years	50–59 years	60–69 years	70–79 years	80 years and older
Hepatitis A	Recommended for some men – talk with your provider (age 18 and older)						
Hepatitis B	Recommended for some men – talk with your provider (age 18 and older)						
Human Papilloma Virus (HPV) HPV4 vaccine HPV9 vaccine	3 doses (age 18–21)	Talk with your provider (age 21–26)	Not recommended (age 27 and older)				
Influenza (Flu) Injectable, Inhaled	Recommended every year (age 18 and older)						
Measles, Mumps, and Rubella (MMR)	Recommended for some men – talk with your provider (age 18 and older)						
Meningococcal Disease	Recommended for some men – talk with your provider (age 18 and older)						
Pneumococcal Disease PPSV23 vaccine PCV13 vaccine	Recommended for some men – talk with your provider (age 18–64)					Recommended. 1 dose each of 2 vaccines (age 65 and older)	
Tdap (Tetanus, Diphtheria & Pertussis)	Recommended. 1 dose (age 18 and older)						
Td (Tetanus and diphtheria)	Recommended. Booster every 10 years (10 years after last Tdap or Td) (age 18 and older)						
Varicella Zoster RZV (Shingles)	Not recommended (age 18–49)			Recommended 2 doses (age 50 and older), with second dose 2-6 months after first dose			

Figure 5.5. *Screening Tests for Men*

HEALTH CONDITION	18–29 years	30–39 years	40–49 years	50–59 years	60–69 years	70–79 years	80 years and older
Aspirin to Prevent Heart Attack	Not recommended (age 18–44)			Recommended for some men – talk with your provider (age 45–79)			NR (age 80 and older)

Figure 5.6. *Medications for Men*

HEALTH CONDITION	18–29 years	30–39 years	40–49 years	50–59 years	60–69 years	70–79 years	80 years and older
Tobacco Use	Recommended every visit (if using tobacco) (age 18 and older)						
Alcohol Use	Talk with your provider about healthy alcohol use (age 18 and older)						
Healthy Diet and Physical Activity	Talk with your provider about a healthy diet and physical activity (age 18 and older)						

Figure 5.7. *Health Counseling for Men*

HEALTH CONDITION	18–29 years	30–39 years	40–49 years	50–59 years	60–69 years	70–79 years	80 years and older
Hepatitis A	Recommended for some men – talk with your provider (age 18 and older)						
Hepatitis B	Recommended for some men – talk with your provider (age 18 and older)						
Human Papilloma Virus (HPV) HPV4 vaccine HPV9 vaccine	3 doses (age 18–21)	Talk with your provider (age 21–26)	Not recommended (age 27 and older)				
Influenza (Flu) Injectable, Inhaled	Recommended every year (age 18 and older)						
Measles, Mumps, and Rubella (MMR)	Recommended for some men – talk with your provider (age 18 and older)						
Meningococcal Disease	Recommended for some men – talk with your provider (age 18 and older)						
Pneumococcal Disease PPSV23 vaccine PCV13 vaccine	Recommended for some men – talk with your provider (age 18–64)					Recommended. 1 dose each of 2 vaccines (age 65 and older)	
Tdap (Tetanus, Diphtheria & Pertussis)	Recommended. 1 dose (age 18 and older)						
Td (Tetanus and diphtheria)	Recommended. Booster every 10 years (10 years after last Tdap or Td) (age 18 and older)						
Varicella Zoster RZV (Shingles)	Not recommended (age 18–49)			Recommended 2 doses (age 50 and older), with second dose 2–6 months after first dose			

Figure 5.8. *Vaccines for Men*

Medium Gray: *Recommended*
Light Gray: *Recommended for some men—talk with your provider*
Dark Gray: *Not recommended (NR)*

Section 5.3

Get Your Blood Pressure Checked

This section includes text excerpted from "High Blood Pressure,"
National Heart, Lung, and Blood Institute (NHLBI), May 1, 2018.

High blood pressure is a common disease in which blood flows through blood vessels, or arteries, at higher than normal pressures. Blood pressure is the force of blood pushing against the walls of your arteries as the heart pumps blood. High blood pressure, sometimes called hypertension, is when this force against the artery walls is too high. Your doctor may diagnose you with high blood pressure if you have consistently high blood pressure readings.

To control or lower high blood pressure, your doctor may recommend that you adopt heart-healthy lifestyle changes, such as heart-healthy eating patterns like the dietary approaches to stop hypertension (DASH) eating plan, alone or with medicines. Controlling or lowering blood pressure can also help prevent or delay high blood pressure complications, such as chronic kidney disease, heart attack, heart failure, stroke, and possibly vascular dementia.

Screening and Prevention

Everyone age 3 or older should have their blood pressure checked by a healthcare provider at least once a year. Your doctor will use a blood pressure test to see if you have consistently high blood pressure readings. Even small increases in systolic blood pressure can weaken and damage your blood vessels. Your doctor will recommend heart-healthy lifestyle changes to help control your blood pressure and prevent you from developing high blood pressure.

Screening for Consistently High Blood Pressure Readings

Your doctor will use a blood pressure test to see if you have higher than normal blood pressure readings. The reading is made up of two numbers, with the systolic number above the diastolic number. These numbers are measures of pressure in millimeters of mercury (mm Hg).

Your blood pressure is considered high when you have consistent systolic readings of 140 mm Hg or higher or diastolic readings of 90 mm Hg or higher. Based on research, your doctor may also consider you to have high blood pressure if you are an adult or child age 13 or older who has consistent systolic readings of 130–139 mm Hg or diastolic readings of 80–89 mm Hg and you have other cardiovascular risk factors.

For children younger than 13, blood pressure readings are compared to readings common for children of the same, age, sex, and height.

Talk to your doctor if your blood pressure readings are consistently higher than normal. Note that readings above 180 over 120 mm Hg are dangerously high and require immediate medical attention.

A blood pressure test is easy and painless and can be done in a doctor's office or clinic. A healthcare provider will use a gauge, stethoscope, or electronic sensor and a blood pressure cuff to measure your blood pressure. To prepare, take the following steps:

- Do not exercise, drink coffee, or smoke cigarettes for 30 minutes before the test.

- Go to the bathroom before the test.

- For at least 5 minutes before the test, sit in a chair and relax.

- Make sure your feet are flat on the floor.

- Do not talk while you are relaxing or during the test.

- Uncover your arm for the cuff.

- Rest your arm on a table so it is supported and at the level of your heart.

If it is the first time your provider has measured your blood pressure, you may have readings taken on both arms.

Even after taking these steps, your blood pressure reading may not be accurate for other reasons.

- You are excited or nervous. The phrase "white coat hypertension" refers to blood pressure readings that are only high when taken in a doctor's office compared with readings taken in other places. Doctors can detect this type of high blood pressure by reviewing readings from the office and from other places.

- If your blood pressure tends to be lower when measured at the doctor's office. This is called masked high blood pressure. When this happens, your doctor will have difficulty detecting high blood pressure.

- The wrong blood pressure cuff was used. Your readings can appear different if the cuff is too small or too large. It is important for your healthcare team to track your readings over time and ensure the correct pressure cuff is used for your sex and age.

Your doctor may run additional tests to confirm an initial reading. To gather more information about your blood pressure, your doctor may recommend wearing a blood pressure monitor to record readings over 24 hours. Your doctor may also teach you how to take blood pressure readings at home.

Healthy Lifestyle Changes to Prevent High Blood Pressure

Healthy lifestyle changes can help prevent high blood pressure from developing. Healthy lifestyle changes include choosing a heart-healthy eating pattern such as the DASH eating plan, being physically active, aiming for a healthy weight, quitting smoking, and managing stress.

Look For

- **Diagnosis** will discuss tests and procedures that your doctor may use to diagnose high blood pressure.

- **Living With** will explain what your doctor may recommend to prevent high blood pressure from recurring, getting worse, or causing complications.

- **Research for Your Health** will discuss how current researches are used and advances are made in the research to prevent high blood pressure.

Diagnosis

Your doctor may diagnose you with high blood pressure based on your medical history and if your blood pressure readings are consistently at high levels. Diagnoses for children younger than 13 are based on typical readings for their sex, height, and age.

Confirming High Blood Pressure

To diagnose high blood pressure, your doctor will take two or more readings at separate medical appointments.

Your doctor may diagnose you with high blood pressure when you have consistent systolic readings of 140 mm Hg or higher or diastolic readings of 90 mm Hg or higher. Based on research, your doctor may also consider you to have high blood pressure if you are an adult or child age 13 or older who has consistent systolic readings of 130–139 mm Hg or diastolic readings of 80–89 mm Hg and you have other cardiovascular risk factors.

For children younger than 13, blood pressure readings are compared to readings common for children of the same, age, sex, and height.

Talk to your doctor if your blood pressure readings are consistently higher than normal. Note that readings above 180 over 120 mm Hg are dangerously high and require immediate medical attention.

Depending on the cause, your doctor could diagnose you with primary or secondary high blood pressure.

- Primary high blood pressure. Primary, or essential, high blood pressure is the most common type of high blood pressure. This type of high blood pressure tends to develop over years as a person ages.

- Secondary high blood pressure. Secondary high blood pressure is caused by another medical condition or occurs as a side effect of a medicine. Your blood pressure may improve once the cause is treated or removed.

Medical History

Your doctor will want to understand your risk factors, general information about your health—such as your eating patterns, your physical activity levels, and your family's health history.

Tests to Identify Other Medical Conditions

Your doctor may order additional tests to see if another condition or medicine is causing your high blood pressure. Doctors can use this information to develop your treatment plan.

Section 5.4

Talk with Your Doctor about Depression

This section includes text excerpted from "Talk with Your Doctor about Depression," Office of Disease Prevention and Health Promotion (ODPHP), U.S. Department of Health and Human Services (HHS), July 20, 2017.

The Basics

If you think you might be depressed, talk with a doctor about how you are feeling.

What Is Depression?

Depression is an illness that involves the brain. It can affect your thoughts, mood, and daily activities. Depression is more than feeling sad for a few days.

Depression can be mild or severe. Mild depression can become more serious if it's not treated.

If you are diagnosed with depression, you aren't alone. Depression is a common illness that affects millions of adults in the United States every year.

The good news is that depression can be treated. Getting help is the best thing you can do for yourself and your loved ones. You can feel better.

What Are the Signs of Depression?

It's normal to feel sad sometimes, but if you feel sad or "down" on most days for more than two weeks at a time, you may be depressed. Depression affects people differently. Some signs of depression are:

- Losing interest in activities you used to enjoy
- Feeling hopeless or empty
- Forgetting things or having trouble making decisions
- Sleeping too much or too little
- Gaining or losing weight without meaning to
- Thinking about suicide or death

How Is Depression Treated?

Depression can be treated with talk therapy, medicines (called antidepressants), or both. Your doctor may refer you to a mental health professional for talk therapy or medicine.

Take Action

Depression is a real illness. If you think you might be depressed, see your doctor.

Talk to a Doctor about How You Are Feeling

Get a medical checkup. Ask to see a doctor or nurse who can screen you for depression.

The doctor or nurse may also check to see if you have another health condition (like thyroid disease) that can cause depression or make it worse. If you have one of these health conditions, it's important to get treatment right away.

What about Cost?

Under the Affordable Care Act (ACA), the healthcare reform law passed in 2010, insurance plans must cover screening for depression. This means you may be able to get screened at no cost to you.

If you don't have insurance, you can still get healthcare. Find a health center near you and make an appointment.

Get Treatment for Depression

When you have depression, seeking help is the best thing you can do. Depression can be treated with talk therapy, medicines, or both.

Ask your doctor for a referral to a mental health professional or use this treatment locator to find mental health services near you. Some programs offer free or low-cost treatment if you don't have insurance.

Here are some places you can go to for help with depression:

- Doctor's office or health clinic

- Family service or social service agency

- Psychologist

- Counselor or social worker

- Psychotherapist

Remember, even if asking for help seems scary, it's an important step toward feeling better.

Get Support

If you have depression, it can also help to reach out for social support. You don't have to face depression alone. A trusted family member, friend, or faith leader can help support you as you seek out medical treatment.

Get Active

Getting active can lower your stress level and help your treatment work better. It can also help keep you from getting depressed again. But it's important to know that physical activity isn't a treatment for depression.

Section 5.5

Get Tested for Cholesterol

This section includes text excerpted from "Get Your Cholesterol Checked," Office of Disease Prevention and Health Promotion (ODPHP), U.S. Department of Health and Human Services (HHS), January 25, 2018.

The Basics

It's important to get your cholesterol checked regularly. Too much cholesterol in your blood can cause a heart attack or a stroke.

The good news is that it's easy to get your cholesterol checked. If your cholesterol is high, you can take steps to lower it—like eating healthy, getting more physical activity, and taking medicine if your doctor recommends it.

How Often Do I Need to Get My Cholesterol Checked?

The general recommendation is to get your cholesterol checked every 4–6 years. Some people may need to get their cholesterol checked more or less often depending on their risk for developing heart disease. Talk to your doctor about what's best for you.

What Is Cholesterol?

Cholesterol is a waxy substance (material) that's found naturally in your blood. Your body makes cholesterol and uses it to do important things, like making hormones and digesting fatty foods.

You also get cholesterol by eating foods like egg yolks, fatty meats, and regular cheese.

If you have too much cholesterol in your body, it can build up inside your blood vessels and make it hard for blood to flow through them. Over time, this can lead to heart disease and heart attack or stroke.

How Can I Tell If I Have High Cholesterol?

There are no signs or symptoms of high cholesterol. That's why it's so important to get your cholesterol checked.

How Can I Get My Cholesterol Checked?

Your doctor will check your cholesterol levels with a blood test called a lipid profile. For the test, a nurse will take a small sample of blood from your finger or arm.

Be sure to find out how to get ready for the test. For example, you may need to fast (not eat or drink anything except water) for 9–12 hours before the test.

There are other blood tests that can check cholesterol, but a lipid profile gives the most information.

What Do the Test Results Mean?

If you get a lipid profile test, the results will show 4 numbers. A lipid profile measures:

- Total cholesterol

- Low-density lipoprotein (LDL) (bad) cholesterol

- High-density lipoprotein (HDL) (good) cholesterol

- Triglycerides

Total cholesterol is a measure of all the cholesterol in your blood. It's based on the LDL, HDL, and triglycerides numbers.

LDL cholesterol is the "bad" type of cholesterol that can block your arteries—so a lower level is better for you.

HDL cholesterol is the "good" type of cholesterol. It helps clear LDL cholesterol out of your arteries, so a higher level is better for you. Having a low HDL cholesterol level can increase your risk for heart disease.

Triglycerides are a type of fat in your blood that can increase your risk for heart attack and stroke.

What Can Cause Unhealthy Cholesterol Levels?

LDL cholesterol levels tend to increase as people get older. Other causes of high LDL (bad) cholesterol levels include:

- Family history of high LDL cholesterol

- High blood pressure or type 2 diabetes

- Smoking

- Being overweight

- Not getting enough physical activity

- Eating too much saturated fat, trans fat, and cholesterol—and not enough fruits and vegetables

- Taking certain medicines, like medicines to lower blood pressure

Causes of low HDL (good) cholesterol levels include:

- Smoking

- Being overweight

- Not getting enough physical activity

- Eating too much sugar and starch (called carbohydrates)

- Not eating enough fruits, vegetables, and unsaturated fat (like olive oil)

What If My Cholesterol Levels Aren't Healthy?

As your LDL cholesterol gets higher, so does your risk of heart disease. Take these steps to lower your cholesterol and reduce your risk of heart disease:

- Eat heart-healthy foods.

- Get active.

- Stay at a healthy weight.

- If you smoke, quit.

- If you have type 2 diabetes or high blood pressure, take steps to manage it.

- Ask your doctor about taking medicine to lower your risk of heart attack and stroke.

Take Action

Find out what your cholesterol levels are. If your cholesterol is high or you are at risk for heart disease, take steps to control your cholesterol levels.

Make an Appointment to Get Your Cholesterol Checked

Call your doctor's office or health center to schedule the test. Be sure to ask for a complete lipid profile—and find out what instructions you'll need to follow before the test. For example, you may need to fast (not eat or drink anything except water) for 9–12 hours before the test.

What about Cost?

Cholesterol testing is covered under the Affordable Care Act (ACA), the healthcare reform law passed in 2010. Depending on your insurance plan, you may be able to get your cholesterol checked at no cost to you.

Keep Track of Your Cholesterol Levels

Remember to ask the doctor or nurse for your cholesterol levels each time you get your cholesterol checked. Write the levels down to keep track of your progress.

Eat Heart-Healthy Foods

Making healthy changes to your diet can help lower your cholesterol. Try to:

- Eat less saturated fat, which comes from animal products (like regular cheese, fatty meats, and dairy desserts) and tropical oils (like palm, palm kernel, and coconut oil). Use healthy oils (like olive, peanut, or canola oil) instead.

- Choose foods with healthy fat, such as olives, avocados, nuts, and fish. Stay away from trans fats, which may be in foods like stick margarines, coffee creamers, and some desserts.

- Limit foods that are high in cholesterol, including fatty meats and organ meat (like liver and kidney).

- Limit foods that are high in sodium (salt) or added sugar.

- Choose low-fat or fat-free milk, cheese, and yogurt.

- Eat more foods that are high in fiber, like oatmeal, oat bran, beans, and lentils.

- Eat more vegetables and fruits.

Get Active

Getting active can help you lose weight, lower your LDL (bad) cholesterol, and raise your HDL (good) cholesterol. Aim for 2 hours and 30 minutes a week of moderate activity, such as:

- Walking fast
- Biking slowly
- Light gardening

Or aim for 1 hour and 15 minutes a week of vigorous activity, such as:

- Jogging or running
- Swimming
- Aerobics

Quit Smoking

Quitting smoking will help lower your cholesterol. If you smoke, make a plan to quit today. Call 800-QUIT-NOW (800-784-8669) for free support and to set up your quit plan.

Chapter 6

Preventive Care and Screening for Seniors

Chapter Contents

Section 6.1

Bone Density Test

This section includes text excerpted from "Get a Bone Density Test," Office of Disease Prevention and Health Promotion (ODPHP), U.S. Department of Health and Human Services (HHS), June 28, 2018.

The Basics

A bone density test measures how strong bones are. The test will tell you if you have osteoporosis, or weak bones.

Women are at higher risk for osteoporosis than men, and this risk increases with age.

- If you are a woman age 65 or older, schedule a bone density test

- If you are a woman age 50–64, ask your doctor if you need a bone density test

- If you are at risk for osteoporosis, your doctor or nurse may recommend you get a bone density test every 2 years

Men can get osteoporosis, too. If you are a man over age 65 and you are concerned about your bone strength, talk with your doctor or nurse.

What Is Osteoporosis?

Osteoporosis is a bone disease. It means your bones are weak and more likely to break. People with osteoporosis most often break bones in the hip, spine, and wrist. There are no signs or symptoms of osteoporosis. You might not know you have the disease until you break a bone. That's why it's so important to get a bone density test to measure your bone strength.

What Happens during a Bone Density Test?

A bone density test is like an X-ray or scan of your body. A bone density test doesn't hurt, and you don't need to do anything to prepare for it. It only takes about 15 minutes.

Am I at Risk for Osteoporosis?

Anyone can get osteoporosis, but it's most common in older women. The older you are, the greater your risk for osteoporosis.

These things can also increase your risk for osteoporosis:

- Hormone changes (especially for women who have gone through menopause)

- Not getting enough calcium and Vitamin D

- Taking certain medicines

- Smoking cigarettes or drinking too much alcohol

- Not getting enough physical activity

What If I Have Osteoporosis?

If you have osteoporosis, you can still slow down bone loss. Finding and treating this disease early can keep you healthier and more active, lowering your chances of breaking a bone.

Depending on the results of your bone density test, you may need to:

- Add more calcium and vitamin D to your diet

- Exercise more to strengthen your bones

- Take medicine to stop bone loss

Your doctor can tell you what steps are right for you. It doesn't matter how old you are—it's not too late to build stronger bones.

Take Action

Take these steps to protect your bone health.

Schedule a Bone Density Test, If Your Doctor Recommends It

Ask your doctor if you are at risk for osteoporosis and find out when to start getting bone density tests.

What about Cost?

Screening for osteoporosis is covered under the Affordable Care Act (ACA), the healthcare reform law passed in 2010. Depending on your insurance plan, you may be able to get screened at no cost to you.

- If you don't have health insurance, you can still get a bone density test

- You need both vitamin D and calcium for strong bones

Get Enough Calcium

Calcium helps keep your bones strong. Good sources of calcium include:

- Low-fat or fat-free milk, cheese, and yogurt
- Almonds
- Broccoli and greens
- Tofu with added calcium
- Orange juice with added calcium
- Calcium pills

Get Enough Vitamin D

Vitamin D helps your body absorb (take in) calcium. Your body makes vitamin D when you are out in the sun. You can also get vitamin D from:

- Salmon or tuna
- Fat-free or low-fat milk and yogurt with added vitamin D
- Breakfast cereals and juices with added vitamin D
- Vitamin D pills

Get Active

Physical activity can help slow down bone loss. Weight-bearing activities (like running or doing jumping jacks) help keep your bones strong.

- Aim for 2 hours and 30 minutes a week of moderate aerobic activity. If you are new to exercise, start with 10 minutes of activity at a time.
- Do strengthening activities at least 2 days a week. These include lifting weights or using resistance bands (long rubber strips that stretch).
- Find an exercise buddy or go walking with friends. You will be more likely to stick with it if you exercise with other people.

Find Activities That Work for You

You don't need special equipment or a gym membership to stay active. Check with your local community center or senior center to find fun, low-cost, or free exercise options. If you have a health condition or a disability, be as active as you can be. Your doctor can help you choose activities that are right for you.

Stay Away from Cigarettes and Alcohol

Smoking cigarettes and drinking too much alcohol can weaken your bones.

- Try to quit smoking.
- If you drink alcohol, drink only in moderation. This means no more than 1 drink a day for women and no more than 2 drinks a day for men.

Take Steps to Prevent Falls

Falls can be especially serious for people with weak bones. You can make small changes to lower your risk of falling, like doing exercises that improve your balance. For example, try walking backward or standing up from a sitting position without using your hands.

Section 6.2

Hearing Test

This section includes text excerpted from "Get Your Hearing Checked," Office of Disease Prevention and Health Promotion (ODPHP), U.S. Department of Health and Human Services (HHS), June 18, 2018.

The Basics

If you are worried that you might have hearing loss, you aren't alone. Many people lose their hearing slowly as they age.

- Almost 1 in 4 Americans between ages 65 and 74 have hearing loss

- Almost 1 in 2 Americans over age 75 have hearing loss

It's also possible to develop hearing loss due to noise. This is true at any age—and it can happen suddenly or over time. At least 10 million Americans under age 70 may have a hearing problem caused by being around loud noise. Start by talking with your doctor. Your doctor may refer you to a hearing specialist for a hearing test.

Hearing Problems Are Serious

Hearing loss can be frustrating and even dangerous. If you have hearing loss, you may:

- Have trouble hearing doorbells or alarms
- Miss important directions or warnings
- Feel alone or depressed
- Have other health problems

The good news is that if you have a hearing problem, there are things you can do to hear better. That's why it's important to get your hearing checked.

How Do I Know If I Have Hearing Loss?

If you have hearing loss, you may have trouble hearing or understanding family members, friends, or coworkers. It may also help to ask yourself these questions:

- Do I often ask people to repeat themselves?
- Do I hear ringing in my ears?
- Do I have trouble hearing the TV or radio when others don't?
- Do I have trouble hearing when there's noise in the background?

What Can I Do If I Have Hearing Loss?

There are many products, tools, and devices that can help with hearing loss:

- Special phones and smartphone apps that make sounds louder
- Tools to help you hear in places like a classroom or theater (called assistive listening devices)

- Television (TV) settings that also show text (called closed captioning)

- Flashing lights to let you know when an alarm or doorbell is ringing

- Hearing aids you wear in or behind your ear

If you think you have hearing loss, a doctor can help you figure out which options are right for you.

Take Action

Take steps to find out if you have hearing loss.

Ask Your Doctor about Getting Your Hearing Tested

If you are worried about your hearing, talk with your doctor. Your doctor or nurse may refer you to a specialist for a hearing test—or for help with your hearing.

What about Cost?

Check with your insurance provider to find out if your plan covers the cost of a hearing test. Medicare may also cover hearing tests with a referral from your doctor.

Talk to Your Friends and Family

If you have trouble hearing, your friends and family need to know. They can make small changes to help you hear better when they talk. Ask them to:

- Find a quiet place to talk where there isn't a lot of background noise

- Face you, speak louder, and talk clearly

- Keep their hands away from their mouths while they talk

- Avoid eating or chewing gum while talking with you

- Repeat what they said if you didn't hear it the first time

- Write down important information for you

Protect Your Ears from Loud Noises

Loud noises can cause hearing loss—no matter how old you are. To help prevent damage to your hearing:

- Wear earplugs or special earmuffs if you are going to be around loud sounds, like at a construction site or a concert.

- Keep the volume low when you listen to music through earbuds or headphones.

Section 6.3

Vision Test

This section includes text excerpted from "Get Your Eyes Tested," Office of Disease Prevention and Health Promotion (ODPHP), U.S. Department of Health and Human Services (HHS), December 21, 2017.

The Basics

Have your eyes tested (examined) regularly to help find problems early, when they may be easier to treat. The doctor will also do tests to make sure you are seeing as clearly as possible.

How Often Do I Need an Eye Exam?

How often you need an eye exam depends on your risk for eye disease. Talk to your doctor about how often to get your eyes tested.

Get an eye exam every 1–2 years if you:

- Are over age 60

- Are African American and over age 40

- Have a family history of glaucoma

People with Diabetes May Need Eye Exams More Often

If you have diabetes, it's important to get your eyes tested at least once a year. Talk to your doctor about what's right for you.

What Happens during an Eye Exam?

- The doctor will ask you questions about your health and vision

- You will read charts with letters and numbers so the doctor can check your vision

- The doctor will do tests to look for problems with your eyes, including glaucoma

- The doctor will put drops in your eyes to dilate (enlarge) your pupils. A dilated eye exam is the only way to find some types of eye disease.

Am I at Risk for a Vision Problem?

As you get older, your eyes change. This increases your chance of developing a vision problem. You may be at higher risk if one of your parents had a vision problem, like needing to wear glasses.

Common vision problems are:

- Nearsightedness—a condition that makes faraway objects look blurry

- Farsightedness—a condition that makes nearby objects look blurry

- Astigmatism—a condition that makes things look blurry or distorted at all distances

- Presbyopia—a condition that older adults can get that makes it hard to see things up close

Am I at Risk for Eye Disease?

Getting older increases your risk of certain eye diseases. You may be at higher risk if you have diabetes or high blood pressure—or if you have a family member with diabetes or an eye disease.

Eye diseases like glaucoma can lead to vision loss and blindness if they aren't caught and treated early.

Depending on your age and medical history, the doctor may look for eye problems that are common in older adults, including:

- Cataracts

- Glaucoma

- Age-related macular degeneration (AMD)

77

- Diabetic eye disease

- Low vision

- Dry eye

What's the Difference between a Vision Screening and an Eye Exam?

A vision screening is a short checkup for your eyes. It usually takes place during a regular doctor visit. Vision screenings can only find certain eye problems.

An eye exam takes more time than a vision screening, and it's the only way to find some types of eye disease.

These two kinds of doctors can perform eye exams:

1. Optometrist

2. Ophthalmologist

Take Action

Protect your vision. Get regular eye exams so you can find problems early, when they may be easier to treat.

Schedule an Eye Exam

Ask your doctor or health center for the name of an eye care professional.

When you go for your exam, be sure to:

- Ask the doctor for a dilated eye exam.

- Tell the doctor if anyone in your family has eye problems or diabetes.

What about Cost?

Check with your insurance plan about costs and copayments. Medicare covers eye exams for:

- People with diabetes

- People who are at high risk for glaucoma

- Some people who have age-related macular degeneration

If you don't have insurance, look for free or low-cost eye care programs where you live.

Tell a Doctor about Problems

See an eye doctor right away if you have any of these problems:

- Sudden loss of vision
- Flashes of light
- Tiny spots that float across your eye
- Eye pain
- Redness or swelling

Get Regular Physical Exams

Get regular checkups to help you stay healthy. Ask your doctor or nurse how you can prevent type 2 diabetes and high blood pressure. These diseases can cause eye problems if they aren't treated.

Lower Your Risk of Falling

Poor vision or the wrong glasses can increase your risk of falling. One in 3 older adults will fall each year. Falling can cause serious injuries and health problems, especially for people over age 64.

Section 6.4

Recommended Immunizations for Seniors

This section includes text excerpted from "Get Shots to Protect Your Health (Adults Age 50 or Older)," Office of Disease Prevention and Health Promotion (ODPHP), U.S. Department of Health and Human Services (HHS), February 21, 2018.

The Basics

Older adults need to get shots (vaccines) to prevent serious diseases. Protect your health by getting all your shots on schedule.

If you are age 50 or older:

- Get shots to prevent shingles. Shingles causes a rash and can lead to pain that lasts for months.

If you are age 65 or older:

- Get shots to prevent pneumococcal disease. Pneumococcal disease can include pneumonia, meningitis, and blood infections.

It's also important for all adults to:

- Get a flu vaccine every year. The seasonal flu vaccine is the best way to protect yourself and others from the flu.

- Get the Tdap shot to protect against tetanus, diphtheria, and whooping cough (pertussis). Everyone needs to get the Tdap shot once.

- After you get a Tdap shot, get a Td shot every 10 years to keep you protected against tetanus and diphtheria.

Ask your doctor or nurse about other shots you may need to stay healthy.

Why Do I Need to Get These Shots?

Shots help protect you against diseases that can be serious and sometimes deadly. Many of these diseases are common.

Even if you have always gotten your shots on schedule, you still need to get some shots as an older adult. This is because:

- Older adults are more likely to get certain diseases.

- Older adults are more at risk for serious complications from infections.

- The protection from some shots can wear off over time.

Getting Your Shots Also Protects Other People

When you get shots, you don't just protect yourself—you also protect others. This is especially important if you spend time around anyone with a long-term health problem or a weak immune system (the system in the body that fights infections). Protect yourself and those around you by staying up to date on your shots.

Do I Need Any Other Shots to Help Me Stay Healthy?

You may need other shots if you:

- Didn't get all of your shots as a child

- Have a health condition that weakens your immune system (like cancer or human immunodeficiency virus (HIV))

- Have a long-term (chronic) health problem like diabetes or heart, lung, or liver disease

- Are a man who has sex with men

- Smoke

- Spend time with infants or young children

- Work or spend time in a school, hospital, prison, or health clinic

- Travel outside the United States

Ask your doctor or nurse if you need any other shots.

Take Action

Talk with a doctor, nurse, or pharmacist about getting up to date on your shots.

Make a Plan to Get Your Shots

Schedule an appointment with your doctor or nurse to get the shots you need. You may also be able to get shots at your local pharmacy.

Get a Seasonal Flu Shot Every Year

Remember, everyone age 6 months and older needs to get the seasonal flu vaccine every year.

What about Cost?

Under the Affordable Care Act (ACA), the healthcare reform law passed in 2010, most private insurance plans must cover recommended shots for adults. Depending on your insurance plan, you may be able to get your shots at no cost to you.

Medicare also covers most recommended shots for older adults, depending on your plan.

If you don't have insurance, you still may be able to get free shots.

- Call your state health department to find a free or low-cost vaccination program.

- Find a health center near you and ask about affordable vaccine services.

Keep a Copy of Your Vaccination Record

Ask your doctor to print out a record of all the shots you've had. Keep this record in a safe place. You may need it for certain jobs or if you travel outside the United States.

Chapter 7

Genetic Testing

Chapter Contents

Section 7.1

Frequently Asked Questions about Genetic Testing

This section includes text excerpted from "What Is Genetic Testing?" Genetics Home Reference (GHR), National Institutes of Health (NIH), June 26, 2018.

What Is Genetic Testing?

Genetic testing is a type of medical test that identifies changes in chromosomes, genes, or proteins. The results of a genetic test can confirm or rule out a suspected genetic condition or help determine a person's chance of developing or passing on a genetic disorder. More than 1,000 genetic tests are currently in use, and more are being developed.

Several methods can be used for genetic testing:

- Molecular genetic tests (or gene tests) study single genes or short lengths of deoxyribonucleic acid (DNA) to identify variations or mutations that lead to a genetic disorder.

- Chromosomal genetic tests analyze whole chromosomes or long lengths of DNA to see if there are large genetic changes, such as an extra copy of a chromosome, that cause a genetic condition.

- Biochemical genetic tests study the amount or activity level of proteins; abnormalities in either can indicate changes to the DNA that result in a genetic disorder.

Genetic testing is voluntary. Because testing has benefits as well as limitations and risks, the decision about whether to be tested is a personal and complex one. A geneticist or genetic counselor can help by providing information about the pros and cons of the test and discussing the social and emotional aspects of testing.

What Are the Types of Genetic Tests?

Genetic testing can provide information about a person's genes and chromosomes. Available types of testing include:

Newborn Screening

Newborn screening is used just after birth to identify genetic disorders that can be treated early in life. Millions of babies are tested each year in the United States. All states currently test infants for phenyl-ketonuria (PKU) (a genetic disorder that causes intellectual disability (ID) if left untreated) and congenital hypothyroidism (CH) (a disorder of the thyroid gland). Most states also test for other genetic disorders.

Diagnostic Testing

Diagnostic testing is used to identify or rule out a specific genetic or chromosomal condition. In many cases, genetic testing is used to confirm a diagnosis when a particular condition is suspected based on physical signs and symptoms. Diagnostic testing can be performed before birth or at any time during a person's life, but is not available for all genes or all genetic conditions. The results of a diagnostic test can influence a person's choices about healthcare and the management of the disorder.

Carrier Testing

Carrier testing is used to identify people who carry one copy of a gene mutation that, when present in two copies, causes a genetic disorder. This type of testing is offered to individuals who have a family history of a genetic disorder and to people in certain ethnic groups with an increased risk of specific genetic conditions. If both parents are tested, the test can provide information about a couple's risk of having a child with a genetic condition.

Prenatal Testing

Prenatal testing is used to detect changes in a fetus's genes or chromosomes before birth. This type of testing is offered during pregnancy if there is an increased risk that the baby will have a genetic or chromosomal disorder. In some cases, prenatal testing can lessen a couple's uncertainty or help them make decisions about a pregnancy. It cannot identify all possible inherited disorders and birth defects, however.

Preimplantation Testing

Preimplantation testing, also called preimplantation genetic diagnosis (PGD), is a specialized technique that can reduce the risk of having a child with a particular genetic or chromosomal disorder. It is used to detect genetic changes in embryos that were created using assisted reproductive techniques such as in-vitro fertilization (IVF). IVF involves removing egg cells from a woman's ovaries and fertilizing them with sperm cells outside the body. To perform preimplantation testing, a small number of cells are taken from these embryos and tested for certain genetic changes. Only embryos without these changes are implanted in the uterus to initiate a pregnancy.

Predictive and Presymptomatic Testing

Predictive and presymptomatic types of testing are used to detect gene mutations associated with disorders that appear after birth, often later in life. These tests can be helpful to people who have a family member with a genetic disorder, but who have no features of the disorder themselves at the time of testing. Predictive testing can identify mutations that increase a person's risk of developing disorders with a genetic basis, such as certain types of cancer. Presymptomatic testing can determine whether a person will develop a genetic disorder, such as hereditary hemochromatosis (HFE) (an iron overload disorder), before any signs or symptoms appear. The results of predictive and presymptomatic testing can provide information about a person's risk of developing a specific disorder and help with making decisions about medical care.

Forensic Testing

Forensic testing uses DNA sequences to identify an individual for legal purposes. Unlike the tests described above, forensic testing is not used to detect gene mutations associated with disease. This type of testing can identify crime or catastrophe victims, rule out or implicate a crime suspect, or establish biological relationships between people (for example, paternity).

How Is Genetic Testing Done?

Once a person decides to proceed with genetic testing, a medical geneticist, primary care doctor, specialist, or nurse practitioner can order the test. Genetic testing is often done as part of a genetic consultation.

Genetic tests are performed on a sample of blood, hair, skin, amniotic fluid (the fluid that surrounds a fetus during pregnancy), or other tissue. For example, a procedure called a buccal smear uses a small brush or cotton swab to collect a sample of cells from the inside surface of the cheek. The sample is sent to a laboratory where technicians look for specific changes in chromosomes, DNA, or proteins, depending on the suspected disorder. The laboratory reports the test results in writing to a person's doctor or genetic counselor, or directly to the patient if requested.

Newborn screening tests are done on a small blood sample, which is taken by pricking the baby's heel. Unlike other types of genetic testing, a parent will usually only receive the result if it is positive. If the test result is positive, additional testing is needed to determine whether the baby has a genetic disorder.

Before a person has a genetic test, it is important that he or she understands the testing procedure, the benefits and limitations of the test, and the possible consequences of the test results. The process of educating a person about the test and obtaining permission is called informed consent.

What Is Informed Consent?

Before a person has a genetic test, it is important that he or she fully understands the testing procedure, the benefits and limitations of the test, and the possible consequences of the test results. The process of educating a person about the test and obtaining permission to carry out testing is called informed consent. "Informed" means that the person has enough information to make an educated decision about testing; "consent" refers to a person's voluntary agreement to have the test done.

In general, informed consent can only be given by adults who are competent to make medical decisions for themselves. For children and others who are unable to make their own medical decisions (such as people with impaired mental status), informed consent can be given by a parent, guardian, or other person legally responsible for making decisions on that person's behalf.

Informed consent for genetic testing is generally obtained by a doctor or genetic counselor during an office visit. The healthcare provider will discuss the test and answer any questions. If the person wishes to have the test, he or she will then usually read and sign a consent form.

Several factors are commonly included on an informed consent form:

- A general description of the test, including the purpose of the test and the condition for which the testing is being performed.

- How the test will be carried out (for example, a blood sample).

- What the test results mean, including positive and negative results, and the potential for uninformative results or incorrect results such as false positives or false negatives.

- Any physical or emotional risks associated with the test.

- Whether the results can be used for research purposes.

- Whether the results might provide information about other family members' health, including the risk of developing a particular condition or the possibility of having affected children.

- How and to whom test results will be reported and under what circumstances results can be disclosed (for example, to health insurance providers).

- What will happen to the test specimen after the test is complete.

- Acknowledgment that the person requesting testing has had the opportunity to discuss the test with a healthcare professional.

- The individual's signature, and possibly that of a witness.

The elements of informed consent may vary, because some states have laws that specify factors that must be included. (For example, some states require disclosure that the test specimen will be destroyed within a certain period of time after the test is complete.)

Informed consent is not a contract, so a person can change his or her mind at any time after giving initial consent. A person may choose not to go through with genetic testing even after the test sample has been collected. A person simply needs to notify the healthcare provider if he or she decides not to continue with the testing process.

How Can Consumers Be Sure a Genetic Test Is Valid and Useful?

Before undergoing genetic testing, it is important to be sure that the test is valid and useful. A genetic test is valid if it provides an accurate result. Two main measures of accuracy apply to genetic tests: analytical validity and clinical validity. Another measure of the quality of a genetic test is its usefulness, or clinical utility.

- Analytical validity refers to how well the test predicts the presence or absence of a particular gene or genetic change. In other words, can the test accurately detect whether a specific genetic variant is present or absent?

- Clinical validity refers to how well the genetic variant being analyzed is related to the presence, absence, or risk of a specific disease.

- Clinical utility refers to whether the test can provide information about diagnosis, treatment, management, or prevention of a disease that will be helpful to a consumer.

All laboratories that perform health-related testing, including genetic testing, are subject to federal regulatory standards called the Clinical Laboratory Improvement Amendments (CLIA) or even stricter state requirements. CLIA standards cover how tests are performed, the qualifications of laboratory personnel, and quality control and testing procedures for each laboratory. By controlling the quality of laboratory practices, CLIA standards are designed to ensure the analytical validity of genetic tests.

CLIA standards do not address the clinical validity or clinical utility of genetic tests. The U.S. Food and Drug Administration (FDA) requires information about clinical validity for some genetic tests. Additionally, the state of New York requires information on clinical validity for all laboratory tests performed for people living in that state. Consumers, health providers, and health insurance companies are often the ones who determine the clinical utility of a genetic test.

It can be difficult to determine the quality of a genetic test sold directly to the public. Some providers of direct-to-consumer (DTC) genetic tests are not CLIA-certified, so it can be difficult to tell whether their tests are valid. If providers of DTC genetic tests offer easy-to-understand information about the scientific basis of their tests, it can help consumers make more informed decisions. It may also be helpful to discuss any concerns with a health professional before ordering a DTC genetic test.

What Do the Results of Genetic Tests Mean?

The results of genetic tests are not always straightforward, which often makes them challenging to interpret and explain. Therefore, it is important for patients and their families to ask questions about the potential meaning of genetic test results both before and after the test is performed. When interpreting test results, healthcare professionals consider a person's medical history, family history, and the type of genetic test that was done.

A positive test result means that the laboratory found a change in a particular gene, chromosome, or protein of interest. Depending on the purpose of the test, this result may confirm a diagnosis, indicate that a person is a carrier of a particular genetic mutation, identify an increased risk of developing a disease (such as cancer) in the future, or suggest a need for further testing. Because family members have some genetic material in common, a positive test result may also have implications for certain blood relatives of the person undergoing testing. It is important to note that a positive result of a predictive or presymptomatic genetic test usually cannot establish the exact risk of developing a disorder. Also, health professionals typically cannot use a positive test result to predict the course or severity of a condition.

A negative test result means that the laboratory did not find a change in the gene, chromosome, or protein under consideration. This result can indicate that a person is not affected by a particular disorder, is not a carrier of a specific genetic mutation, or does not have an increased risk of developing a certain disease. It is possible, however, that the test missed a disease-causing genetic alteration because many tests cannot detect all genetic changes that can cause a particular disorder. Further testing may be required to confirm a negative result.

In some cases, a test result might not give any useful information. This type of result is called uninformative, indeterminate, inconclusive, or ambiguous. Uninformative test results sometimes occur because everyone has common, natural variations in their DNA, called polymorphisms, that do not affect health. If a genetic test finds a change in DNA that has not been associated with a disorder in other people, it can be difficult to tell whether it is a natural polymorphism or a disease-causing mutation. An uninformative result cannot confirm or rule out a specific diagnosis, and it cannot indicate whether a person has an increased risk of developing a disorder. In some cases, testing other affected and unaffected family members can help clarify this type of result.

What Is the Cost of Genetic Testing, and How Long Does It Take to Get the Results?

The cost of genetic testing can range from under $100 to more than $2,000, depending on the nature and complexity of the test. The cost increases if more than one test is necessary or if multiple family members must be tested to obtain a meaningful result. For newborn screening, costs vary by state. Some states cover part of the total cost, but most charge a fee of $15 to $60 per infant.

From the date that a sample is taken, it may take a few weeks to several months to receive the test results. Results for prenatal testing are usually available more quickly because time is an important consideration in making decisions about a pregnancy.

The doctor or genetic counselor who orders a particular test can provide specific information about the cost and time frame associated with that test.

Will Health Insurance Cover the Costs of Genetic Testing?

In many cases, health insurance plans will cover the costs of genetic testing when it is recommended by a person's doctor. Health insurance providers have different policies about which tests are covered, however. A person interested in submitting the costs of testing may wish to contact his or her insurance company beforehand to ask about coverage.

Some people may choose not to use their insurance to pay for testing because the results of a genetic test can affect a person's insurance coverage. Instead, they may opt to pay out-of-pocket for the test. People considering genetic testing may want to find out more about their state's privacy protection laws before they ask their insurance company to cover the costs.

What Are the Benefits of Genetic Testing?

Genetic testing has potential benefits whether the results are positive or negative for a gene mutation. Test results can provide a sense of relief from uncertainty and help people make informed decisions about managing their healthcare. For example, a negative result can eliminate the need for unnecessary checkups and screening tests in some cases. A positive result can direct a person toward available prevention, monitoring, and treatment options. Some test results can also help people make decisions about having children. Newborn screening can identify genetic disorders early in life so treatment can be started as early as possible.

What Are the Risks and Limitations of Genetic Testing?

The physical risks associated with most genetic tests are very small, particularly for those tests that require only a blood sample or buccal smear (a method that samples cells from the inside surface of the cheek). The procedures used for prenatal testing carry a small but real risk of losing the pregnancy (miscarriage) because they require a sample of amniotic fluid or tissue from around the fetus.

Many of the risks associated with genetic testing involve the emotional, social, or financial consequences of the test results. People may feel angry, depressed, anxious, or guilty about their results. In some cases, genetic testing creates tension within a family because the results can reveal information about other family members in addition to the person who is tested. The possibility of genetic discrimination in employment or insurance is also a concern.

Genetic testing can provide only limited information about an inherited condition. The test often can't determine if a person will show symptoms of a disorder, how severe the symptoms will be, or whether the disorder will progress over time. Another major limitation is the lack of treatment strategies for many genetic disorders once they are diagnosed.

A genetics professional can explain in detail the benefits, risks, and limitations of a particular test. It is important that any person who is considering genetic testing understand and weigh these factors before making a decision.

How Does Genetic Testing in a Research Setting Differ from Clinical Genetic Testing?

The main differences between clinical genetic testing and research testing are the purpose of the test and who receives the results. The goals of research testing include finding unknown genes, learning how genes work, developing tests for future clinical use, and advancing the understanding of genetic conditions. The results of testing done as part of a research study are usually not available to patients or their healthcare providers. Clinical testing, on the other hand, is done to find out about an inherited disorder in an individual patient or family. People receive the results of a clinical test and can use them to help them make decisions about medical care or reproductive issues.

It is important for people considering genetic testing to know whether the test is available on a clinical or research basis. Clinical and research testing both involve a process of informed consent in which patients learn about the testing procedure, the risks and benefits of the test, and the potential consequences of testing.

Section 7.2

Genetic Consultation

This section includes text excerpted from "What Is a
Genetic Consultation?" Genetics Home Reference (GHR),
National Institutes of Health (NIH), July 3, 2018.

What Is a Genetic Consultation?

A genetic consultation is a health service that provides information and support to people who have, or may be at risk for, genetic disorders. During a consultation, a genetics professional meets with an individual or family to discuss genetic risks or to diagnose, confirm, or rule out a genetic condition.

Genetics professionals include medical geneticists (doctors who specialize in genetics) and genetic counselors (certified healthcare workers with experience in medical genetics and counseling). Other healthcare professionals such as nurses, psychologists, and social workers trained in genetics can also provide genetic consultations.

Consultations usually take place in a doctor's office, hospital, genetics center, or other type of medical center. These meetings are most often in-person visits with individuals or families, but they are occasionally conducted in a group or over the telephone.

Why Might Someone Have a Genetic Consultation?

Individuals or families who are concerned about an inherited condition may benefit from a genetic consultation. The reasons that a person might be referred to a genetic counselor, medical geneticist, or other genetics professional include:

- A personal or family history of a genetic condition, birth defect, chromosomal disorder, or hereditary cancer.

- Two or more pregnancy losses (miscarriages), a stillbirth, or a baby who died.

- A child with a known inherited disorder, a birth defect, intellectual disability (ID), or developmental delay.

- A woman who is pregnant or plans to become pregnant at or after age 35. (Some chromosomal disorders occur more frequently in children born to older women.)

- Abnormal test results that suggest a genetic or chromosomal condition.

- An increased risk of developing or passing on a particular genetic disorder on the basis of a person's ethnic background.

- People related by blood (for example, cousins) who plan to have children together. (A child whose parents are related may be at an increased risk of inheriting certain genetic disorders.)

A genetic consultation is also an important part of the decision-making process for genetic testing. A visit with a genetics professional may be helpful even if testing is not available for a specific condition, however.

What Happens during a Genetic Consultation?

A genetic consultation provides information, offers support, and addresses a patient's specific questions and concerns. To help determine whether a condition has a genetic component, a genetics professional asks about a person's medical history and takes a detailed family history (a record of health information about a person's immediate and extended family). The genetics professional may also perform a physical examination and recommend appropriate tests.

If a person is diagnosed with a genetic condition, the genetics professional provides information about the diagnosis, how the condition is inherited, the chance of passing the condition to future generations, and the options for testing and treatment.

During a consultation, a genetics professional will:

- interpret and communicate complex medical information

- help each person make informed, independent decisions about their healthcare and reproductive options

- respect each person's individual beliefs, traditions, and feelings

A genetics professional will NOT:

- tell a person which decision to make

- advise a couple not to have children

- recommend that a woman continue or end a pregnancy

- tell someone whether to undergo testing for a genetic disorder

How Can I Find a Genetics Professional in My Area?

To find a genetics professional in your community, you may wish to ask your doctor for a referral. If you have health insurance, you can also contact your insurance company to find a medical geneticist or genetic counselor in your area who participates in your plan.

Several organizations have tips for finding a healthcare professional:

- The Genetic and Rare Diseases Information Center (GARD), a service of the National Institutes of Health (NIH), provides a guide to finding specialists in particular genetic and rare conditions.

- The Tuberous Sclerosis (TS) Alliance provides advice on finding and choosing a doctor. Although this advice is written for adults with tuberous sclerosis, much of it applies to people with any chronic health condition.

Additional resources for locating a genetics professional in your community are available online:

- The National Society of Genetic Counselors (NSGC) offers a searchable directory of genetic counselors in the United States and Canada. You can search by location, name, area of practice/ specialization, and/or ZIP Code.

- The American Board of Genetic Counseling (ABGC) provides a searchable directory of certified genetic counselors worldwide. You can search by practice area, name, organization, or location.

- The Canadian Association of Genetic Counsellors (CAGC) has a searchable directory of genetic counselors in Canada. You can search by name, distance from an address, province, or services.

- The American College of Medical Genetics and Genomics (ACMG) has a searchable database of medical genetics clinic services in the United States.

- The National Cancer Institute (NCI) provides a Cancer Genetics Services Directory, which lists professionals who provide services related to cancer genetics. You can search by type of cancer or syndrome, location, and/or provider name.

What Is the Prognosis of a Genetic Condition?

The prognosis of a genetic condition includes its likely course, duration, and outcome. When health professionals refer to the prognosis of a disease, they may also mean the chance of recovery; however, most genetic conditions are life-long and are managed rather than cured.

Disease prognosis has multiple aspects, including:

- How long a person with the disorder is likely to live (life expectancy)

- Whether the signs and symptoms worsen (and how quickly) or are stable over time

- Quality of life, such as independence in daily activities

- Potential for complications and associated health issues

The prognosis of a genetic condition depends on many factors, including the specific diagnosis and an individual's particular signs and symptoms. Sometimes the associated genetic change, if known, can also give clues to the prognosis. Additionally, the course and outcome of a condition depends on the availability and effectiveness of treatment and management approaches. The prognosis of very rare diseases can be difficult to predict because so few affected individuals have been identified. Prognosis may also be difficult or impossible to establish if a person's diagnosis is unknown.

The prognoses of genetic disorders vary widely, often even among people with the same condition. Some genetic disorders cause physical and developmental problems that are so severe they are incompatible with life. These conditions may cause a miscarriage of an affected embryo or fetus, or an affected infant may be stillborn or die shortly after birth. People with less severe genetic conditions may live into childhood or adulthood but have a shortened lifespan due to health problems related to their disorder. Genetic conditions with a milder course may be associated with a normal lifespan and few related health issues.

The prognosis of a disease is based on probability, which means that it is likely but not certain that the disorder will follow a particular course. Your healthcare provider is the best resource for information about the prognosis of your specific genetic condition. He or she can assess your medical history and signs and symptoms to give you the most accurate estimate of your prognosis.

How Are Genetic Conditions Diagnosed?

A doctor may suspect a diagnosis of a genetic condition on the basis of a person's physical characteristics and family history, or on the results of a screening test.

Genetic testing is one of several tools that doctors use to diagnose genetic conditions. The approaches to making a genetic diagnosis include:

- **A physical examination:** Certain physical characteristics, such as distinctive facial features, can suggest the diagnosis of a genetic disorder. A geneticist will do a thorough physical examination that may include measurements such as the distance around the head (head circumference), the distance between the eyes, and the length of the arms and legs. Depending on the situation, specialized examinations such as nervous system (neurological) or eye (ophthalmologic) exams may be performed. The doctor may also use imaging studies including X-rays, computerized tomography (CT) scans, or magnetic resonance imaging (MRI) to see structures inside the body.

- **Personal medical history:** Information about an individual's health, often going back to birth, can provide clues to a genetic diagnosis. A personal medical history includes past health issues, hospitalizations and surgeries, allergies, medications, and the results of any medical or genetic testing that has already been done.

- **Family medical history:** Because genetic conditions often run in families, information about the health of family members can be a critical tool for diagnosing these disorders. A doctor or genetic counselor will ask about health conditions in an individual's parents, siblings, children, and possibly more distant relatives. This information can give clues about the diagnosis and inheritance pattern of a genetic condition in a family.

- **Laboratory tests, including genetic testing:** Molecular, chromosomal, and biochemical genetic testing are used to diagnose genetic disorders. Other laboratory tests that measure the levels of certain substances in blood and urine can also help suggest a diagnosis.

Genetic testing is currently available for many genetic conditions. However, some conditions do not have a genetic test; either the genetic cause of the condition is unknown or a test has not yet been developed. In these cases, a combination of the approaches listed above may be used to make a diagnosis. Even when genetic testing is available, the tools listed above are used to narrow down the possibilities (known as a differential diagnosis) and choose the most appropriate genetic tests to pursue.

A diagnosis of a genetic disorder can be made anytime during life, from before birth to old age, depending on when the features of the condition appear and the availability of testing. Sometimes, having a diagnosis can guide treatment and management decisions. A genetic diagnosis can also suggest whether other family members may be affected by or at risk of a specific disorder. Even when no treatment is available for a particular condition, having a diagnosis can help people know what to expect and may help them identify useful support and advocacy resources.

How Are Genetic Conditions Treated or Managed?

Many genetic disorders result from gene changes that are present in essentially every cell in the body. As a result, these disorders often affect many body systems, and most cannot be cured. However, approaches may be available to treat or manage some of the associated signs and symptoms.

For a group of genetic conditions called inborn errors of metabolism, which result from genetic changes that disrupt the production of specific enzymes, treatments sometimes include dietary changes or replacement of the particular enzyme that is missing. Limiting certain substances in the diet can help prevent the buildup of potentially toxic substances that are normally broken down by the enzyme. In some cases, enzyme replacement therapy can help compensate for the enzyme shortage. These treatments are used to manage existing signs and symptoms and may help prevent future complications.

For other genetic conditions, treatment and management strategies are designed to improve particular signs and symptoms associated with the disorder. These approaches vary by disorder and are specific to an individual's health needs. For example, a genetic disorder associated with a heart defect might be treated with surgery to repair the defect or with a heart transplant. Conditions that are characterized by defective blood cell formation, such as sickle cell disease, can sometimes be treated with a bone marrow transplant. Bone marrow transplantation can allow the formation of normal blood cells and, if done early in life, may help prevent episodes of pain and other future complications.

Some genetic changes are associated with an increased risk of future health problems, such as certain forms of cancer. One well-known example is familial breast cancer related to mutations in the *BRCA1* and *BRCA2* genes. Management may include more frequent cancer screening or preventive (prophylactic) surgery to remove the tissues at highest risk of becoming cancerous.

Genetic disorders may cause such severe health problems that they are incompatible with life. In the most severe cases, these conditions may cause a miscarriage of an affected embryo or fetus. In other cases, affected infants may be stillborn or die shortly after birth. Although few treatments are available for these severe genetic conditions, health professionals can often provide supportive care, such as pain relief or mechanical breathing assistance, to the affected individual.

Most treatment strategies for genetic disorders do not alter the underlying genetic mutation; however, a few disorders have been treated with gene therapy. This experimental technique involves changing a person's genes to prevent or treat a disease. Gene therapy, along with many other treatment and management approaches for genetic conditions, are under study in clinical trials.

Section 7.3

Genetic Testing for Breast Cancer Risk

This section includes text excerpted from "BRCA Mutations: Cancer Risk and Genetic Testing," National Cancer Institute (NCI), January 30, 2018.

What Are BRCA1 *and* BRCA2 *?*

BRCA1 and *BRCA2* are human genes that produce tumor suppressor proteins. These proteins help repair damaged deoxyribonucleic acid (DNA) and, therefore, play a role in ensuring the stability of each cell's genetic material. When either of these genes is mutated, or altered, such that its protein product is not made or does not function correctly, DNA damage may not be repaired properly. As a result, cells are more likely to develop additional genetic alterations that can lead to cancer.

Specific inherited mutations in *BRCA1* and *BRCA2* most notably increase the risk of female breast and ovarian cancers, but they have also been associated with increased risks of several additional types of cancer. People who have inherited mutations in *BRCA1* and *BRCA2* tend to develop breast and ovarian cancers at younger ages than people who do not have these mutations.

A harmful *BRCA1* or *BRCA2* mutation can be inherited from a person's mother or father. Each child of a parent who carries a mutation in one of these genes has a 50 percent chance (or 1 chance in 2) of inheriting the mutation. The effects of mutations in *BRCA1* and *BRCA2* are seen even when a person's second copy of the gene is normal.

How Much Does Having a BRCA1 *or* BRCA2 *Gene Mutation Increase a Woman's Risk of Breast and Ovarian Cancer?*

A woman's lifetime risk of developing breast and/or ovarian cancer is greatly increased if she inherits a harmful mutation in *BRCA1* or *BRCA2*.

Breast cancer: About 12 percent of women in the general population will develop breast cancer sometime during their lives. By contrast, a recent large study estimated that about 72 percent of women who inherit a harmful *BRCA1* mutation and about 69 percent of women who inherit a harmful *BRCA2* mutation will develop breast cancer by the age of 80.

Like women from the general population, those with harmful *BRCA1* or *BRCA2* mutations also have a high risk of developing a new primary cancer in the opposite (contralateral) breast in the years following a breast cancer diagnosis. It has been estimated that, by 20 years after the first breast cancer diagnosis, about 40 percent of women who inherit a harmful *BRCA1* mutation and about 26 percent of women who inherit a harmful *BRCA2* mutation will develop cancer in their other breast.

Ovarian cancer: About 1.3 percent of women in the general population will develop ovarian cancer sometime during their lives. By contrast, it is estimated that about 44 percent of women who inherit a harmful *BRCA1* mutation and about 17 percent of women who inherit a harmful *BRCA2* mutation will develop ovarian cancer by the age of 80.

What Other Cancers Have Been Linked to Mutations in BRCA1 *and* BRCA2 *?*

Harmful mutations in *BRCA1* and *BRCA2* increase the risk of several cancers in addition to breast and ovarian cancer. These include fallopian tube cancer and peritoneal cancer. Men with *BRCA2* mutations, and to a lesser extent *BRCA1* mutations, are also at increased risk of breast cancer and prostate cancer. Both men and women with harmful *BRCA1* or *BRCA2* mutations are at increased risk of pancreatic cancer.

Certain mutations in *BRCA2* (also known as *FANCD1*), if they are inherited from both parents, can cause a rare form of Fanconi anemia (subtype FA-D1), a syndrome that is associated with childhood solid tumors and development of acute myeloid leukemia. Likewise, certain mutations in *BRCA1* (also known as FANCS), if they are inherited from both parents, can cause another Fanconi anemia subtype.

Are Mutations in BRCA1 *and* BRCA2 *More Common in Certain Racial/Ethnic Populations Than Others?*

Yes. For example, people of Ashkenazi Jewish descent have a higher prevalence of harmful *BRCA1* and *BRCA2* mutations than people in the general U.S. population. Other ethnic and geographic populations around the world, such as the Norwegian, Dutch, and Icelandic peoples, also have a higher prevalence of specific harmful *BRCA1* and *BRCA2* mutations.

In addition, the prevalence of specific harmful *BRCA1* and *BRCA2* mutations may vary among individual racial and ethnic groups in the United States, including African Americans, Hispanics, Asian Americans, and non-Hispanic whites.

This question is under intensive study, since identifying population-specific mutations in these genes can greatly simplify the genetic testing for *BRCA1* and *BRCA2* mutations.

Are Genetic Tests Available to Detect BRCA1 *and* BRCA2 *Mutations?*

Yes, several different tests are available. Some tests look for a specific harmful *BRCA1* or *BRCA2* gene mutation that has already been identified in another family member. Other tests check for all of the known harmful mutations in both genes. Multigene (panel) testing uses next-generation sequencing to look for harmful mutations in many genes that are associated with an increased risk of breast and ovarian cancer, including *BRCA1* and *BRCA2*, at the same time.

DNA (usually from a blood or saliva sample) is needed for all of these tests. The sample is sent to a laboratory for analysis. It usually takes about a month to get the test results.

Who Should Consider Genetic Testing for BRCA1 *and* BRCA2 *Mutations?*

Because harmful *BRCA1* and *BRCA2* gene mutations are relatively rare in the general population, most experts agree that mutation testing of individuals who do not have cancer should be performed only when the person's individual or family history suggests the possible presence of a harmful mutation in *BRCA1* or *BRCA2*.

The U.S. Preventive Services Task Force (USPSTF) recommends that women who have family members with breast, ovarian, fallopian tube, or peritoneal cancer be evaluated to see if they have a family history that is associated with an increased risk of a harmful mutation in one of these genes.

Several screening tools are available to help healthcare providers with this evaluation. These tools assess personal or family history factors that are associated with an increased likelihood of having a harmful mutation in *BRCA1* or *BRCA2*, such as:

- Breast cancer diagnosed before age 50 years

- Cancer in both breasts in the same woman

- Both breast and ovarian cancers in either the same woman or the same family

- Multiple breast cancers in the family

- Two or more primary types of *BRCA1*- or *BRCA2*-related cancers in a single family member

- Cases of male breast cancer

- Ashkenazi Jewish ethnicity

When an individual has a family history that is suggestive of the presence of a *BRCA1* or *BRCA2* mutation, it may be most informative to first test a family member who has cancer, if that person is still alive and willing to be tested. If that person has a harmful *BRCA1* or *BRCA2* mutation, then other family members may want to consider genetic counseling to learn more about their potential risks and whether genetic testing for mutations in *BRCA1* and *BRCA2* might be appropriate for them.

If it can't be determined whether the family member with cancer has a harmful *BRCA1* or *BRCA2* mutation, members of a family whose history is suggestive of the presence of a *BRCA1* or *BRCA2* gene mutation may still want to consider genetic counseling for possible testing.

Some individuals—for example, those who were adopted at birth— may not know their family history. If a woman with an unknown family history has an early-onset breast cancer or ovarian cancer or a man with an unknown family history is diagnosed with breast cancer, that individual may want to consider genetic counseling and testing for a *BRCA1* or *BRCA2* mutation.

Professional societies do not recommend that children under age 18, even those with a family history suggestive of a harmful *BRCA1* or *BRCA2* mutation, undergo genetic testing for *BRCA1* or *BRCA2* This is because there are no risk-reduction strategies that are specifically meant for children, and children's risks of developing a cancer type associated with a *BRCA1* or *BRCA2* mutation are extremely low.

Should People Considering Genetic Testing for BRCA1 *and* BRCA2 *Mutations Talk with a Genetic Counselor?*

Genetic counseling is generally recommended before and after any genetic test for an inherited cancer syndrome. This counseling should be performed by a healthcare professional who is experienced in cancer genetics. Genetic counseling usually covers many aspects of the testing process, including:

- A hereditary cancer risk assessment based on an individual's personal and family medical history

- Discussion of:

  - The appropriateness of genetic testing

  - The medical implications of a positive or a negative test result

  - The possibility that a test result might not be informative (that is, it might find an alteration whose effect on cancer risk is not known)

  - The psychological risks and benefits of genetic test results

  - The risk of passing a mutation to children

- Explanation of the specific test(s) that might be used and the technical accuracy of the test(s)

Does Health Insurance Cover the Cost of BRCA1 *and* BRCA2 *Mutation Testing?*

People considering *BRCA1* and *BRCA2* mutation testing may want to confirm their insurance coverage for genetic counseling and testing.

The Affordable Care Act considers genetic counseling and *BRCA1* and *BRCA2* mutation testing a covered preventive service for women who have not already been diagnosed with a cancer related to a mutation in *BRCA1* or *BRCA2* and who meet the USPSTF recommendations for testing.

Medicare covers *BRCA1* and *BRCA2* mutation testing for women who have signs and symptoms of breast, ovarian, or other cancers that are related to mutations in *BRCA1* and *BRCA2* but not for unaffected women.

Some of the genetic testing companies that offer testing for *BRCA1* and *BRCA2* mutations may offer testing at no charge to patients who lack insurance and meet specific financial and medical criteria.

What Do BRCA1 *or* BRCA2 *Genetic Test Results Mean?*

BRCA1 and *BRCA2* gene mutation testing can give several possible results: a positive result, a negative result, or an ambiguous or uncertain result.

Positive result. A positive test result indicates that a person has inherited a known harmful mutation in *BRCA1* or *BRCA2* and, therefore, has an increased risk of developing certain cancers. However, a positive test result cannot tell whether or when an individual will actually develop cancer. Some women who inherit a harmful *BRCA1* or *BRCA2* mutation never develop breast or ovarian cancer.

A positive test result may also have important implications for family members, including future generations.

Both men and women who inherit a harmful *BRCA1* or *BRCA2* mutation, whether or not they develop cancer themselves, may pass the mutation on to their sons and daughters. Each child has a 50 percent chance of inheriting a parent's mutation.

If a person learns that he or she has inherited a harmful *BRCA1* or *BRCA2* mutation, this will mean that each of his or her full siblings has a 50 percent chance of having inherited the mutation as well.

Negative result. A negative test result can be more difficult to understand than a positive result because what the result means depends in part on an individual's family history of cancer and whether a *BRCA1* or *BRCA2* mutation has been identified in a blood relative.

If a close (first- or second-degree) relative of the tested person is known to carry a harmful *BRCA1* or *BRCA2* mutation, a negative test result is clear: it means that person does not carry the harmful mutation that is responsible for their family's cancer risk, and thus cannot pass it on to their children. Such a test result is called a true negative. A person with such a test result is currently thought to have the same risk of cancer as someone in the general population.

If the tested person has a family history that suggests the possibility of having a harmful mutation in *BRCA1* or *BRCA2* but complete gene testing identifies no such mutation in the family, a negative result is less clear. The likelihood that genetic testing will miss a known harmful *BRCA1* or *BRCA2* mutation is very low, but it could happen. Moreover, scientists continue to discover new *BRCA1* and *BRCA2* mutations and have not yet identified all potentially harmful ones. Therefore, it is possible that a person in this scenario with a "negative" test result may actually have a harmful *BRCA1* or *BRCA2* mutation that has not previously been identified.

It is also possible for people to have a mutation in a gene other than *BRCA1* or *BRCA2* that increases their cancer risk but is not detectable by the test used. It is important that people considering genetic testing for *BRCA1* and *BRCA2* mutations discuss these potential uncertainties with a genetic counselor before undergoing testing.

Ambiguous or uncertain result. Sometimes, a genetic test finds a change in *BRCA1* or *BRCA2* that has not been previously associated with cancer. This type of test result may be described as "ambiguous" (often referred to as "a genetic variant of uncertain significance") because it isn't known whether this specific genetic change is harmful. One study found that 10 percent of women who underwent *BRCA1* and *BRCA2* mutation testing had this type of ambiguous result.

As more research is conducted and more people are tested for *BRCA1* and *BRCA2* mutations, scientists will learn more about these changes and cancer risk. Genetic counseling can help a person understand what an ambiguous change in *BRCA1* or *BRCA2* may mean in terms of cancer risk. Over time, additional studies of variants of uncertain significance may result in a specific mutation being reclassified as either clearly harmful or clearly not harmful.

How Can a Person Who Has a Harmful BRCA1 or BRCA2 Gene Mutation Manage Their Risk of Cancer?

Several options are available for managing cancer risk in individuals who have a known harmful *BRCA1* or *BRCA2* mutation. These include enhanced screening, prophylactic (risk-reducing) surgery, and chemoprevention.

Enhanced screening. Some women who test positive for *BRCA1* and *BRCA2* mutations may choose to start breast cancer screening at younger ages, and/or have more frequent screening, than women at average risk of breast cancer. For example, some experts recommend that women who carry a harmful *BRCA1* or *BRCA2* mutation undergo clinical breast examinations beginning at age 25 to 35 years. And some expert groups recommend that women who carry such a mutation have a mammogram every year, beginning at age 25–35 years.

Enhanced screening may increase the chance of detecting breast cancer at an early stage, when it may have a better chance of being treated successfully. Studies have shown that magnetic resonance imaging (MRI) may be better able than mammography to find tumors, particularly in younger women at high risk of breast cancer. However, mammography can also identify some breast cancers that are not identified by MRI. Also, MRI may be less specific (that is, lead to more false-positive results) than mammography.

Several organizations, such as the American Cancer Society (ACS) and the National Comprehensive Cancer Network (NCCN), now recommend annual screening with both mammography and MRI for women who have a high risk of breast cancer. Women who test positive for a *BRCA1* or *BRCA2* mutation should ask their healthcare provider about the possible harms of diagnostic tests that involve radiation (mammograms or X-rays).

No effective ovarian cancer screening methods currently exist. Some groups recommend transvaginal ultrasound, blood tests for the antigen *CA-125* (cancer antigen 125), and clinical examinations for ovarian cancer screening in women with harmful *BRCA1* or *BRCA2* mutations, but none of these methods appears to detect ovarian tumors at an early enough stage to reduce the risk of dying from ovarian cancer. For a screening method to be considered effective, it must have demonstrated reduced mortality from the disease of interest. This standard has not yet been met for ovarian cancer screening.

The benefits of screening for breast and other cancers in men who carry harmful mutations in *BRCA1* or *BRCA2* are also not known, but some expert groups recommend that men who are known to carry a harmful mutation undergo regular breast exams as well as testing for prostate cancer.

Prophylactic (risk-reducing) surgery. Prophylactic surgery involves removing as much of the "at-risk" tissue as possible. Women may choose to have both breasts removed (bilateral prophylactic mastectomy) to reduce their risk of breast cancer. Surgery to remove a woman's ovaries and fallopian tubes (bilateral prophylactic salpingo-oophorectomy (BSO)) can help reduce her risk of ovarian cancer. (Ovarian cancers often originate in the fallopian tubes, so it is essential that they be removed along with the ovaries.) Removing the ovaries may also reduce the risk of breast cancer in premenopausal women by eliminating a source of hormones that can fuel the growth of some types of breast cancer.

Whether bilateral prophylactic mastectomy reduces breast cancer risk in men with a harmful *BRCA1* or *BRCA2* mutation or a family history of breast cancer isn't known. Therefore, bilateral prophylactic mastectomy for men at high risk of breast cancer is considered an experimental procedure, and insurance companies will not normally cover it.

Prophylactic surgery does not guarantee that cancer will not develop because not all at-risk tissue can be removed by these procedures. That is why these surgical procedures are often described as "risk-reducing" rather than "preventive." Some women have developed breast cancer, ovarian cancer, or primary peritoneal carcinomatosis (a type of cancer similar to ovarian cancer) even after risk-reducing surgery. Nevertheless, these surgical procedures confer substantial benefits. For example, research demonstrates that women who underwent BSO had a nearly 80 percent reduction in risk of dying from ovarian cancer, a 56 percent reduction in risk of dying from breast cancer, and a 77 percent reduction in risk of dying from any cause during the studies' follow-up periods.

The reduction in breast and ovarian cancer risk from removal of the ovaries and fallopian tubes appears to be similar for carriers of *BRCA1* and *BRCA2* mutations.

Chemoprevention. Chemoprevention is the use of medicines to try to reduce the risk of cancer. Although two chemopreventive drugs (tamoxifen and raloxifene) have been approved by the U.S. Food and Drug Administration (FDA) to reduce the risk of breast cancer in women at increased risk, the role of these drugs in women with harmful BRCA1 or BRCA2 mutations is not yet clear. However, these medications may be an option for women who don't choose, or can't undergo, surgery.

Data from three studies suggest that tamoxifen may be able to help lower the risk of breast cancer in women who carry harmful mutations in *BRCA2*, as well as the risk of cancer in the opposite breast among *BRCA1* and *BRCA2* mutation carriers previously diagnosed with breast cancer. Studies have not examined the effectiveness of raloxifene in *BRCA1* and *BRCA2* mutation carriers specifically.

Oral contraceptives (birth control pills) are thought to reduce the risk of ovarian cancer by about 50 percent both in the general population and in women with harmful *BRCA1* or *BRCA2* mutations.

What Are Some of the Benefits of Genetic Testing for Breast and Ovarian Cancer Risk?

There can be benefits to genetic testing, regardless of whether a person receives a positive or a negative result.

The potential benefits of a true negative result include a sense of relief regarding the future risk of cancer, learning that one's children are not at risk of inheriting the family's cancer susceptibility, and the possibility that special checkups, tests, or preventive surgeries may not be needed.

A positive test result may bring relief by resolving uncertainty regarding future cancer risk and may allow people to make informed decisions about their future healthcare, including taking steps to reduce their cancer risk. In addition, people who have a positive test result may choose to participate in medical research that could, in the long run, help reduce deaths from hereditary breast and ovarian cancer.

What Are Some of the Possible Harms of Genetic Testing for BRCA Gene Mutations?

The direct medical harms of genetic testing are minimal, but knowledge of test results may have harmful effects on a person's emotions, social relationships, finances, and medical choices.

People who receive a positive test result may feel anxious, depressed, or angry, particularly immediately after they learn the result. People who learn that they carry a BRCA mutation may have difficulty making choices about whether to have preventive surgery or about which surgery to have.

People who receive a negative test result may experience "survivor guilt," caused by the knowledge that they likely do not have an increased risk of developing a disease that affects one or more loved ones.

Because genetic testing can reveal information about more than one family member, the emotions caused by test results can create tension within families. Test results can also affect personal life choices, such as decisions about career, marriage, and childbearing.

Violations of privacy and of the confidentiality of genetic test results are additional potential risks. However, the federal Health Insurance Portability and Accountability Act (HIPAA) and various state laws protect the privacy of a person's genetic information. Moreover, the federal Genetic Information Nondiscrimination Act (GINA), along with many state laws, prohibits discrimination based on genetic information in relation to health insurance and employment, although it does not cover life insurance, disability insurance, or long-term care insurance (LTCI).

Finally, there is a small chance that test results may not be accurate, leading people to make medical decisions based on incorrect information. Although it is rare that results are inaccurate, people with these concerns should address them during genetic counseling.

What Are the Implications of Having a Harmful BRCA1 *or* BRCA2 *Mutation for Breast and Ovarian Cancer Prognosis and Treatment?*

Some studies have investigated whether there are clinical differences between breast and ovarian cancers that are associated with harmful *BRCA1* or *BRCA2* mutations and cancers that are not associated with these mutations.

- There is evidence that, over the long term, women who carry these mutations are more likely to develop a second cancer in either the same (ipsilateral) breast or the opposite (contralateral) breast than women who do not carry these mutations. Thus, some women with a harmful *BRCA1* or *BRCA2* mutation who develop breast cancer in one breast opt for a bilateral mastectomy, even if they would otherwise be candidates for breast-conserving surgery (BCS). Because of the increased risk of a second breast cancer among *BRCA1* and *BRCA2* mutation carriers, some doctors recommend that women with early-onset breast cancer and those whose family history is consistent with a mutation in one of these genes have genetic testing when breast cancer is diagnosed.

• Breast cancers in women with a harmful *BRCA1* mutation tend to be "triple-negative cancers" (that is, the breast cancer cells do not have estrogen receptors, progesterone receptors, or large amounts of HER2/neu protein), which generally have poorer prognosis than other breast cancers.

• Because the *BRCA1* and BRCA2 genes are involved in DNA repair, some investigators have suggested that cancer cells with a harmful mutation in either of these genes may be more sensitive to anticancer agents that act by damaging DNA, such as cisplatin. A class of drugs called poly (ADP-ribose) polymerase (PARP) inhibitors, which block the repair of DNA damage, have been found to arrest the growth of cancer cells that have *BRCA1* or *BRCA2* mutations. Several PARP inhibitors, including olaparib (Lynparza™) and rucaparib (Rubraca®), have been approved by the U.S. Food and Drug Administration (FDA) for the treatment of advanced ovarian cancers in women with a *BRCA1* or *BRCA2* mutation. Olaparib is also approved for the treatment of HER2-negative metastatic breast cancers in women with a *BRCA1* or *BRCA2* mutation.

Do Inherited Mutations in Other Genes Increase the Risk of Breast and/or Ovarian Tumors?

Yes. Although harmful mutations in *BRCA1* and *BRCA2* are responsible for the disease in nearly half of families with multiple cases of breast cancer and up to 90 percent of families with both breast and ovarian cancer, mutations in a number of other genes have been associated with increased risks of breast and/or ovarian cancers. These other genes include several that are associated with the inherited disorders Cowden syndrome (CS), Peutz-Jeghers syndrome (PJS), Li-Fraumeni syndrome (LFS), and Fanconi anemia (FA), which increase the risk of many cancer types.

Most mutations in these other genes do not increase breast cancer risk to the same extent as mutations in *BRCA1* and *BRCA2*. However, researchers have reported that inherited mutations in the *PALB2* gene are associated with a risk of breast cancer nearly as high as that associated with inherited *BRCA1* and *BRCA2* mutations. They estimated that 33 percent of women who inherit a harmful mutation in PALB2 will develop breast cancer by age 70 years.

Recently, mutations in other genes that increase breast and ovarian cancer risk have been identified. These include mutations in the genes *TP53, CDH1,* and *CHEK2,* which increase the risk of breast cancer, and in *RAD51C, RAD51D,* and *STK11,* which increase the risk of ovarian cancer. Genetic testing for these other mutations is available as part of multigene (panel) testing. However, expert groups have not yet developed specific guidelines for who should be tested, or for the management of breast or ovarian cancer risk in people with these other high-risk mutations.

Chapter 8

Required Medical Screening of Immigrants to the United States

What Is the Purpose of the Medical Examination?

The purpose of the medical examination is to identify applicants with inadmissible health-related conditions for the U.S. Department of State (DOS) and U.S. Citizenship and Immigration Services (USCIS). The health-related grounds for inadmissibility include persons who have a communicable disease of public health significance, who fail to present documentation of having received vaccination against vaccine-preventable diseases, who have or have had a physical or mental disorder with associated harmful behavior, or who are a drug abuser or an addict.

Who Is Required to Have a Medical Examination for Migration to the United States?

All immigrants, refugees and certain nonimmigrants, including fiancés, coming to the United States must have a physical and mental

---

This chapter includes text excerpted from "Medical Examination: Frequently Asked Questions (FAQs)," Centers for Disease Control and Prevention (CDC), February 22, 2017.

Table 8.1. Medical Examination for Migration to the United States

Category	Medical Examination	Examination Site	Examination Location
Immigrants	Yes	Panel Physicians	Overseas
Refugees	Yes	Panel Physicians	Overseas
Status adjusters	Yes	Civil Surgeons	U.S.
Nonimmigrants	No	—	—
Short-term Transit	No	—	—
Others*	No	—	—

(Source: U.S. Department of Homeland Security (DHS).)
*Others include migrants who entered the United States without inspection, including those who entered with and without proper documentation.

examination abroad by a panel physician. Persons in the United States applying for adjustment of status to a permanent resident of the United States must have a physical and mental examination in the United States by a civil surgeon.

What Does a Medical Examination Entail?

The medical examination procedure consists of a physical examination, an evaluation (skin test/chest X-ray examination) for tuberculosis (TB), and blood test for syphilis. The vaccination requirements include vaccines recommended by the Advisory Committee on Immunization Practices (ACIP).

Additional immigration information and regulations are available on the USCIS website (www.uscis.gov/portal/site/uscis).

What Vaccines/Boosters Are Required for Immigrants and Those Applying for Adjustment of Status in the United States?

As part of the medical examination for immigration, all immigrants are required to have an assessment for the following vaccine-preventable diseases (VPDs): mumps, measles, rubella, polio, tetanus and diphtheria toxoids, pertussis, Haemophilus influenzae type b (Hib), rotavirus, hepatitis A, hepatitis B, meningococcal disease, varicella, influenza, and pneumococcal pneumonia. Persons already in the United States applying for adjustment of status for permanent residency, including refugees, are also required to be assessed for these VPDs.

Each set of technical instructions for medical examination of aliens has an addendum regarding the vaccination requirements for immigrants.

Part Two

Laboratory Tests

Chapter 9

Understanding Laboratory Tests

What Are Lab Tests?

Laboratory tests are medical procedures that are intended for use on samples of blood, urine, or other tissues or substances taken from the body to help diagnose disease or other conditions.

Why Does Your Doctor Use Lab Tests?

Your doctor uses laboratory tests to help

- Identify changes in your health condition before any symptoms occur,

- Diagnose or aid in diagnosing a disease or condition,

- Plan your treatment for a disease or condition,

- Evaluate your response to a treatment, or

- Monitor the course of a disease over time.

This chapter includes text excerpted from "Tests Used in Clinical Care," U.S. Food and Drug Administration (FDA), March 26, 2018.

How Are Lab Tests Analyzed?

After your doctor collects a sample from your body, it is sent to a laboratory. Laboratories perform tests on the sample to see if it contains different substances, and how much. Depending on the test, the presence, absence, or amount of an analyte may mean you do have a particular condition or it may mean that you do not have the particular condition. Sometimes laboratories compare your results to results obtained from previous tests, to see if there has been a change in your condition.

What Do Lab Tests Show?

Some types of lab tests show whether or not your results fall within normal ranges. Normal test values are usually given as a range, rather than as a specific number, because normal values vary from person to person. What is normal for one person may not be normal for another person.

Other types of lab tests show whether there is a particular substance present or absent, in your body such as a mutation in a gene or an infectious organism, which indicate whether you have a disease, an infection, or may or may not respond to a therapy.

Some laboratory tests are precise, reliable indicators of specific health problems, while others provide more general information that gives doctors clues to your possible health problems. Information obtained from laboratory tests may help doctors decide whether other tests or procedures are needed to make a diagnosis or to develop or revise a previous treatment plan. All laboratory test results must be interpreted within the context of your overall health and should be used along with other examinations or tests.

What Factors Affect Your Lab Test Results?

Many factors can affect test results, including:

- Sex
- Age
- Race
- Medical history
- General health
- Specific foods

- Drugs you are taking
- How closely your follow preparatory instructions
- Variations in laboratory techniques
- Variations from one laboratory to another.

Chapter 10

Point-of-Care Diagnostic Testing

What Is Point-of-Care Testing?

Point-of-care (POC) testing allows patient diagnoses in the physician's office, an ambulance, the home, the field, or in the hospital. The results of care are timely, and allow rapid treatment to the patient. Empowering clinicians to make decisions at the "point-of-care" has the potential to significantly impact healthcare delivery and to address the challenges of health disparities. The success of a potential shift from curative medicine, to predictive, personalized, and preemptive medicine could rely on the development of portable diagnostic and monitoring devices for point-of-care testing (POCT).

This chapter contains text excerpted from the following sources: Text under the heading "What Is Point-of-Care Testing?" is excerpted from "Point-of-Care Diagnostic Testing," National Institutes of Health (NIH), October 2010. Reviewed July 2018; Text beginning with the heading "PATH Toward New Point-of-Care Diagnostics for Low-Resource Settings" is excerpted from "PATH Toward New Point-of-Care Diagnostics for Low-Resource Settings," National Institute of Biomedical Imaging and Bioengineering (NIBIB), September 30, 2010. Reviewed July 2018; Text under the heading "Point-of-Care Diagnostic Test for Anthrax" is excerpted from "HHS Advances Point-Of-Care Diagnostic Test for Anthrax," U.S. Department of Health and Human Services (HHS), September 26, 2017.

PATH toward New POC Diagnostics for Low-Resource Settings

- Imagine you come down with a fever and the nearest hospital is hours away. The local doctor makes an educated guess as to what you have based on your symptoms. If the doctor is wrong, you may receive the wrong treatment while the illness continues ravaging your body, possibly until it is too late.

Bringing Diagnostics to the Patient

- This low-cost disposable cartridge system can simultaneously test blood samples for multiple infections including, human immunodeficiency virus (HIV), syphilis, and Hepatitis B and C. In collaboration with PATH, mBio Diagnostics™, Inc. is scheduled to field test the device in late 2010. Image provided courtesy of Michael J. Lockhead, Ph.D., mBio Diagnostics™, Inc.

- This scenario is the reality for millions of people living in low-resource settings, where centralized diagnostics laboratories are few and far between, and people must make the difficult choice between losing a day's wages to reach a hospital or working to feed their children. A prudent solution to this problem is to bring diagnostic tests to the patients instead of bringing patients (or their samples) to the laboratory so that appropriate treatment can be promptly administered. Sometimes patients who wait days or weeks for test results never return for treatment; POC diagnostics can reduce or possibly eliminate this "loss to follow-up" problem.

- The approach, known as "point-of-care" (POC) diagnostics, is used in the United States for relatively few specific applications, such as blood glucose tests for diabetics, home pregnancy tests, and strep throat tests at the doctor's office, as well as tests for sexually transmitted diseases administered in health clinics and during "home visits" to disadvantaged communities. Future applications of POC technology might take the form of an inexpensive lab-in-a-box that could be stored long-term for immediate use in the event of a natural disaster, such as flooding or earthquake. Another possible application is a home test kit that tracks your biomarker signature and flags the doctor if there is a worrisome trend, such as indications of early-stage cancer or heart disease.

Transforming Healthcare Delivery in Developing Countries

- In the United States, most diagnostics are performed in large, factory-like centralized laboratories. The picture is quite different in developing countries, where there are scant resources to set up and maintain laboratories and keep samples refrigerated during transportation. In situations like this, "POC methodology has the opportunity to transform healthcare in developing countries, enabling them to build lean, efficient systems based on decentralized healthcare delivery rather than emulating the sometimes wasteful systems of the developed world," says Bernhard Weigl, Ph.D., M.Sc., Group Leader, Diagnostic Development Teams, Program for Appropriate Technology in Health (PATH) and Director, National Institute of Biomedical Imaging and Bioengineering (NIBIB) Center for POC Diagnostics for Global Health.

- The principal mission of the Center for Point-of-Care Diagnostics for Global Health (managed by PATH) is to improve access to POC diagnostic tests in low-resource settings around the world. "PATH works with companies to move their technologies more quickly toward a robust commercial product that serves public health needs," says Matthew Steele, Ph.D., M.P.H., Senior Program Officer and Clinical and Field Research Coordinator at PATH. The Center's clinical user needs assessment team proposes POC diagnostic technologies for evaluation and development based on analysis of the most pressing healthcare challenges. The team considers how a product would fit into a particular country—what characteristics would make it useful; how people would interpret the results; and how doctors would react if they had a diagnosis but no way of treating the patient.

- Working closely with technology developers, the Center conducts laboratory and clinical testing of prototype POC diagnostic technologies. Projects are selected based on clinical need and understanding the constraints on their use. "We initially strive to understand how people conceptualize the product and how mature the product is in the pipeline; and also consider key factors associated with the success of the future commercial product related to intellectual property, leadership, and financial liquidity of the manufacturer," explains Steele. The Center is currently evaluating several prototype POC technologies for measuring levels of CD4 immune cells in the blood; CD4 cells are used to establish eligibility for antiviral treatments for HIV patients. An HIV/syphilis disposable cartridge test for pregnant women is scheduled for testing in Kenya in late 2010. The device has the potential for detecting over 10 diseases at the same time.

• The Center's Exploratory Technology Core, led by Gonzalo Domingo, Ph.D., supports development of new diagnostic technologies—a portable, no-power device for extracting viral RNA from the blood to monitor the status of HIV infection in patients, a small collection/processing container for detecting tuberculosis from sputum, and a test strip for simultaneous visual detection of multiple pathogen test results without the need for instrumentation. The two-year projects are selected through a competitive review process that takes into account technical merit, market viability of the technology, appropriateness for low-resource settings, and the research team's competency to do the work. In addition to monitoring the projects' progress, PATH provides technical input on feasibility and performance criteria. "Because we insist on meeting the clinical and user specifications from the beginning, the transition to field testing should be smoother," explains Domingo.

PATH Connects Users with Developers

Running on mechanical pressure provided by a bicycle pump, this portable system extracts RNA from a patient's blood sample and stores it on a sample stabilization "straw." Stored samples will not require a cold chain of transportation. The device will be useful in monitoring the status of HIV infection. Image provided courtesy of Catherine Klapperich, Ph.D., Boston University.

Running on mechanical pressure provided by a bicycle pump, this portable system extracts RNA from a patient's blood sample and stores it on a sample stabilization "straw." Stored samples will not require a cold chain of transportation. The device will be useful in monitoring the status of HIV infection. Image provided courtesy of Catherine Klapperich, Ph.D., Boston University.

In addition to supporting and monitoring development of new diagnostic technologies, PATH also offers training programs that bring together diagnostics users from developing countries and developers of new diagnostics in developed countries. "The diagnostics users learn from developers about the new opportunities they could introduce in their countries, and conversely the developers learn from the users what kind[s] of diagnostics are needed," says Weigl.

PATH is working with local ministries of health and noncommercial laboratories to obtain co-funding for diagnosing neglected diseases such as Chagas. Approximately 100,000 new cases of this parasitic disease occur each year in Latin America. At present, Chagas can be diagnosed only in a lab, and many people in remote areas go undiagnosed. PATH has developed a low-cost (less than $2) diagnostic strip test for Chagas. The strip test, which does not require laboratory instrumentation, provides an immediate diagnosis, overcoming the problem of transporting samples to remote laboratories and helping more people receive the treatment they need.

Although the greatest demand for POC diagnostics for low-resource settings still lies in the infectious disease arena (HIV, tuberculosis, malaria), there is an emerging need for chronic disease (e.g., diabetes) testing. "POC could be the main way people diagnose diseases in developing countries. Implementing POC diagnostics everywhere would eliminate the need for centralized laboratory testing. In countries where central labs were never built in the first place, they may never actually be needed," indicates Weigl.

This work is supported in part by the National Institute of Biomedical Imaging and Bioengineering. The Center for POC Diagnostics for Global Health is one of four centers in the national Point-of-Care Technologies Research Network, which NIBIB created to drive development of appropriate diagnostic technologies through collaborations that merge scientific and technological capabilities with clinical need. The Network provides an opportunity for collaboration through multidisciplinary partnerships, coordination of developments, clinical evaluations, and educational activities to advance POC testing in varied health settings.

Point-of-Care Diagnostic Test for Anthrax

- A point-of-care diagnostic test that may be able to determine within 15 minutes whether a patient has been infected with the bacterium that causes anthrax is moving forward in research and development with the support of the U.S. Department of Health and Human Services' (HHS) Office of the Assistant Secretary for Preparedness and Response (ASPR).

- A three-year, $8.1 million contract with the Biomedical Advanced Research and Development Authority (BARDA), part of ASPR, and InBios International, Inc. of Seattle, Washington, will allow for studies needed to apply for licensure from the U.S. Food and Drug Administration (FDA).

- The contract also requires the company to perform studies necessary to support its submission for pre-Emergency Use Authorization from the FDA.

- "Inhalational anthrax is a deadly disease and a significant biological threat to our nation," said BARDA Director Rick Bright, Ph.D. "To save lives during an anthrax emergency, healthcare providers must be able to screen patients rapidly to provide treatment as quickly as possible. That's our goal in supporting development of point-of-care tests like this."

- InBios' test, a lateral flow immunoassay, determines whether a patient has been infected with anthrax-causing Bacillus anthracis bacteria by identifying specific proteins from the bacteria in a few drops of a person's blood. In studies to date, the test has identified the bacterial proteins within about 15 minutes.

- The test has the potential for use in hospital emergency rooms, local health clinics, and at a patient's bedside. It also could be used by first responders.

- Protecting health after anthrax exposure requires not only detecting but also preventing and treating anthrax infections. To meet this national health security need, BARDA's portfolio includes supporting three anthrax antitoxin drugs approved by the FDA. BARDA also supports advanced development of vaccines to prevent illness after exposure to anthrax and improvements to the only anthrax vaccine licensed for use postexposure so that fewer doses are needed to protect human health.

Chapter 11

Common Blood Tests

What Are Blood Tests?

Blood tests help doctors check for certain diseases and conditions. They also help check the function of your organs and show how well treatments are working.

Specifically, blood tests can help doctors:

- Evaluate how well organs—such as the kidneys, liver, thyroid, and heart—are working

- Diagnose diseases and conditions such as cancer, human immunodeficiency virus/acquired immunodeficiency syndrome (HIV/AIDS), diabetes, anemia, and coronary heart disease (CHD)

- Find out whether you have risk factors for heart disease

- Check whether medicines you're taking are working

- Assess how well your blood is clotting

Blood tests are very common. When you have routine checkups, your doctor may recommend blood tests to see how your body is working.

Many blood tests don't require any special preparations. For some, you may need to fast (not eat any food) for 8–12 hours before the test. Your doctor will let you know how to prepare for blood tests.

This chapter includes text excerpted from "Blood Tests," National Heart, Lung, and Blood Institute (NHLBI), August 4, 2015.

During a blood test, a small sample of blood is taken from your body. It's usually drawn from a vein in your arm using a needle. A finger prick also might be used.

The procedure usually is quick and easy, although it may cause some short-term discomfort. Most people don't have serious reactions to having blood drawn.

Laboratory (lab) workers draw the blood and analyze it. They use either whole blood to count blood cells, or they separate the blood cells from the fluid that contains them. This fluid is called plasma or serum.

The fluid is used to measure different substances in the blood. The results can help detect health problems in early stages, when treatments or lifestyle changes may work best.

Doctors can't diagnose many diseases and medical problems with blood tests alone. Your doctor may consider other factors to confirm a diagnosis. These factors can include your signs and symptoms, your medical history, your vital signs (blood pressure, breathing, pulse, and temperature), and results from other tests and procedures.

Blood tests have few risks. Most complications are minor and go away shortly after the tests are done.

Types

Some of the most common blood tests are:

- A complete blood count (CBC)
- Blood chemistry tests
- Blood enzyme tests
- Blood tests to assess heart disease risk

Complete Blood Count (CBC)

The complete blood count (CBC) is one of the most common blood tests. It's often done as part of a routine checkup.

The CBC can help detect blood diseases and disorders, such as anemia, infections, clotting problems, blood cancers, and immune system disorders. This test measures many different parts of your blood, as discussed in the following paragraphs.

Red Blood Cells (RBCs)

Red blood cells (RBCs) carry oxygen from your lungs to the rest of your body. Abnormal RBC levels may be a sign of anemia, dehydration (too little fluid in the body), bleeding, or another disorder.

130

White Blood Cells (WBCs)

White blood cells (WBCs) are part of your immune system, which fights infections and diseases. Abnormal WBC levels may be a sign of infection, blood cancer, or an immune system disorder.

A CBC measures the overall number of WBCs in your blood. A CBC with differential looks at the amounts of different types of WBCs in your blood.

Platelets

Platelets are blood cell fragments that help your blood clot. They stick together to seal cuts or breaks on blood vessel walls and stop bleeding.

Abnormal platelet levels may be a sign of a bleeding disorder (not enough clotting) or a thrombotic disorder (too much clotting).

Hemoglobin

Hemoglobin is an iron-rich protein in red blood cells that carries oxygen. Abnormal hemoglobin levels may be a sign of anemia, sickle cell anemia, thalassemia, or other blood disorders.

If you have diabetes, excess glucose in your blood can attach to hemoglobin and raise the level of hemoglobin A1c.

Hematocrit

Hematocrit is a measure of how much space RBCs take up in your blood. A high hematocrit level might mean you're dehydrated. A low hematocrit level might mean you have anemia. Abnormal hematocrit levels also may be a sign of a blood or bone marrow disorder.

Mean Corpuscular Volume (MCV)

Mean corpuscular volume (MCV) is a measure of the average size of your RBCs. Abnormal MCV levels may be a sign of anemia or thalassemia.

Blood Chemistry Tests / Basic Metabolic Panel (BMP)

The basic metabolic panel (BMP) is a group of tests that measures different chemicals in the blood. These tests usually are done on the fluid (plasma) part of blood. The tests can give doctors information about your muscles (including the heart), bones, and organs, such as the kidneys and liver.

131

The BMP includes blood glucose, calcium, and electrolyte tests, as well as blood tests that measure kidney function. Some of these tests require you to fast (not eat any food) before the test, and others don't. Your doctor will tell you how to prepare for the test(s) you're having.

Blood Glucose

Glucose is a type of sugar that the body uses for energy. Abnormal glucose levels in your blood may be a sign of diabetes.

For some blood glucose tests, you have to fast before your blood is drawn. Other blood glucose tests are done after a meal or at any time with no preparation.

Calcium

Calcium is an important mineral in the body. Abnormal calcium levels in the blood may be a sign of kidney problems, bone disease, thyroid disease, cancer, malnutrition, or another disorder.

Electrolytes

Electrolytes are minerals that help maintain fluid levels and acid-base balance in the body. They include sodium, potassium, bicarbonate, and chloride.

Abnormal electrolyte levels may be a sign of dehydration, kidney disease, liver disease, heart failure, high blood pressure, or other disorders.

Kidneys

Blood tests for kidney function measure levels of blood urea nitrogen (BUN) and creatinine. Both of these are waste products that the kidneys filter out of the body. Abnormal BUN and creatinine levels may be signs of a kidney disease or disorder.

Blood Enzyme Tests

Enzymes are chemicals that help control chemical reactions in your body. There are many blood enzyme tests. The following paragraphs focuses on blood enzyme tests used to check for heart attack. These include troponin and creatine kinase (CK) tests.

Troponin

Troponin is a muscle protein that helps your muscles contract. When muscle or heart cells are injured, troponin leaks out and its levels in your blood rise.

For example, blood levels of troponin rise when you have a heart attack. For this reason, doctors often order troponin tests when patients have chest pain or other heart attack signs and symptoms.

Creatine Kinase (CK)

A blood product called CK-MB (creatine kinase-muscle/brain) is released when the heart muscle is damaged. High levels of CK-MB in the blood can mean that you've had a heart attack.

Blood Tests to Assess Heart Disease Risk

A lipoprotein panel is a blood test that can help show whether you're at risk for coronary heart disease (CHD). This test looks at substances in your blood that carry cholesterol.

A lipoprotein panel gives information about your:

- **Total cholesterol**

- **Low-density lipoprotein (LDL) ("bad") cholesterol.** This is the main source of cholesterol buildup and blockages in the arteries.

- **High-density lipoprotein (HDL) ("good") cholesterol.** This type of cholesterol helps decrease blockages in the arteries.

- **Triglycerides.** Triglycerides are a type of fat in your blood.

A lipoprotein panel measures the levels of LDL and HDL cholesterol and triglycerides in your blood. Abnormal cholesterol and triglyceride levels may be signs of increased risk for CHD.

Most people will need to fast for 9–12 hours before a lipoprotein panel.

Blood Clotting Tests

Blood clotting tests sometimes are called a coagulation panel. These tests check proteins in your blood that affect the blood clotting process. Abnormal test results might suggest that you're at risk of bleeding or developing clots in your blood vessels.

Your doctor may recommend these tests if he or she thinks you have a disorder or disease related to blood clotting.

Blood clotting tests also are used to monitor people who are taking medicines to lower the risk of blood clots. Warfarin and heparin are two examples of such medicines.

What to Expect with Blood Tests

What to Expect before Blood Tests

Many blood tests don't require any special preparation and take only a few minutes.

Other blood tests require fasting (not eating any food) for 8–12 hours before the test. Your doctor will tell you how to prepare for your blood test(s).

What to Expect during Blood Tests

Blood usually is drawn from a vein in your arm or other part of your body using a needle. It also can be drawn using a finger prick.

The person who draws your blood might tie a band around the upper part of your arm or ask you to make a fist. Doing this can make the veins in your arm stick out more, which makes it easier to insert the needle.

The needle that goes into your vein is attached to a small test tube. The person who draws your blood removes the tube when it's full, and the tube seals on its own. The needle is then removed from your vein. If you're getting a few blood tests, more than one test tube may be attached to the needle before it's withdrawn.

Some people get nervous about blood tests because they're afraid of needles. Others may not want to see blood leaving their bodies.

If you're nervous or scared, it can help to look away or talk to someone to distract yourself. You might feel a slight sting when the needle goes in or comes out.

Drawing blood usually takes less than three minutes.

What to Expect after Blood Tests

Once the needle is withdrawn, you'll be asked to apply gentle pressure with a piece of gauze or bandage to the place where the needle was inserted. This helps stop bleeding. It also helps prevent swelling and bruising.

Most of the time, you can remove the pressure after a minute or two. You may want to keep a bandage on for a few hours.

Usually, you don't need to do anything else after a blood test. Results can take anywhere from a few minutes to a few weeks to come back. Your doctor should get the results. It's important that you follow up with your doctor to discuss your test results.

What Are the Risks of Blood Tests?

The main risks of blood tests are discomfort and bruising at the site where the needle goes in. These complications usually are minor and go away shortly after the tests are done.

What Do Blood Tests Show?

Blood tests show whether the levels of different substances in your blood fall within a normal range.

For many blood substances, the normal range is the range of levels seen in 95 percent of healthy people in a certain group. For many tests, normal ranges vary depending on your age, gender, race, and other factors.

Your blood test results may fall outside the normal range for many reasons. Abnormal results might be a sign of a disorder or disease. Other factors—such as diet, menstrual cycle, physical activity level, alcohol intake, and medicines (both prescription and over-the-counter (OTC))—also can cause abnormal results.

Your doctor should discuss any unusual or abnormal blood test results with you. These results may or may not suggest a health problem.

Many diseases and medical problems can't be diagnosed with blood tests alone. However, blood tests can help you and your doctor learn more about your health. Blood tests also can help find potential problems early, when treatments or lifestyle changes may work best.

Result Ranges for Common Blood Tests

NOTE: All values mentioned are for adults only. They don't apply to children. Talk to your child's doctor about values on blood tests for children.

Complete Blood Count (CBC)

The table below shows some normal ranges for different parts of the complete blood count (CBC) test. Some of the normal ranges differ between men and women. Other factors, such as age and race, also may affect normal ranges.

Your doctor should discuss your results with you. He or she will advise you further if your results are outside the normal range for your group.

Table 11.1. Ranges for Different Parts of the Complete Blood Count (CBC)

Test	Normal Range Results*
Red blood cell (RBC) (varies with altitude)	Male: 5–6 million cells/mcL Female: 4–5 million cells/mcL
White blood cell (WBC)	4,500–10,000 cells/mcL
Platelets	140,000–450,000 cells/mcL
Hemoglobin (varies with altitude)	Male: 14–17 gm/dL Female: 12–15 gm/dL
Hematocrit (varies with altitude)	Male: 41–50 percent Female: 36–44 percent
Mean corpuscular volume (MCV)	80–95 femtoliter[†]

* Cells/mcL = cells per microliter; gm/dL = grams per deciliter.
[†] A femtoliter is a measure of volume.

Blood Glucose

This table below shows the ranges for blood glucose levels after 8–12 hours of fasting (not eating). It shows the normal range and the abnormal ranges that are a sign of prediabetes or diabetes.

Table 11.2. Ranges for Blood Glucose Levels

Plasma Glucose Results (mg/dL)*	Diagnosis
70–99	Normal
100–125	Prediabetes
126 and above	Diabetes[†]

* mg/dL = milligrams per deciliter.
[†] The test is repeated on another day to confirm the results.

Lipoprotein Panel

The table below shows ranges for total cholesterol, low-density lipoprotein (LDL) ("bad") cholesterol, and high-density lipoprotein

(HDL) ("good") cholesterol levels after 9–12 hours of fasting. High blood cholesterol is a risk factor for coronary heart disease.

Your doctor should discuss your results with you. He or she will advise you further if your results are outside the desirable range.

Table 11.3. Ranges for Total Cholesterol Levels

Total Cholesterol Level	Total Cholesterol Category
Less than 200 mg/dL	Desirable
200–239 mg/dL	Borderline high
240 mg/dL and above	High

Table 11.4. Ranges for LDL ("Bad") Cholesterol Levels

LDL Cholesterol Level	LDL Cholesterol Category
Less than 100 mg/dL	Optimal
100–129 mg/dL	Near optimal/above optimal
130–159 mg/dL	Borderline high
160–189 mg/dL	High
190 mg/dL and above	Very high

Table 11.5. Ranges for HDL ("Good") Cholesterol Levels

HDL Cholesterol Level	HDL Cholesterol Category
Less than 40 mg/dL	A major risk factor for heart disease
40–59 mg/dL	The higher, the better
60 mg/dL and above	Considered protective against heart disease

Chapter 12

Biopsies

Chapter Contents

Section 12.1

Biopsy Basics

This section contains text excerpted from the following
sources: Text in this section begins with excerpts from "Biopsy,"
MedlinePlus, National Institutes of Health (NIH), May 2, 2017;
Text under the heading "Types of Biopsies" is excerpted from "
All about Biopsies," National Cancer Institute (NCI),
February 21, 2013. Reviewed July 2018.

A biopsy is a procedure that removes cells or tissue from your body.
A doctor called a pathologist looks at the cells or tissue under a microscope to check for damage or disease. The pathologist may also do
other tests on it.

Biopsies can be done on all parts of the body. In most cases, a biopsy
is the only test that can tell for sure if a suspicious area is cancer. But
biopsies are performed for many other reasons too.

Types of Biopsies

1. **Excisional biopsy.** A whole organ or a whole lump is
    removed (excised). These are less common now, since
    the development of fine needle aspiration. Some types of
    tumors(such as lymphoma, a cancer of the lymphocyte
    blood cells) have to be examined whole to allow an accurate
    diagnosis, so enlarged lymph nodes are good candidates for
    excisional biopsies.

    Some surgeons prefer excisional biopsies of most breast lumps
    to ensure the greatest diagnostic accuracy. Some organs, such
    as the spleen, are dangerous to cut into without removing the
    whole organ, so excisional biopsies are preferred for these.

2. **Incisional biopsy.** Only a portion of the lump is removed
    surgically. This type of biopsy is most commonly used for
    tumors of the soft tissues (muscle, fat, connective tissue) to
    distinguish benign conditions from malignant soft tissue
    tumors, called sarcomas.

3. **Endoscopic biopsy.** This is probably the most commonly
    performed type of biopsy. It is done through a fiberoptic
    endoscope the doctor inserts into the gastrointestinal tract
    (alimentary tract endoscopy), urinary bladder (cystoscopy),

abdominal cavity (laparoscopy), joint cavity (arthroscopy), mid-portion of the chest (mediastinoscopy), or trachea and bronchial system (laryngoscopy and bronchoscopy), either through a natural body orifice or a small surgical incision.

4. **Colposcopic biopsy.** This is a gynecologic procedure that typically is used to evaluate a patient who has had an abnormal Pap smear. The colposcope is actually a close-focusing telescope that allows the physician to see in detail abnormal areas on the cervix of the uterus, so that a good representation of the abnormal area can be removed and sent to the pathologist.

5. **Fine needle aspiration (FNA) biopsy.** This is an extremely simple technique that has been used in Sweden for decades but has only been developed widely in the United States over the last 10 years. A needle no wider than that typically used to give routine injections (about 22 gauge) is inserted into a lump (tumor), and a few tens to thousands of cells are drawn up (aspirated) into a syringe. These are smeared on a slide, stained, and examined under a microscope by the pathologist.

6. **Punch biopsy.** This technique is typically used by dermatologists to sample skin rashes and small masses. After a local anesthetic is injected, a biopsy punch, which is basically a small (3 or 4 mm in diameter) version of a cookie cutter, is used to cut out a cylindrical piece of skin. The hole is typically closed with a suture and heals with minimal scarring.

7. **Bone marrow biopsy.** In cases of abnormal blood counts, such as unexplained anemia, high white cell count, and low platelet count, it is necessary to examine the cells of the bone marrow. In adults, the sample is usually taken from the pelvic bone, typically from the posterior superior iliac spine. This is the prominence of bone on either side of the pelvis underlying the "bikini dimples" on the lower back/upper buttocks. Hematologists do bone marrow biopsies all the time, but most internists and pathologists and many family practitioners are also trained to perform this procedure.

Section 12.2

Breast Biopsy

This section includes text excerpted from "Breast
Changes and Conditions," National Cancer
Institute (NCI), September 22, 2017.

You may have just received an abnormal mammogram result, or
perhaps you or your healthcare provider found a breast lump or other
breast change. Keep in mind that breast changes are very common,
and most are not cancer.

This section is about various types of breast biopsies that are used
to diagnose breast conditions.

What Is Breast Biopsy?

Biopsy is a procedure that removes a sample of breast tissue or
an entire lump so that it can be checked for signs of disease. Imaging
procedures (such as ultrasound, magnetic resonance imaging (MRI),
or X-rays) are often used during a biopsy to guide the surgeon. A
pathologist then examines the sample under a microscope or performs
other tests on it.

Common Types of Breast Biopsies

The following are some of the common types of breast biopsies
include:

- **Core needle biopsy (CNB).** The use of a wide needle to remove
  small tissue sample(s) that are about the size of a grain of rice.
  It may cause a temporary bruise. Also called core biopsy.

- **Fine-needle aspiration (FNA) biopsy.** The use of a thin
  needle to drain fluid and/or to remove cells.

- **Surgical biopsy.** The removal of part, or all, of a lump so it can
  be checked for signs of cancer. An incisional biopsy removes a
  sample of breast tissue. An excisional biopsy removes an entire
  lump or suspicious area. Wire localization (also called needle
  localization and needle (wire) localization) may be used to mark
  the area of abnormal tissue before the biopsy.

- **Vacuum-assisted biopsy.** The removal of a small sample of
  breast tissue using a probe that is connected to a vacuum device.

The small cut made in the breast is much smaller than with surgical biopsy. This procedure causes little scarring, and no stitches are needed. It may also be called vacuum-assisted core biopsy.

Where Is Biopsy Performed?

Biopsies are usually done in a doctor's office or a clinic on an outpatient basis. This means you will go home the same day as the procedure. Local anesthesia is used for many biopsies, so you'll be awake but won't feel pain during the procedure. General anesthesia is commonly used for surgical biopsies, which means you'll be asleep during the procedure.

How Is a Biopsy Done?

A breast biopsy is a procedure to remove a sample of breast cells or tissue, or an entire lump. A pathologist then looks at the sample under a microscope to check for signs of disease. A biopsy is the only way to find out if cells are cancer. Print out and take this list of questions with you when you talk with your healthcare provider.

Questions to Ask If a Biopsy Is Recommended

The following questions can help you to check with your healthcare provider on why a biopsy has been recommended for you:

- Why is a biopsy needed? What will it tell us?
- What type of biopsy will I have? How will the biopsy be done?
- Where will the biopsy be done? How long will it take?
- How much breast tissue will be removed?
- Will it hurt?
- Will I be awake?
- What tests will be done on the breast tissue?
- When will I know the results?
- Will there be side effects?
- How should I care for the biopsy site?
- Will I need to rest after the biopsy?

Questions to Ask about Your Biopsy Results

The following set of questions will help you to get a better understanding of your biopsy results:

- What were the results of the biopsy?

- What do the biopsy results mean?

- What are the next steps? Do I need more tests?

- Who should I talk with next?

- Do I have an increased risk of breast cancer?

- Who can give me a second opinion on my biopsy results?

Section 12.3

Kidney Biopsy

This section includes text excerpted from "Kidney Biopsy,"
National Institute of Diabetes and Digestive and Kidney
Diseases (NIDDK), November 2015.

What Is a Kidney Biopsy?

A kidney biopsy is a procedure that involves taking a small piece of kidney tissue for examination with a microscope. A pathologist—a doctor who specializes in diagnosing diseases—examines the kidney tissue sample in a lab. The pathologist looks for signs of kidney disease or infection. If the kidney has been transplanted and is not working, a kidney biopsy may help identify the cause.

One of the following specialists will perform the kidney biopsy at a hospital or an outpatient center:

A **nephrologist**—a doctor who specializes in treating kidney disease

A **urologist**—a doctor who specializes in treating urologic and sexual problems

A **transplant surgeon**—a doctor who specializes in performing organ transplants

An **interventional radiologist**—a doctor who performs procedures using imaging equipment

Why Is a Kidney Biopsy Performed?

A healthcare provider will perform a kidney biopsy to evaluate any of the following conditions:

Hematuria—blood in the urine, which can be a sign of kidney disease or other urinary problems

Albuminuria—a condition in which the urine has more-than-normal amounts of a protein called albumin. Albuminuria may be a sign of kidney disease.

Changes in kidney function, which can cause the buildup of waste products in the blood
The kidney tissue sample can show inflammation, scarring, infection, or unusual deposits of a protein called immunoglobulin. If a person has chronic kidney disease—any condition that causes reduced kidney function over a period of time—the biopsy may show how quickly the disease is advancing. A biopsy can also help explain why a transplanted kidney is not working properly.

Healthcare providers may use a kidney biopsy to diagnose cancer. If cancer is present, there is a small chance that the biopsy needle will spread the cancer. In addition, the biopsy specimen is very small and may miss the cancer and, therefore, may not provide the right diagnosis.

What Should a Person Do Days before a Kidney Biopsy?

Days before the procedure, a person should prepare for a kidney biopsy by:

- Talking with a healthcare provider
- Arranging for a ride home

Talking with a Healthcare Provider

People should talk with their healthcare provider about medical conditions they have and all prescribed and over-the-counter (OTC) medications, vitamins, and supplements they take, including:

- Aspirin or medications that contain aspirin

- Nonsteroidal anti-inflammatory medications such as ibuprofen and naproxen

- Blood thinners

- Arthritis medications

People should also tell their healthcare provider about any allergies they have to medications or foods.

The healthcare provider should discuss the risks of the procedure, and the person should ask questions or bring up concerns. Two weeks before the biopsy, the healthcare provider may instruct a person to stop taking certain medications that cause thinning of the blood because this may increase the risk of bleeding after the kidney biopsy. The healthcare provider may also tell the person not to eat or drink anything for 8 hours before the biopsy.

Arranging for a Ride Home after the Procedure

For safety reasons, people can't drive for 24 hours after the procedure because they are given a sedative to help them relax just before the procedure. A healthcare provider will ask a person to make advance arrangements for getting home after the procedure.

What Can a Person Expect on the Day of the Kidney Biopsy?

A person should arrive 90 minutes to 2 hours before the kidney biopsy to have time for several preliminary procedures, including:

- Signing a consent form

- Having blood tests

- Receiving intravenous (IV) fluids and medications

Signing a Consent Form

A healthcare provider will ask the person to sign a consent form that states that he or she understands the risks of the procedure and gives permission for the healthcare provider to perform the kidney biopsy.

Having Blood Tests

Shortly before the procedure, a healthcare provider will perform blood and urine tests to make sure the person doesn't have a condition that would make having a biopsy risky, such as a bleeding problem or high blood potassium.

Receiving Intravenous (IV) Fluids and Medications

A nurse or technician will insert an IV line into a vein in the person's arm to give fluids and medications, including sedatives.

How Is a Kidney Biopsy Performed?

The procedure typically takes about an hour and includes the following steps:

- **Physical examination.** Most people will lie on their abdomen on an examination table. The technician will place a firm pillow or sandbag under a person's body to support the abdomen and help push the kidneys up toward the person's back and the surface of the skin. People who have a transplanted kidney lie on their backs because surgeons place transplanted kidneys in the front-lower part of the abdomen, to one side of the bladder.

- **Sedation.** A nurse or technician will give the person sedatives through the IV.

- **Local anesthesia.** The healthcare provider will mark the point where the needle will enter the skin, clean the area, and inject a local anesthetic to numb the area.

- **Guiding biopsy needle into the kidney.** Next, the healthcare provider uses imaging techniques, such as ultrasound, to guide the biopsy needle into the kidney. Ultrasound uses a device called a transducer that bounces safe, painless sound waves off organs to create an image of their structure. Sometimes the healthcare provider uses a computerized tomography (CT) scan or magnetic resonance imaging (MRI) to guide the needle into the kidney.

- **Removal of kidney tissue.** The healthcare provider will ask the person to hold his or her breath and stay still as the healthcare provider inserts the biopsy needle and removes the kidney tissue. When the healthcare provider takes the biopsy, the instrument will make a clicking or popping noise. The healthcare provider may need to insert the needle three or four times. People most often will need to hold their breath for about 30 seconds or a little longer for each insertion.

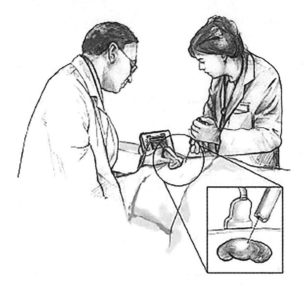

Figure 12.1. *Kidney Biopsy*

The healthcare provider uses imaging techniques such as ultrasound to guide the biopsy needle into the kidney.

For people with bleeding problems, the healthcare provider uses a laparoscope—a thin tube with a video camera. This procedure is surgery that requires general anesthesia. The surgeon makes a small incision into the back and inserts the laparoscope to see the kidney. The surgeon can insert tiny tools through the laparoscope to collect tissue samples and can watch after the procedure through the camera to make sure that if there is any bleeding, he or she can stop it.

What Can a Person Expect after a Kidney Biopsy?

After a kidney biopsy, a person can expect to:

- Lie on his or her back in the clinic or hospital for a few hours. During this time, the staff will monitor the person's blood pressure, pulse, urine, and blood test results.

- Go home the same day, in most cases; however, a person will need to rest at home for 12–24 hours after the biopsy. Sometimes a person may need to stay overnight at the hospital.

- Have some pain or soreness near the point where the needle went through the skin.

- Receive written instructions for ensuring a healthy recovery from the procedure. Most people need to wait 2 weeks before resuming strenuous activities, such as heavy lifting or participating in contact sports.

A healthcare provider most often receives the complete biopsy results from the pathologist in about a week. In urgent cases, a person may receive a preliminary report within 24 hours. The healthcare provider will review the results with the person during a follow-up visit.

What Are the Risks of a Kidney Biopsy?

The risks of a kidney biopsy include:

- Bleeding—the most common complication of a kidney biopsy. Bleeding may come from the kidney or the puncture site. Bleeding from the kidney rarely requires a blood transfusion.

- Infection—a rare complication of a kidney biopsy. Healthcare providers prescribe bacteria-fighting medications called antibiotics to treat infections.

Seek Immediate Care

People who have any of the following symptoms after a kidney biopsy should seek immediate medical attention:

- Unable to urinate

- Frequent or urgent need to urinate

- Burning sensation when urinating

- Urine that is dark red or brown. Blood that makes the urine pink or slightly cloudy is normal for 24 hours after the procedure.

- Blood or pus from the biopsy site that saturates the bandage

- Worsening pain at the biopsy site

- Fever

- Feeling faint or dizzy

Section 12.4

Liver Biopsy

This section includes text excerpted from "Liver Biopsy," National Institute of Diabetes and Digestive and Kidney Diseases (NIDDK), May 2014. Reviewed July 2018.

What Is a Liver Biopsy?

A liver biopsy is a procedure that involves taking a small piece of liver tissue for examination with a microscope for signs of damage or disease. The three types of liver biopsy are the following:

Percutaneous biopsy—the most common type of liver biopsy—involves inserting a hollow needle through the abdomen into the liver. The abdomen is the area between the chest and hips.

Transvenous biopsy involves making a small incision in the neck and inserting a needle through a hollow tube called a sheath through the jugular vein to the liver.

Laparoscopic biopsy involves inserting a laparoscope, a thin tube with a tiny video camera attached, through a small incision to look inside the body to view the surface of organs. The healthcare provider will insert a needle through a plastic, tube-like instrument called a cannula to remove the liver tissue sample.

What Is the Liver and What Does It Do?

The liver is the body's largest internal organ. The liver is called the body's metabolic factory because of the important role it plays in metabolism—the way cells change food into energy after food is digested and absorbed into the blood. The liver has many functions, including:

- Taking up, storing, and processing nutrients from food— including fat, sugar, and protein—and delivering them to the rest of the body when needed

- Making new proteins, such as clotting factors and immune factors

- Producing bile, which helps the body absorb fats, cholesterol, and fat-soluble vitamins

- Removing waste products the kidneys cannot remove, such as fats, cholesterol, toxins, and medications

A healthy liver is necessary for survival. The liver can regenerate most of its own cells when they become damaged.

Why Is a Liver Biopsy Performed?

A healthcare provider will perform a liver biopsy to:

- Diagnose liver diseases that cannot be diagnosed with blood or imaging tests

- Estimate the degree of liver damage, a process called staging

- Help determine the best treatment for liver damage or disease

How Does a Person Prepare for a Liver Biopsy?

A person prepares for a liver biopsy by:

- Talking with a healthcare provider

- Having blood tests

- Arranging for a ride home

- Fasting before the procedure

Talking with a healthcare provider. People should talk with their healthcare provider about medical conditions they have and all prescribed and over-the-counter (OTC) medications, vitamins, and supplements they take, including:

- Antibiotics

- Antidepressants

- Aspirin

- Asthma medications

- Blood pressure medications

- Blood thinners

- Diabetes medications

- Dietary supplements

- Nonsteroidal anti-inflammatory drugs (NSAIDs) such as ibuprofen and naproxen

The healthcare provider may tell the person to stop taking medications temporarily that affect blood clotting or interact with anesthesia, which people sometimes receive during a liver biopsy.

Having blood tests. A person will have a test to show how well his or her blood clots. A person will have a test to show how well his or her blood clots. A technician or nurse draws a blood sample during an office visit or at a commercial facility and sends the sample to a lab for analysis. People with severe liver disease often have blood-clotting problems that can increase their chance of bleeding after the biopsy. A healthcare provider may give the person a medication called clotting factor concentrates just before a liver biopsy to reduce the chance of bleeding.

Arranging for a ride home after the procedure. For safety reasons, most people cannot drive home after the procedure. A healthcare provider will ask a person to make advance arrangements for getting home after the procedure.

Fasting before the procedure. A healthcare provider will ask a person not to eat or drink for 8 hours before the procedure if the provider anticipates using anesthesia or sedation.

How Is a Liver Biopsy Performed?

A healthcare provider performs the liver biopsy at a hospital or an outpatient center and determines which type of biopsy is best for the person.

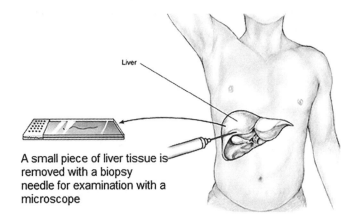

Liver

A small piece of liver tissue is removed with a biopsy needle for examination with a microscope

Figure 12.2. *Percutaneous Liver Biopsy*

Percutaneous liver biopsy is the most common type of liver biopsy.

Percutaneous Liver Biopsy

A person lies face up on a table and rests the right hand above the head. A healthcare provider gives the person a local anesthetic on the area where he or she will insert the biopsy needle. If needed, the healthcare provider will give the person sedatives and pain medication.

The healthcare provider either taps on the abdomen to locate the liver or uses one of the following imaging techniques:

- **Ultrasound**. Ultrasound uses a device, called a transducer, that bounces safe, painless sound waves off organs to create an image of their structure.

- **Computerized tomography (CT) scan.** A CT scan uses a combination of X-rays and computer technology to create images. For a CT scan, a technician may give the person a solution to drink and an injection of a special dye, called contrast medium. CT scans require the person to lie on a table that slides into a tunnel-shaped device where the technician takes the X-rays.

Research has shown fewer complications after biopsy when health-care providers use ultrasound to locate the liver compared with tapping on the abdomen. Healthcare providers may select ultrasound over a CT scan because it is quicker and less expensive, and can show the biopsy needle in real time.

The healthcare provider will:

- Make a small incision in the right side of the person's abdomen, either toward the bottom of or just below the rib cage

- Insert the biopsy needle

- Ask the person to exhale and hold his or her breath while the healthcare provider inserts the needle and quickly removes a sample of liver tissue

- Insert and remove the needle several times if multiple samples are needed

- Place a bandage over the incision

After the biopsy, the person must lie on his or her right side for up to 2 hours to reduce the chance of bleeding. Medical staff monitor the person for signs of bleeding for 2–4 more hours.

Transvenous Liver Biopsy

When a person's blood clots slowly or the person has ascites—a buildup of fluid in the abdomen—the healthcare provider may perform a transvenous liver biopsy.

For this procedure, the person lies face up on an X-ray table, and a healthcare provider applies local anesthetic to one side of the neck. The healthcare provider will give sedatives and pain medication if the person needs them.

The healthcare provider will:

- Make a small incision in the neck

- Insert a sheath into the jugular vein and thread the sheath down the jugular vein, along the side of the heart, and into one of the veins in the liver

- Inject contrast medium into the sheath and take an X-ray. The contrast medium makes the blood vessels and the location of the sheath clearly visible on the X-ray images.

- Thread a biopsy needle through the sheath and into the liver and quickly remove a liver tissue sample

- Insert and remove the biopsy needle several times if multiple samples are needed

- Carefully withdraw the sheath and close the incision with a bandage

Medical staff monitor the person for 4–6 hours afterward for signs of bleeding.

Laparoscopic Liver Biopsy

Healthcare providers use this type of biopsy to obtain a tissue sample from a specific area or from multiple areas of the liver, or when the risk of spreading cancer or infection exists. A healthcare provider may take a liver tissue sample during laparoscopic surgery performed for other reasons, including liver surgery.

The person lies on his or her back on an operating table. A nurse or technician will insert an intravenous (IV) needle into the person's arm to give anesthesia. The healthcare provider will:

- Make a small incision in the abdomen, just below the rib cage

- Insert a thin tube into the incision and fill the abdomen with gas to provide space to work inside the abdominal cavity and to see the liver

- Insert a biopsy needle through the cannula and into the liver and quickly remove a liver tissue sample

- Insert and remove the biopsy needle several times if multiple samples are needed

- Remove the thin tube and close the incisions with dissolvable stitches

The healthcare provider can easily spot any bleeding from the procedure with the camera on the laparoscope and treat it using an electric probe. The person stays at the hospital or an outpatient center for a few hours while the anesthesia wears off.

What Can a Person Expect after a Liver Biopsy?

After a liver biopsy, a person can expect:

- Full recovery in 1–2 days

- To avoid intense activity, exercise, or heavy lifting for up to one week

- Soreness around the biopsy or incision site for about a week. Acetaminophen (Tylenol) or other pain medications that do not interfere with blood clotting may help. People should check with their healthcare provider before taking any pain medications.

- A member of the healthcare team to review the discharge instructions with the person—or with an accompanying friend or family member if the person is still groggy—and provide a written copy. The person should follow all instructions given.

Liver biopsy results take a few days to come back. The liver sample goes to a pathology lab where a technician stains the tissue. Staining highlights important details within the liver tissue and helps identify any signs of liver disease. The pathologist—a doctor who specializes in diagnosing diseases—looks at the tissue with a microscope and sends a report to the person's healthcare provider.

What Are the Risks of Liver Biopsy?

The risks of a liver biopsy include:

- Pain and bruising at the biopsy or incision site—the most common complication after a liver biopsy. Most people experience mild pain that does not require medication; however, some people need medications to relieve the pain.

- Prolonged bleeding from the biopsy or incision site or internal bleeding. A person may require hospitalization, transfusions, and sometimes surgery or another procedure to stop the bleeding.

- Infection of the biopsy site or incision site that may cause sepsis. Sepsis is an illness in which the body has a severe response to bacteria or a virus.

- Pneumothorax, also called collapsed lung, which occurs when air or gas builds up in the pleural space. The pleural space is thin layers of tissue that wrap around the outside of the lungs and line the inside of the chest cavity. Pneumothorax may happen when the biopsy needle punctures the pleural space.

- Hemothorax, or the buildup of blood in the pleural space

- Puncture of other organs

Seek Immediate Care

People who have any of the following symptoms after a liver biopsy should seek immediate medical attention:

- Chest pain

- Difficulty breathing

- Increasing abdominal pain

- Dizziness

- Bleeding from the incision or biopsy site

- Abdominal swelling or bloating

- Fever

- Swelling or redness at the incision or biopsy site

- Nausea or vomiting

Section 12.5

Sentinel Lymph Node Biopsy

This section includes text excerpted from "Sentinel Lymph Node Biopsy," National Cancer Institute (NCI), August 11, 2011. Reviewed July 2018.

What Are Lymph Nodes?

Lymph nodes are small round organs that are part of the body's lymphatic system. They are found widely throughout the body and are connected to one another by lymph vessels. Groups of lymph nodes are located in the neck, underarms, chest, abdomen, and groin. A clear fluid called lymph flows through lymph vessels and lymph nodes.

Lymph originates from a fluid, known as interstitial fluid, that has diffused, or "leaked," out of small blood vessels called capillaries. This fluid contains many substances, including blood plasma, proteins, glucose, and oxygen. It bathes most of the body's cells, providing them with the oxygen and nutrients they need for growth and survival. Interstitial fluid also picks up waste products from cells as well as other materials, such as bacteria and viruses, to help remove them from the body's tissues. Interstitial fluid eventually collects in lymph vessels, where it becomes known as lymph. Lymph flows through the body's lymph vessels to reach two large ducts at the base of the neck, where it is emptied into the bloodstream.

Lymph nodes are important parts of the body's immune system. They contain B lymphocytes, T lymphocytes, and other types of immune system cells. These cells monitor lymph for the presence of "foreign" substances, such as bacteria and viruses. If a foreign substance is detected, some of the cells will become activated and an immune response will be triggered.

Lymph nodes are also important in helping to determine whether cancer cells have developed the ability to spread to other parts of the body. Many types of cancer spread through the lymphatic system, and one of the earliest sites of spread for these cancers is nearby lymph nodes.

What Is a Sentinel Lymph Node?

A sentinel lymph node is defined as the first lymph node to which cancer cells are most likely to spread from a primary tumor. Sometimes, there can be more than one sentinel lymph node.

What Is a Sentinel Lymph Node Biopsy (SLNB)?

A sentinel lymph node biopsy (SLNB) is a procedure in which the sentinel lymph node is identified, removed, and examined to determine whether cancer cells are present.

A negative SLNB result suggests that cancer has not developed the ability to spread to nearby lymph nodes or other organs. A positive SLNB result indicates that cancer is present in the sentinel lymph node and may be present in other nearby lymph nodes (called regional lymph nodes) and, possibly, other organs. This information can help a doctor determine the stage of the cancer (extent of the disease within the body) and develop an appropriate treatment plan.

What Happens during an SLNB?

A surgeon injects a radioactive substance, a blue dye, or both near the tumor to locate the position of the sentinel lymph node. The surgeon then uses a device that detects radioactivity to find the sentinel node or looks for lymph nodes that are stained with the blue dye. Once the sentinel lymph node is located, the surgeon makes a small incision (about 1/2 inch) in the overlying skin and removes the node.

The sentinel node is then checked for the presence of cancer cells by a pathologist. If cancer is found, the surgeon may remove additional lymph nodes, either during the same biopsy procedure or during a follow-up surgical procedure. SLNBs may be done on an outpatient basis or may require a short stay in the hospital.

SLNB is usually done at the same time the primary tumor is removed. However, the procedure can also be done either before or after removal of the tumor.

What Are the Benefits of SLNB?

In addition to helping doctors stage cancers and estimate the risk that tumor cells have developed the ability to spread to other parts of the body, SLNB may help some patients avoid more extensive lymph node surgery. Removing additional nearby lymph nodes to look for cancer cells may not be necessary if the sentinel node is negative for cancer. All lymph node surgery can have adverse effects, and some of these effects may be reduced or avoided if fewer lymph nodes are removed. The potential adverse effects of lymph node surgery include the following:

- Lymphedema, or tissue swelling. During SLNB or more extensive lymph node surgery, lymph vessels leading to and from the sentinel node or group of nodes are cut, thereby disrupting the normal flow of lymph through the affected area. This disruption may lead to an abnormal buildup of lymph fluid. In addition to swelling, patients with lymphedema may experience pain or discomfort in the affected area, and the overlying skin may become thickened or hard. In the case of extensive lymph node surgery in an armpit or groin, the swelling may affect an entire arm or leg. In addition, there is an increased risk of infection in the affected area or limb. Very rarely, chronic lymphedema due to extensive lymph node removal may cause a cancer of the lymphatic vessels called lymphangiosarcoma.

- Seroma, or the buildup of lymph fluid at the site of the surgery

- Numbness, tingling, or pain at the site of the surgery

- Difficulty moving the affected body part

Is SLNB Associated with Other Harms?

SLNB, like other surgical procedures, can cause short-term pain, swelling, and bruising at the surgical site and increase the risk of infection. In addition, some patients may have skin or allergic reactions to the blue dye used in SLNB. Another potential harm is a false-negative biopsy result—that is, cancer cells are not seen in the sentinel lymph node although they are present and may have already spread to other regional lymph nodes or other parts of the body. A false-negative biopsy result gives the patient and the doctor a false sense of security about the extent of cancer in the patient's body.

Is SLNB Used to Help Stage All Types of Cancer?

No. SLNB is most commonly used to help stage breast cancer and melanoma. However, it is being studied with other cancer types, including colorectal cancer, gastric cancer, esophageal cancer, head and neck cancer, thyroid cancer, and nonsmall cell lung cancer.

Section 12.6

Other Biopsies

Text under the heading "Fine-Needle Aspiration (FNA) Biopsy of the Thyroid and Surgical Biopsy" is excerpted from "Thyroid Cancer Treatment (Adult) (PDQ®)–Patient Version," National Cancer Institute (NCI), May 23, 2018; Text under the heading "Muscle Biopsy" is excerpted from "Muscle Biopsy Evaluation in Neuromuscular Disorders," National Library of Medicine (NLM), October 1, 2015; Text under the heading "FNA Biopsy of the Lung" is excerpted from "Small Cell Lung Cancer Treatment (PDQ®)–Patient Version," National Cancer Institute (NCI), May 11, 2018; Text under the heading "Bone Marrow Aspiration and Biopsy" is excerpted from "Myelodysplastic Syndromes Treatment (PDQ®)–Patient Version," National Cancer Institute (NCI), June 14, 2018; Text under the heading "Skin Biopsy" is excerpted from "Skin Cancer Treatment (PDQ®)–Patient Version," National Cancer Institute (NCI), August 28, 2017.

Fine-Needle Aspiration (FNA) Biopsy of the Thyroid and Surgical Biopsy

Fine-needle aspiration (FNA) biopsy of the thyroid and surgical biopsy are two of the tests that are used to examine the thyroid, neck, and blood are used to detect (find) and diagnose thyroid cancer.

FNA biopsy of the thyroid. The removal of thyroid tissue using a thin needle. The needle is inserted through the skin into the thyroid. Several tissue samples are removed from different parts of the thyroid. A pathologist views the tissue samples under a microscope to look for cancer cells. Because the type of thyroid cancer can be hard to diagnose, patients should ask to have biopsy samples checked by a pathologist who has experience diagnosing thyroid cancer.

Surgical biopsy. The removal of the thyroid nodule or one lobe of the thyroid during surgery so the cells and tissues can be viewed under a microscope by a pathologist to check for signs of cancer. Because the type of thyroid cancer can be hard to diagnose, patients should ask to have biopsy samples checked by a pathologist who has experience diagnosing thyroid cancer.

Muscle Biopsy

Muscle biopsy is an important tool for the evaluation and diagnosis of patients presenting to clinic with acute or progressive weakness who are suspected of having an underlying neuromuscular disorder. Alongside the clinical examination, electrodiagnostic, laboratory and molecular genetic testing, muscle biopsy has a critical role, providing diagnostic evidence that either establishes a disease etiology or focuses the differential diagnosis. For example, in the setting of rapidly progressive muscle weakness, a muscle biopsy is the most expeditious diagnostic study to allow the clinician to distinguish between a necrotizing, metabolic or inflammatory myopathy and facilitate rapid, appropriate therapeutic management. Or, as in the case of a young boy who presents with progressive proximal weakness and hyperCKemia, and whose genetic tests do not confirm a dystrophinopathy, immunohistochemical staining on the muscle biopsy specimen can often identify the pathologic protein defect and pave the way for genetic confirmation of the disease.

FNA Biopsy of the Lung

FNA biopsy of the lung is one of the test that is used for examining the lungs to detect (find), diagnose, and stage small cell lung cancer. It deals with the removal of tissue or fluid from the lung, using a thin needle. A computerized tomography (CT) scan, ultrasound, or other imaging procedure is used to find the abnormal tissue or fluid in the lung. A small incision may be made in the skin where the biopsy needle is inserted into the abnormal tissue or fluid. A sample is removed with the needle and sent to the laboratory. A pathologist then views the sample under a microscope to look for cancer cells. A chest X-ray is done after the procedure to make sure no air is leaking from the lung into the chest.

Bone Marrow Aspiration and Biopsy

This test is used for examining the blood and bone marrow to detect (find) and diagnose myelodysplastic syndromes. The bone marrow aspiration and biopsy involves the removal of bone marrow, blood, and a small piece of bone by inserting a hollow needle into the hipbone or breastbone. A pathologist views the bone marrow, blood, and bone under a microscope to look for abnormal cells.

Skin Biopsy

Skin biopsy is one of the procedures that is performed to examine the skin for the diagnosis of nonmelanoma skin cancer and actinic keratosis. All or part of the abnormal-looking growth is cut from the skin and viewed under a microscope by a pathologist to check for signs of cancer. There are four main types of skin biopsies:

1. **Shave biopsy.** A sterile razor blade is used to "shave-off" the abnormal-looking growth.

2. **Punch biopsy.** A special instrument called a punch or a trephine is used to remove a circle of tissue from the abnormal-looking growth.

3. **Incisional biopsy.** A scalpel is used to remove part of a growth.

4. **Excisional biopsy.** A scalpel is used to remove the entire growth.

Chapter 13

Bone Marrow Tests

What Are Bone Marrow Tests?

Bone marrow is a soft, spongy tissue found in the center of most bones. Bone marrow makes different types of blood cells. These include:

- Red blood cells (RBCs) (also called erythrocytes), which carry oxygen from your lungs to every cell in your body

- White blood cells (WBCs) (also called leukocytes), which help you fight infections

- Platelets, which help with blood clotting

Bone marrow tests check to see if your bone marrow is working correctly and making normal amounts of blood cells. The tests can help diagnose and monitor various bone marrow disorders, blood disorders, and certain types of cancer. There are two types of bone marrow tests:

- Bone marrow aspiration, which removes a small amount of bone marrow fluid

- Bone marrow biopsy, which removes a small amount of bone marrow tissue

Bone marrow aspiration and bone marrow biopsy tests are usually performed at the same time.

This chapter includes text excerpted from "Bone Marrow Test," MedlinePlus, National Institutes of Health (NIH), April 11, 2018.

Other names: bone marrow examination

What Are They Used For?

Bone marrow tests are used to:

- Find out the cause of problems with RBCs, WBCs, or platelets
- Diagnose and monitor blood disorders, such as anemia, polycythemia vera (PV), and thrombocytopenia
- Diagnose bone marrow disorders
- Diagnose and monitor certain types of cancers, including leukemia, multiple myeloma, and lymphoma
- Diagnose infections that may have started or spread to the bone marrow

Why Do I Need a Bone Marrow Test?

Your healthcare provider may order a bone marrow aspiration and a bone marrow biopsy if other blood tests show your levels of RBCs, WBCs, or platelets are not normal. Too many or too few of these cells may mean you have a medical disorder, such as cancer that starts in your blood or bone marrow. If you are being treated for another type of cancer, these tests can find out if the cancer has spread to your bone marrow.

What Happens during a Bone Marrow Test?

Bone marrow aspiration and bone marrow biopsy tests are usually given at the same time. A doctor or other healthcare provider will perform the tests. Before the tests, the provider may ask you to put on a hospital gown. The provider will check your blood pressure, heart rate, and temperature. You may be given a mild sedative, a medicine that will help you relax. During the test:

- You'll lie down on your side or your stomach, depending on which bone will be used for testing. Most bone marrow tests are taken from the hip bone.
- Your body will be covered with cloth, so that only the area around the testing site is showing.
- The site will be cleaned with an antiseptic.

- You will get an injection of a numbing solution. It may sting.
- Once the area is numb, the healthcare provider will take the sample. You will need to lie very still during the tests.
- For a bone marrow aspiration, which is usually performed first, the healthcare provider will insert a needle through the bone and pull out bone marrow fluid and cells. You may feel a sharp but brief pain when the needle is inserted.
- For a bone marrow biopsy, the healthcare provider will use a special tool that twists into the bone to take out a sample of bone marrow tissue. You may feel some pressure on the site while the sample is being taken.
- It takes about 10 minutes to perform both tests.
- After the test, the healthcare provider will cover the site with a bandage.
- Plan to have someone drive you home, since you may be given a sedative before the tests, which may make you drowsy.

Will I Need to Do Anything to Prepare for the Test?

You will be asked to sign a form that gives permission to perform bone marrow tests. Be sure to ask your provider any questions you have about the procedure.

Are There Any Risks to the Test?

Many people feel a little uncomfortable after bone marrow aspiration and bone marrow biopsy testing. After the test, you may feel stiff or sore at the injection site. This usually goes away in a few days. Your healthcare provider may recommend or prescribe a pain reliever to help. Serious symptoms are very rare, but may include:

- Long-lasting pain or discomfort around the injection site
- Redness, swelling, or excessive bleeding at the site
- Fever

If you have any of these symptoms, call your healthcare provider.

What Do the Results Mean?

It may take several days or even several weeks to get your bone marrow test results. The results may show whether you have a bone marrow disease, a blood disorder, or cancer. If you are being treated for cancer, the results may show:

- Whether your treatment is working

- How advanced your disease is

If your results are not normal, your healthcare provider will likely order more tests or discuss treatment options. If you have questions about your results, talk to your healthcare provider.

Chapter 14

Drug Testing

What Is a Drug Test?

A drug test looks for the presence of one or more illegal or prescription drugs in your urine, blood, saliva, hair, or sweat. Urine testing is the most common type of drug screening. The drugs most often tested for include:

- Marijuana

- Opioids, such as heroin, codeine, oxycodone, morphine, hydrocodone, and fentanyl

- Amphetamines, including methamphetamine

- Cocaine

- Steroids

- Barbiturates, such as phenobarbital and secobarbital

- Phencyclidine (PCP)

Other names: drug screen, drug test, drugs of abuse testing, substance abuse testing, toxicology screen, tox screen, sports doping tests

---

This chapter includes text excerpted from "Drug Testing," MedlinePlus, National Institutes of Health (NIH), October 11, 2017.

What Is It Used For?

Drug screening is used to find out whether or not a person has taken a certain drug or drugs. It may be used for:

Employment. Employers may test you before hiring and/or after hiring to check for on-the-job drug use.

Sports organizations. Professional and collegiate athletes usually need to take a test for performance-enhancing drugs or other substances.

Legal or forensic purposes. Testing may be part of a criminal or motor vehicle accident investigation. Drug screening may also be ordered as part of a court case.

Monitoring opioid use. If you've been prescribed an opioid for chronic pain, your healthcare provider may order a drug test to make sure you are taking the right amount of your medicine.

Why Do I Need a Drug Test?

You may have to take a drug test as a condition of your employment, in order to participate in organized sports, or as part of a police investigation or court case. Your healthcare provider may order drug screening if you have symptoms of drug abuse. These symptoms include:

- Slowed or slurred speech
- Dilated or small pupils
- Agitation
- Panic
- Paranoia
- Delirium
- Difficulty breathing
- Nausea
- Changes in blood pressure or heart rhythm

What Happens during a Drug Test?

A drug test generally requires that you give a urine sample in a lab. You will be given instructions to provide a "clean catch" sample. The clean catch method includes the following steps:

1. Wash your hands.

2. Clean your genital area with a cleansing pad given to you by your provider. Men should wipe the tip of their penis. Women should open their labia and clean from front to back.

3. Start to urinate into the toilet.

4. Move the collection container under your urine stream.

5. Collect at least an ounce or two of urine into the container, which should have markings to indicate the amounts.

6. Finish urinating into the toilet.

7. Return the sample container to the lab technician or healthcare provider.

In certain instances, a medical technician or other staff member may need to be present while you provide your sample.

For a blood test for drugs, you will go to a lab to provide your sample. During the test, a healthcare professional will take a blood sample from a vein in your arm, using a small needle. After the needle is inserted, a small amount of blood will be collected into a test tube or vial. You may feel a little sting when the needle goes in or out. This usually takes less than five minutes.

Will I Need to Do Anything to Prepare for the Test?

Be sure to tell the testing provider or your healthcare provider if you are taking any prescription drugs, over-the-counter (OTC) medicines, or supplements because they may give you a positive result for certain illegal drugs. Also, you should avoid foods with poppy seeds, which can cause a positive result for opioids.

Are There Any Risks to the Test?

There are no known physical risks to having a drug test, but a positive result may affect other aspects of your life, including your job, your eligibility to play sports, and the outcome of a court case.

What Do the Results Mean?

If your results are negative, it means no drugs were found in your body, or the level of drugs was below an established level, which differs depending on the drug. If your results are positive, it means one or more drugs were found in your body above an established level. However, false positives can happen. So if your first test shows that you have drugs in your system, you will have further testing to figure out whether or not you are actually taking a certain drug or drugs.

Is There Anything Else I Need to Know about a Drug Test?

Before you take a drug test, you should be told what you are being tested for, why you are being tested, and how the results will be used. If you have questions or concerns about your test, talk to your healthcare provider or contact the individual or organization that ordered the test.

Chapter 15

Lumbar Puncture (Spinal Tap)

What Is Lumbar Puncture?

A lumbar puncture (spinal tap) test is a procedure to remove a small sample of cerebral spinal fluid from the lower spine. A needle is inserted between the vertebrae (backbones) in the lower back and into the space containing the spinal fluid which surrounds and cushions the brain and spinal cord.

How Long Does It Take?

About 20–30 minutes. There is an additional recovery period of about 30 minutes after the test, when you will remain at the clinic.

Why Is the Lumbar Puncture Test Performed?

To obtain a specimen of fluid for testing. Cerebrospinal fluid (CSF) bathes the brain and contains proteins that can provide clues about disorders such as Alzheimer disease (AD) or changes in the brain that accompany aging.

This chapter includes text excerpted from "Lumbar Puncture Fact Sheet," National Institute on Aging (NIA), National Institutes of Health (NIH), March 31, 2015.

Does It Hurt?

You may experience pressure when the needle is inserted. You may also feel some very brief leg pain while the needle is positioned because it may briefly touch a floating nerve ending.

How Is It Performed?

- You will lie on your side with your knees drawn up toward your chin as far as possible or you will sit on the edge of an exam table, in a hunched forward position.

- The doctor will cleanse the skin over your spinal column with iodine.

- An injection of local anesthetic may be given at the puncture site.

- A needle is inserted into your spinal fluid space.

- Spinal fluid is collected into specimen tubes for laboratory testing.

- The needle is withdrawn, your back is cleaned, and a bandage is placed over the spot.

After the Test

- You will be asked to lie down for about 30 minutes.

- You will be given something to eat and drink.

- While you are recovering, please report any of the following symptoms to the doctor or nurse:

  - Headache

  - Tingling

  - Numbness or pain in your lower back and legs

  - Problems with urination

  - You will return home after the recovery period.

Instructions to Follow at Home

- Drink at least 6 glasses of fluid (no alcohol) in the next 12 hours.

- Remain quiet for the next 24 hours.

- Avoid any strenuous physical activity for 48 hours—no exercising, heavy lifting, or repeated bending.

- A mild headache may follow a lumbar puncture. It is often relieved by caffeine, aspirin or tylenol, and drinking plenty of fluids.

- If you develop a headache that persists more than 24 hours, in particular one that is worse on sitting or standing, and better when lying down, then call the doctor or study coordinator at the clinic.

Chapter 16

Stool Tests

Chapter Contents

Section 16.1

Stool Culture

"Stool Culture," © 2018 Omnigraphics.
Reviewed July 2018.

What Is a Stool Culture?

A stool culture is a diagnostic test to detect or rule out the presence of bacterial organisms in the stool that can cause gastrointestinal (GI) symptoms, infections, and diseases. The test helps the doctor understand if there are any digestive problems in the GI tract. The laboratory staff may examine the stool under a microscope to check for any signs of ova or parasites using a dye-staining method. The following bacteria are examined in the stool:

- *Campylobacter* species

- *Salmonella* species

- *Shigella* species

The following risk factors may be analyzed if you're considering traveling outside of the United States:

- *Pleisomonas*

- *Vibrio* species

- *Yersinia enterocolitica*

- *Escherichia coli* 0157:H7

- *Aeromonas*

Other tests include a test for *Clostridium difficile* (*C. difficile*) toxin or an ova and parasite examination to look for parasites in the intestine.

How Is a Stool Culture Performed?

A sample of your stool is collected by the doctor. A clean, dry, and airtight container is used to collect the sample. The sample is sent to the laboratory for culturing and examining under a microscope. Special dyes allow the laboratory to identify the type of bacteria in the sample. The lab technician uses a special dish to place the sample. A gel is added to the sample to identify bacterial growth. After examining it, the results of the stool culture is sent to the doctor.

When Is a Stool Culture Performed?

A stool culture is performed when the following signs and symptoms are detected in the digestive tract:

- Diarrhea with blood or mucus
- Abdominal pain and cramping
- Nausea and vomiting
- Fever

Other symptoms that require a stool culture are:

- Severe dehydration, electrolyte imbalance, or other complications
- Symptoms that persist for an extended period of time and require treatment
- When fluids or food are contaminated with pathogenic bacteria
- An outbreak of foodborne or waterborne diseases

What Does the Test Result Mean?

Your doctor will recommend follow-up steps based on the results of your stool sample. For instance, the doctor might look for signs of irritable bowel syndrome (IBS), a parasitic infection, or other problems related to GI infection. Common bacterial infections that are known to cause infections in the United States are:

- *Salmonella*—found in raw eggs, raw poultry, uncooked vegetables, and reptiles. Some people may carry Salmonella in their intestines without being ill themselves. Salmonella is usually transmitted from person to person.
- *Campylobacter*—found in raw or undercooked poultry and unpasteurized milk, and is one of the most common causes of bacterial diarrhea in the United States. Long-term complications might result in arthritis and Guillain-Barre syndrome (GBS).
- *Shigella*—found in contaminated food and water, and it can also pass from one infected person to another when proper sanitation and hygiene are not observed.

177

Other bacterial infections can be identified with a stool culture. Some examples include:

- *Escherichia coli* 0157:H7 and other toxin-producing *E. coli*—found in raw or undercooked beef, spinach, and unpasteurized cider. It causes watery stools and may eventually lead to hemolytic uremic syndrome.

- *Clostridium difficile*—toxin-producing strains that can cause diarrhea and other serious intestinal complications. Tests to detect the presence of these strains are performed separately.

Examples of other less common causes include:

- *Vibrio cholerae* and other *Vibrio* species
- *Yersinia enterocolitica*
- *Aeromonas*
- *Plesiomonas*

References

1. Case-Lo, Christine. "Stool Culture," July 21, 2016.

2. "Fecal Culture," April 30, 2018.

3. "Stool Culture," June 5, 2018.

Section 16.2

Detecting Parasite Antigens

This section includes text excerpted from "Stool Specimens—Detection of Parasite Antigens," Centers for Disease Control and Prevention (CDC), May 3, 2016.

The diagnosis of human intestinal protozoa depends on microscopic detection of the various parasite stages in feces, duodenal fluid, or small intestine biopsy specimens. Since fecal examination is very labor-intensive and requires a skilled microscopist, antigen detection tests have been developed as alternatives using direct fluorescent antibody (DFA), enzyme immunoassay (EIA), and rapid, dipstick-like tests. Antigen detection methods can be performed quickly and do not require an experienced and skilled morphologist. Much work has been accomplished on the development of antigen detection tests, resulting in commercially available reagents for the intestinal parasites *Cryptosporidium* spp., *Entamoeba histolytica, Giardia duodenalis,* and *Trichomonas vaginalis.* In addition, antigen detection tests using blood or serum are available for *Plasmodium* and *Wuchereria bancrofti.*

Specimens for Antigen Detection

Fresh or preserved stool samples are the appropriate specimen for antigen detection testing with most kits, but refer to the recommended collection procedures included with each specific kit.

Amebiasis

EIA kits are commercially available for detection of fecal antigens for the diagnosis of intestinal amebiasis. Organisms of both the pathogenic *E. histolytica* and the nonpathogenic Entamoeba dispar strains are morphologically identical. These assays use monoclonal antibodies that detect the galactose-inhibitable adherence protein in the pathogenic *E. histolytica.* The primary drawback of these assays is the requirement for fresh, unpreserved stool specimens. Several EIA kits for antigen detection of the *E. histolytica / E. dispar* group are available in the United States, but only the TechLab kit is specific for *E. histolytica.*

Cryptosporidiosis

Immunodetection of antigens on the surface of organisms in stool specimens, using monoclonal antibody (mAb)-based DFA assays, is the current test of choice for diagnosis of cryptosporidiosis and provides increased sensitivity over modified acid-fast staining techniques. There are commercial products (DFA, indirect fluorescent antibody (IFA), EIA, and rapid tests) available in the United States for the diagnosis of cryptosporidiosis. Several kits are combined tests for *Cryptosporidium, Giardia,* and *E. histolytica.* Factors such as ease of use, technical skill and time, single versus batch testing, and test cost must be considered when determining the test of choice for individual laboratories. The most sensitive (99%) and specific (100%) method is reported to be the DFA test, which identifies oocysts in concentrated or unconcentrated fecal samples by using a fluorescein isothiocyanate (FITC)-labeled mAb. A combined DFA test for the simultaneous detection of *Cryptosporidium oocysts* and *Giardia* cysts is available.

Some commercial EIA tests are available in the microplate format for the detection of *Cryptosporidium* antigens in fresh or frozen stool samples and also in stool specimens preserved in formalin, or sodium acetate-acetic acid-formalin (SAF) fixed stool specimens. Concentrated or polyvinyl alcohol-treated (PVA) samples are unsuitable for testing with available antigen detection EIA kits. The kits are reportedly superior to microscopy, especially acid-fast staining, and show good correlation with the DFA test. Kit sensitivities and specificities reportedly range from 93–100 percent when used in a clinical setting. Laboratories which use these EIA kits need to be aware of potential problems with false-positive results and take steps to monitor kit performance.

Rapid immunochromatographic assays are available for the combined antigen detection of either *Cryptosporidium* and *Giardia* or *Cryptosporidium*, *Giardia*, and *E. histolytica*. These offer the advantage of short test time and multiple results in one reaction device. Initial evaluations indicate comparable sensitivity and specificity to previously available tests.

The Meridian Merifluor DFA Kit for *Cryptosporidium / Giardia*, modified acid-fast stain for *Cryptosporidium* spp., or Wheatley's trichrome stain for *Giardia* spp. are used at Centers for Disease Control and Prevention (CDC) for routine identification of these parasites. These techniques can be used to confirm suspicious or discrepant diagnostic results.

Giardiasis

Detection of antigens on the surface of organisms in stool specimens is the current test of choice for diagnosis of giardiasis and provides increased sensitivity over more common microscopy techniques. Commercial products (DFA, EIAs, and rapid tests) are available in the United States for the immunodiagnosis of giardiasis. DFA assays may be purchased that employ fluorescein isothiocyanate (FITC)-labeled mAb for detection of *Giardia* cysts alone or in a combined kit for the simultaneous detection of *Giardia* cysts and *Cryptosporidium* oocysts. The sensitivity and specificity of these kits were both 100 percent compared to those of microscopy. They may be used for quantitation of cysts and oocysts, and thus may be useful for epidemiologic and control studies.

Some commercial EIA tests are available in the microplate format for the detection of *Giardia* antigen in fresh or frozen stool samples and also in stool specimens preserved in formalin, MIF, or SAF fixatives. Concentrated or PVA samples are not suitable for testing with EIA kits. EIA kit sensitivity rates were reported as ranging from 94–100 percent while specificity rates were all 100 percent.

Trichomoniasis

Trichomoniasis, an infection caused by *Trichomonas vaginalis*, is a common sexually transmitted disease (STD). Diagnosis is made by detection of trophozoites in vaginal secretions or urethral specimens by wet mount microscopic examination, DFA staining of specimens, or culture. Sensitivity of the assays were reported as 60 percent for wet mounts and 86 percent for DFA when compared to cultures. A kit which employs FITC- or enzyme-labeled mAbs for use in a DFA or EIA procedure is available for detection of whole parasites in fluids. A latex agglutination test for antigen detection in vaginal swab specimens is available; the manufacturer's evaluation indicated good sensitivity and specificity.

Section 16.3

Fecal Occult Blood Test (FOBT)

This section includes text excerpted from "Fecal Occult Blood Test (FOBT)," MedlinePlus, National Institutes of Health (NIH), September 22, 2017.

What Is a Fecal Occult Blood Test (FOBT)?

A fecal occult blood test (FOBT) looks at a sample of your stool (feces) to check for blood. Occult blood means that you can't see it with the naked eye. Blood in the stool means there is likely some kind of bleeding in the digestive tract. It may be caused by a variety of conditions, including:

- Polyps

- Hemorrhoids

- Diverticulosis

- Ulcers

- Colitis, a type of inflammatory bowel disease

Blood in the stool may also be a sign of colorectal cancer, a type of cancer that starts in the colon or rectum. Colorectal cancer is the second leading cause of cancer-related deaths in the United States and the third most common cancer in men and in women. A FOBT is a screening test that may help find colorectal cancer early, when treatment is most effective.

Other names: FOBT, stool occult blood, occult blood test, Hemoccult test, guaiac smear test, gFOBT, immunochemical FOBT, iFOBT; FIT

What Is It Used For?

A FOBT is used as an early screening test for colorectal cancer. It may also be used to diagnose other conditions that cause bleeding in the digestive tract.

Why Do I Need a FOBT?

The National Cancer Institute (NCI) recommends that people get regular screenings for colorectal cancer starting at age 50. The screening may be a fecal occult test, a colonoscopy, or another test. Talk with your healthcare provider about which test is right for you.

If you choose a FOBT, you need to get it every year. If you have a colonoscopy, you only need it every ten years. But it is a more invasive procedure. You may need screening more often if you have certain risk factors. These include:

- A family history of colorectal cancer

- Cigarette smoking

- Obesity

- Excessive alcohol use

What Happens during a FOBT?

A FOBT is a noninvasive test that you can perform at home at your convenience. Your healthcare provider will give you a kit that includes instructions on how to do the test. There are two main types of FOBTs: the guaiac smear method (gFOBT) and the immunochemical method (iFOBT or FIT). Below are typical instructions for each test. Your instructions may vary slightly depending on the manufacturer of the test kit.

For a guaiac smear test (gFOBT), you will most likely need to:

- Collect samples from three separate bowel movements.

- For each sample, collect the stool and store in a clean container. Make sure the sample does not mix in with urine or water from the toilet.

- Use the applicator from your test kit to smear some of the stool on the test card or slide, also included in your kit.

- Label and seal all your samples as directed.

- Mail the samples to your healthcare provider or lab.

For a fecal immunochemical test (FIT), you will most likely need to:

- Collect samples from 2 or 3 bowel movements.

- Collect the sample from the toilet using the special brush or other device that was included in your kit.

- For each sample, use the brush or device to take the sample from the surface of the stool.

- Brush the sample onto a test card.

- Label and seal all your samples as directed.

- Mail the samples to your healthcare provider or lab.

Be sure to follow all the instructions provided in your kit, and talk to your healthcare provider if you have any questions.

Will I Need to Do Anything to Prepare for the Test?

Certain foods and drugs may affect the results of a guaiac smear method (gFOBT) test. Your healthcare provider may ask you to avoid the following:

- Nonsteroidal anti-inflammatory drugs (NSAIDs) such as ibuprofen, naproxen, or aspirin for seven days prior to your test. If you take aspirin for heart problems, talk to your healthcare provider before stopping your medicine. Acetaminophen may be safe to use during this time, but check with your healthcare provider before taking it.

- More than 250 mg of vitamin C daily from supplements, fruit juices, or fruit for seven days prior to your test. Vitamin C can affect the chemicals in the test and cause a negative result even if there is blood present.

- Red meat, such as beef, lamb, and pork, for three days prior to the test. Traces of blood in these meats may cause a false-positive result.

There are no special preparations or dietary restrictions for a FIT.

Are There Any Risks to the Test?

There is no known risk to having a FOBT.

What Do the Results Mean?

If your results are positive for either type of FOBT, it means you likely have bleeding somewhere in your digestive tract. But it does not necessarily mean you have cancer. Other conditions that may produce a positive result on a FOBT include ulcers, hemorrhoids, polyps, and benign tumors. If your test results are positive for blood, your healthcare provider will likely recommend additional testing, such as a colonoscopy, to figure out the exact location and cause of your bleeding. If you have questions about your results, talk to your healthcare provider.

Is There Anything Else I Need to Know about a FOBT?

Regular colorectal cancer screenings, such as the FOBT, are an important tool in the fight against cancer. Studies show that screening tests can help find cancer early, and may reduce deaths from the disease.

Chapter 17

Bacteria Culture Test

What Is a Bacteria Culture Test?

Bacteria are a large group of one-celled organisms. They can live on different places in the body. Some types of bacteria are harmless or even beneficial. Others can cause infections and disease. A bacteria culture test can help find harmful bacteria in your body. During a bacteria culture test, a sample will be taken from your blood, urine, skin, or other part of your body. The type of sample depends on the location of the suspected infection. The cells in your sample will be taken to a lab and put in a special environment in a lab to encourage cell growth. Results are often available within a few days. But some types of bacteria grow slowly, and it may take several days or longer.

What Is It Used For?

Bacteria culture tests are used to help diagnose certain types of infections. The most common types of bacteria tests and their uses are listed below.

Throat Culture

- Used to diagnose or rule out strep throat

This chapter includes text excerpted from "Bacteria Culture Test," Medline-Plus, National Institutes of Health (NIH), April 11, 2018.

- Test procedure:
  - Your healthcare provider will insert a special swab into your mouth to take a sample from the back of the throat and tonsils.

Urine Culture

- Used to diagnose a urinary tract infection and identify the bacteria causing the infection
- Test procedure:
  - You will provide a sterile sample of urine in a cup, as instructed by your healthcare provider.

Sputum Culture

Sputum is a thick mucus that is coughed up from the lungs. It is different from spit or saliva.

- Used to help diagnose bacterial infections in the respiratory tract. These include bacterial pneumonia and bronchitis.
- Test procedure:
  - You may be asked to cough up sputum into a special cup as instructed by your provider; or a special swab may be used to take a sample from your nose.

Blood Culture

- Used to detect the presence of bacteria or fungi in the blood
- Test procedure:
  - A healthcare professional will need a blood sample. The sample is most often taken from a vein in your arm.

Stool Culture

Another name for stool is feces.

- Used to detect infections caused by bacteria or parasites in the digestive system. These include food poisoning and other digestive illnesses.
- Test procedure:
  - You will provide a sample of your feces in a clean container as instructed by your healthcare provider.

Wound Culture

- Used to detect infections on open wounds or on burn injuries
- Test procedure:
  - Your healthcare provider will use a special swab to collect a sample from the site of your wound.

Why Do I Need a Bacteria Culture Test?

Your healthcare provider may order a bacteria culture test if you have symptoms of a bacterial infection. The symptoms vary depending on the type of infection.

Why Do I Have to Wait so Long for My Results?

Your test sample doesn't contain enough cells for your healthcare provider to detect an infection. So your sample will be sent to a lab to allow the cells to grow. If there is an infection, the infected cells will multiply. Most disease-causing bacteria will grow enough to be seen within one to two days, but it can take some organisms five days or longer.

Will I Need to Do Anything to Prepare for the Test?

There are many different types of bacteria culture tests. Ask your healthcare provider if you need to do anything to prepare for your test.

Are There Any Risks to the Test?

There are no known risks to having a swab or blood test or to providing a urine or stool sample.

What Do the Results Mean?

If enough bacteria is found in your sample, it likely means you have a bacterial infection. Your healthcare provider may order additional tests to confirm a diagnosis or determine the severity of the infection. Your provider may also order a "susceptibility test" on your sample. A susceptibility test is used to help determine which antibiotic will be most effective in treating your infection. If you have questions about your results, talk to your healthcare provider.

Chapter 18

Strep Throat Test

Strep throat is a bacterial infection that can easily spread to other people. Children and some adults are more likely to get strep throat than others. It is usually a mild infection, but serious complications can occur. There is a quick test doctors can use to see if you have strep throat. If the test is positive, your doctor can prescribe antibiotics so that you feel better sooner and protect others from getting sick.

Causes

Most sore throats are caused by viruses, but strep throat is caused by bacteria called group A Streptococcus or group A strep.

Spread to Others

Group A strep live in the nose and throat and can easily spread to other people. When someone who is infected coughs or sneezes, the bacteria travel in small droplets of water called respiratory droplets. You can get sick if you breathe in those droplets or if you touch something that has the droplets on it and then touch your mouth or nose. You could also become ill if you drink from the same glass or eat from the same plate as a sick person. It is possible to get strep throat from touching sores on the skin caused by group A strep (impetigo).

This chapter includes text excerpted from "Strep Throat," Centers for Disease Control and Prevention (CDC), September 16, 2016.

Although rare, group A strep can be spread through food if it is not handled properly. Pets or household items, like toys, are not known to spread these bacteria.

Signs and Symptoms

In general, strep throat is a mild infection, but it can be very painful. Symptoms of strep throat usually include:

- Sore throat that can start very quickly

- Pain when swallowing

- Fever

- Red and swollen tonsils, sometimes with white patches or streaks of pus

- Tiny, red spots (petechiae) on the roof of the mouth (the soft or hard palate)

- Swollen lymph nodes in the front of the neck

Other symptoms may include a headache, stomach pain, nausea, or vomiting—especially in children. Cough, runny nose, hoarseness (changes in your voice that makes it sound breathy, raspy, or strained), and conjunctivitis (also called pink eye) are not symptoms of strep throat and suggest that a virus is the cause of the illness. Someone with strep throat may also have a rash known as scarlet fever (also called scarlatina).

It usually takes 2–5 days for someone exposed to group A strep to become ill.

Risk Factors

Anyone can get strep throat, but there are some factors that can increase your risk of getting this common infection.

Strep throat is more common in children than adults. It is most common in children 5 through 15 years old. It is rare in children younger than 3 years old. Parents of school-aged children and adults who are often in contact with children will have a higher risk for strep throat than adults who are not around children very often.

Close contact with another person with strep throat is the most common risk factor for illness. For example, if someone has strep throat, it often spreads to other people in their household.

Infectious illnesses tend to spread wherever large groups of people gather together. Crowded conditions—such as those in schools, daycare centers, or military training facilities—can increase the risk of getting a group A strep infection.

Diagnosis and Testing

Since sore throats can be caused by many viruses and bacteria, it is very important to determine if group A strep is the cause. A rapid strep test or a throat culture is needed. A doctor cannot tell if you have strep throat just by looking at the throat.

A rapid strep test involves swabbing the throat and running a test on the swab to quickly see if group A strep is causing the illness. If the test is positive, doctors can prescribe antibiotics (medicine that kills bacteria in the body). If the rapid strep test is negative, but a doctor still strongly suspects strep throat, then they can take a throat culture swab to see if bacteria grow from the sample. A culture test requires more time to get the results but can be important to use in children and teens because they are at risk of getting rheumatic fever if their strep throat infection is not treated. For adults, it is usually not necessary to do a throat culture following a negative rapid strep test since there is little risk of adults getting rheumatic fever following a strep throat infection.

Treatment

Unlike sore throats caused by viruses, strep throat is treated with antibiotics. Either penicillin or amoxicillin are recommended as a first choice for people who are not allergic to penicillin, but other antibiotics can be used to treat strep throat in people who are allergic to penicillin. Antibiotics help shorten how long someone is sick, prevent spreading the disease to others, and prevent getting complications like rheumatic fever.

Someone who has no symptoms but tests positive for strep throat is known as a "carrier." Carriers usually do not need antibiotics. They are less likely to spread the bacteria to others and very unlikely to get complications. If a carrier gets a sore throat illness caused by a virus, the rapid strep test can be positive even though the illness is not caused by the bacteria that cause strep throat. If someone keeps getting a sore throat after testing positive for strep throat and being treated with the right antibiotics, this may be a clue that the person is a strep carrier. Talk to your healthcare professional if you think you or your child may be a strep carrier.

Complications

Complications can occur after a strep throat infection. This can happen if the bacteria spread to other parts of the body. Complications can include abscesses (pockets of pus) around the tonsils, swollen lymph nodes in the neck, and sinus or ear infections. Other complications can affect the heart (rheumatic fever) or kidneys (poststreptococcal glomerulonephritis (PSGN)).

Prevention

People can get strep throat more than once, so having the infection does not protect you from getting it again in the future. While there is no vaccine to prevent strep throat, there are things you can do to protect yourself and others.

Hygiene

The best way to keep from getting or spreading strep throat is to wash your hands often, especially after coughing or sneezing and before preparing foods or eating. To practice good hygiene you should:

- Cover your mouth and nose with a tissue when you cough or sneeze.
- Put your used tissue in the wastebasket.
- Cough or sneeze into your upper sleeve or elbow, not your hands, if you don't have a tissue.
- Wash your hands often with soap and water for at least 20 seconds.
- Use an alcohol-based hand rub if soap and water are not available.

You should also wash glasses, utensils, and plates after someone who is sick uses them. After they have been washed, these items are safe for others to use.

Antibiotics

Someone with strep throat is usually not able to spread the bacteria to others after they have taken the correct antibiotic for 24 hours or longer. If you are diagnosed with strep throat, you should stay home from work, school, or daycare until you no longer have a fever and have taken antibiotics for at least 24 hours so you don't spread the infection to others.

Chapter 19

Urine Tests

Chapter Contents

Section 19.1

Urine Test: Basics

This section contains text excerpted from the following sources: Text in this section begins with excerpts from "Urine and Urination," MedlinePlus, National Institutes of Health (NIH), May 6, 2016; Text beginning with the heading "What Is Urinalysis?" is excerpted from "Urinalysis," MedlinePlus, National Institutes of Health (NIH), May 5, 2016.

Your kidneys make urine by filtering wastes and extra water from your blood. The waste is called urea. Your blood carries it to the kidneys. From the kidneys, urine travels down two thin tubes called ureters to the bladder. The bladder stores urine until you are ready to urinate. It swells into a round shape when it is full and gets smaller when empty. If your urinary system is healthy, your bladder can hold up to 16 ounces (2 cups) of urine comfortably for 2–5 hours.

You may have problems with urination if you have

- Kidney failure

- Urinary tract infections (UTIs)

- An enlarged prostate

- Bladder control problems like incontinence, overactive bladder, or interstitial cystitis (IC)

- A blockage that prevents you from emptying your bladder

Some conditions may also cause you to have blood or protein in your urine. If you have a urinary problem, see your healthcare provider. Urinalysis and other urine tests can help to diagnose the problem. Treatment depends on the cause.

What Is Urinalysis?

A urinalysis is a test of your urine. It is often done to check for a UTIs, kidney problems, or diabetes. You may also have one during a checkup, if you are admitted to the hospital, before you have surgery, or if you are pregnant. It can also monitor some medical conditions and treatments.

A urinalysis involves checking the urine for

- It's color

- Its appearance (whether it is clear or cloudy)

- Any odor

- The pH level (acidity)

- Whether there are substances that are not normally in urine, such as blood, too much protein, glucose, ketones, and bilirubin

- Whether there are cells, crystals, and casts (tube-shaped proteins)

- Whether it contains bacteria or other germs

Section 19.2

Epithelial Cells in Urine

This section includes text excerpted from "Epithelial Cells in Urine," MedlinePlus, National Institutes of Health (NIH), September 22, 2017.

What Is an Epithelial Cells in Urine Test?

Epithelial cells are a type of cell that lines the surfaces of your body. They are found on your skin, blood vessels, urinary tract, and organs. An epithelial cells in urine test looks at urine under a microscope to see if the number of your epithelial cells is in the normal range. It's normal to have a small amount of epithelial cells in your urine. A large amount may indicate an infection, kidney disease, or other serious medical condition.

Other names: microscopic urine analysis, microscopic examination of urine, urine test, urine analysis, UA.

What Is It Used For?

An epithelial cells in urine test is a part of a urinalysis, a test that measures different substances in your urine. A urinalysis may include a visual examination of your urine sample, tests for certain chemicals, and an examination of urine cells under a microscope. An epithelial cells in urine test is part of a microscopic exam of urine.

Why Do I Need an Epithelial Cells in Urine Test?

Your healthcare provider may have ordered an epithelial cells in urine test as part of your regular checkup or if your visual or chemical urine tests showed abnormal results. You may also need this test if you have symptoms of a urinary or kidney disorder. These symptoms may include:

- Frequent and/or painful urination
- Abdominal pain
- Back pain

What Happens during an Epithelial Cells in Urine Test?

Your healthcare provider will need to collect a sample of your urine. During your office visit, you will receive a container to collect the urine and special instructions to make sure that the sample is sterile. These instructions are often called the "clean catch method." The clean catch method includes the following steps:

1. Wash your hands.
2. Clean your genital area with a cleansing pad given to you by your provider. Men should wipe the tip of their penis. Women should open their labia and clean from front to back.
3. Start to urinate into the toilet.
4. Move the collection container under your urine stream.
5. Collect at least an ounce or two of urine into the container. The container will have markings to indicate the amounts.
6. Finish urinating into the toilet.
7. Return the sample container as instructed by your healthcare provider.

Will I Need to Do Anything to Prepare for the Test?

You don't need any special preparations for the test. If your healthcare provider has ordered other urine or blood tests, you may need to fast (not eat or drink) for several hours before the test. Your health-care provider will let you know if there are any special instructions to follow.

Are There Any Risks to the Test?

There is no known risk to having the test.

What Do the Results Mean?

Results are often reported as an approximate amount, such as "few," moderate," or "many" cells. "Few" cells are generally considered in the normal range. "Moderate" or "many" cells may indicate a medical condition such as:

- Urinary tract infection (UTI)
- Yeast infection
- Kidney disease
- Liver disease
- Certain types of cancer

If your results are not in the normal range, it doesn't necessarily mean that you have a medical condition that requires treatment. You may need more tests before you can get a diagnosis. To learn what your results mean, talk to your healthcare provider.

Is There Anything Else I Need to Know about an Epithelial Cells in Urine Test?

There are three types of epithelial cells that line the urinary tract. They are called transitional cells, renal tubular cells (RTC), and squamous cells. If there are squamous epithelial cells in your urine, it may mean your sample was contaminated. This means that the sample contains cells from the urethra (in men) or the vaginal opening (in women). It can happen if you do not clean well enough when using the clean catch method.

Section 19.3

Mucus in Urine

This section includes text excerpted from "Mucus in Urine," MedlinePlus, National Institutes of Health (NIH), September 22, 2017.

How Do You Test for Mucus in Urine?

Mucus is a thick, slimy substance that coats and moistens certain parts of the body, including the nose, mouth, throat, and urinary tract. A small amount of mucus in your urine is normal. An excess amount may indicate a urinary tract infection (UTI) or other medical condition. A test called urinalysis can detect whether there is too much mucus in your urine.

Other names: microscopic urine analysis, microscopic examination of urine, urine test, urine analysis, UA.

What Is It Used For?

A mucus in urine test may be part of a urinalysis. A urinalysis may include a visual check of your urine sample, tests for certain chemicals, and an examination of urine cells under a microscope. A mucus in urine test is part of a microscopic exam of urine.

Why Do I Need a Mucus in Urine Test?

A urinalysis is often part of a routine checkup. Your healthcare provider may include a mucus in urine test in your urinalysis if you have symptoms of a UTI. These include:

- Frequent urge to urinate, but little urine is passed
- Painful urination
- Dark, cloudy, or reddish-colored urine
- Bad smelling urine
- Weakness
- Fatigue

What Happens during a Mucus in Urine Test?

Your healthcare provider will need to collect a sample of your urine. You will receive a container to collect the urine and special instructions to make sure that the sample is sterile. These instructions are often called the "clean catch method." The clean catch method includes the following steps:

1. Wash your hands.

2. Clean your genital area with a cleansing pad given to you by your provider. Men should wipe the tip of their penis. Women should open their labia and clean from front to back.

3. Start to urinate into the toilet.

4. Move the collection container under your urine stream.

5. Collect at least an ounce or two of urine into the container. The container will have markings to indicate the amounts.

6. Finish urinating into the toilet.

7. Return the sample container as instructed by your healthcare provider.

Will I Need to Do Anything to Prepare for the Test?

You don't need any special preparations for this test. If your healthcare provider has ordered other urine or blood tests, you may need to fast (not eat or drink) for several hours before the test. Your healthcare provider will let you know if there are any special instructions to follow.

Are There Any Risks to the Test?

There is no known risk to having a urinalysis or a test for mucus in urine.

What Do the Results Mean?

If your results show a small or moderate amount of mucus in your urine, it is most likely due to normal discharge. A large amount of mucus may indicate one of the following conditions:

- A UTI
- A sexually transmitted disease (STD)
- Kidney stones
- Irritable bowel syndrome (IBS)
- Bladder cancer

To learn what your results mean, talk to your healthcare provider.

Is There Anything Else I Need to Know about a Mucus in Urine Test?

If a urinalysis is part of your regular checkup, your urine will be tested for a variety of substances along with mucus. These include red and white blood cells (WBCs), proteins, acid and sugar levels, and the concentration of particles in your urine.

If you get frequent UTIs, your healthcare provider may recommend more testing, as well as steps that may help prevent reinfection.

Section 19.4

Bilirubin in Urine

This section includes text excerpted from "Bilirubin in Urine," MedlinePlus, National Institutes of Health (NIH), December 19, 2017.

What Is a Bilirubin in Urine Test?

A bilirubin in urine test measures the levels of bilirubin in your urine. Bilirubin is a yellowish substance made during the body's normal process of breaking down red blood cells (RBCs). Bilirubin is found in bile, a fluid in your liver that helps you digest food. If your liver is healthy, it will remove most of the bilirubin from your body. If your liver is damaged, bilirubin can leak into the blood and urine. Bilirubin in urine may be a sign of liver disease.

Other names: urine test, urine analysis, UA, chemical urinalysis, direct bilirubin

What Is It Used For?

A bilirubin in urine test is often part of a urinalysis, a test that measures different cells, chemicals, and other substances in your urine.

Urinalysis is often included as part of a routine exam. This test may also be used to check for liver problems.

Why Do I Need a Bilirubin in Urine Test?

Your healthcare provider may have ordered a bilirubin in urine test as part of your regular checkup, or if you have symptoms of liver disease. These symptoms include:

- Jaundice, a condition that causes your skin and eyes to turn yellow
- Dark-colored urine
- Abdominal pain
- Nausea and vomiting
- Fatigue

Because bilirubin in urine can indicate liver damage before other symptoms appear, your healthcare provider may order a bilirubin in urine test if you are at a higher risk for liver damage. Risk factors for liver disease include:

- Family history of liver disease
- Heavy drinking
- Exposure or possible exposure to hepatitis virus
- Obesity
- Diabetes
- Taking certain medicines that can cause liver damage

What Happens during a Bilirubin in Urine Test?

Your healthcare provider will need to collect a sample of your urine. During your office visit, you will receive a container to collect the urine and special instructions to make sure that the sample is sterile. These instructions are often called the "clean catch method." The clean catch method includes the following steps:

1. Wash your hands.
2. Clean your genital area with a cleansing pad given to you by your provider. Men should wipe the tip of their penis. Women should open their labia and clean from front to back.

3. Start to urinate into the toilet.

4. Move the collection container under your urine stream.

5. Collect at least an ounce or two of urine into the container, which should have markings to indicate the amounts.

6. Finish urinating into the toilet.

7. Return the sample container to your healthcare provider.

Will I Need to Do Anything to Prepare for the Test?

You don't need any special preparations to test for bilirubin in urine. If your healthcare provider has ordered other urine or blood tests, you may need to fast (not eat or drink) for several hours before the test. Your healthcare provider will let you know if there are any special instructions to follow.

Are There Any Risks to the Test?

There is no known risk to having a urinalysis or a bilirubin in urine test.

What Do the Results Mean?

If bilirubin is found in your urine, it may indicate:

• A liver disease such as hepatitis

• A blockage in the structures that carry bile from your liver

• A problem with liver function

A bilirubin in urine test is only one measure of liver function. If your results are abnormal, your healthcare provider may order additional blood and urine tests, including a liver panel. A liver panel is a series of blood tests that measure various enzymes, proteins, and substances in the liver. It is often used to detect liver disease.

Section 19.5

Blood in Urine

This section includes text excerpted from "Blood in Urine," MedlinePlus, National Institutes of Health (NIH), September 22, 2017.

How Do You Test for Blood in Urine?

A test called a urinalysis can detect whether there is blood in your urine. A urinalysis checks a sample of your urine for different cells, chemicals, and other substances, including blood. Most causes of blood in your urine are not serious, But sometimes red or white blood cells (WBCs) in your urine can mean that you have a medical condition that needs treatment, such as a kidney disease, urinary tract infection (UTI), or liver disease.

Other names: microscopic urine analysis, microscopic examination of urine, urine test, urine analysis, UA

What Is It Used For?

A urinalysis, which includes a test for blood in urine, may be done as part of a regular checkup or to check for disorders of the urinary tract, kidney, or liver.

Why Do I Need a Blood in Urine Test?

Your healthcare provider may have ordered a urinalysis as part of a routine exam. You may also need this test if you have seen blood in your urine or have other symptoms of a urinary disorder. These symptoms include:

• Painful urination

• Frequent urination

• Back pain

• Abdominal pain

What Happens during a Blood in Urine Test?

Your healthcare provider will need to collect a sample of your urine. During your office visit, you will receive a container to collect the urine

203

and special instructions to make sure that the sample is sterile. These instructions are often called the "clean catch method." It includes the following steps:

1. Wash your hands.

2. Clean your genital area with a cleansing pad given to you by your provider. Men should wipe the tip of their penis. Women should open their labia and clean from front to back.

3. Start to urinate into the toilet.

4. Move the collection container under your urine stream.

5. Collect at least an ounce or two of urine into the container, which should have markings to indicate the needed amounts.

6. Finish urinating into the toilet.

7. Return the sample container as instructed by your healthcare provider.

Will I Need to Do Anything to Prepare for the Test?

You don't need any special preparations before getting a test for blood in your urine. If your healthcare provider has ordered other urine or blood tests, you may need to fast (not eat or drink) for several hours before the test. Your healthcare provider will let you know if there are any special instructions to follow.

Are There Any Risks to the Test?

There is no known risk to having a urinalysis or a blood in urine test.

What Do the Results Mean?

There are a variety of factors that can cause red or WBCs to be present in the urine. Many are not cause for concern. Small amounts of blood in the urine may be due to certain medicines, intense exercise, sexual activity, or menstruation. If larger amounts of blood are found, your healthcare provider may request further testing.

Increased red blood cells (RBCs) in urine may indicate:

- A viral infection

- Inflammation of the kidney or bladder

- A blood disorder

- Bladder or kidney cancer

Increased white blood cells (WBCs) in urine may indicate:

- A bacterial UTI. This is the most common cause of a high WBC count in urine.

- Inflammation of the urinary tract or kidneys

To learn what your results mean, talk to your healthcare provider.

Is There Anything Else I Need to Know about a Blood in Urine Test?

A blood in urine test is usually part of a typical urinalysis. In addition to checking for blood, a urinalysis measures other substances in the urine, including proteins, acid and sugar levels, cell fragments, and crystals.

Section 19.6

Crystals in Urine Test

This section includes text excerpted from "Crystals in Urine Test," MedlinePlus, National Institutes of Health (NIH), October 3, 2017.

What Is a Crystals in Urine Test?

Your urine contains many chemicals. Sometimes these chemicals form solids, called crystals. A crystals in urine test looks at the amount, size, and type of crystals in your urine. It's normal to have a few small urine crystals. Larger crystals or specific types of crystals can become kidney stones. Kidney stones are hard, pebble-like substances that can get stuck in the kidneys. A stone can be as small as a grain of sand, as big as a pea, or even larger. While kidney stones rarely cause serious damage, they can be very painful.

Other names: urinalysis (crystals) microscopic urine analysis, microscopic examination of urine

What Is It Used For?

A crystals in urine test is often part of a urinalysis, a test that measures different substances in your urine. A urinalysis may include a visual check of your urine sample, tests for certain chemicals, and an examination of urine cells under a microscope. A crystals in urine test is part of a microscopic exam of urine. It may be used to help diagnose kidney stones or a problem with your metabolism, the process of how your body uses food and energy.

Why Do I Need a Crystals in Urine Test?

A urinalysis is often part of a routine checkup. Your healthcare provider may include a crystals in urine test in your urinalysis if you have symptoms of a kidney stone. These include:

- Sharp pains in your abdomen, side, or groin
- Back pain
- Blood in your urine
- Frequent urge to urinate
- Pain when urinating
- Cloudy or bad-smelling urine
- Nausea and vomiting

What Happens during a Crystals in Urine Test?

You will need to provide a sample of your urine. During your office visit, you will receive a container to collect the urine and special instructions to make sure the sample is sterile. These instructions are often called the "clean catch method." The clean catch method includes the following steps:

1. Wash your hands.

2. Clean your genital area with a cleansing pad. Men should wipe the tip of their penis. Women should open their labia and clean from front to back.

3. Start to urinate into the toilet.

4. Move the collection container under your urine stream.

5. Collect at least an ounce or two of urine into the container, which should have markings to indicate the amount.

6. Finish urinating into the toilet.

7. Return the sample container as instructed by your healthcare provider.

Your healthcare provider may also request that you collect all urine during a 24-hour period. This is called a "24-hour urine sample test." It is used because the amounts of substances in urine, including crystals, can vary throughout the day. Your healthcare provider or a laboratory professional will give you a container to collect your urine and instructions on how to collect and store your samples. A 24-hour urine sample test usually includes the following steps:

- Empty your bladder in the morning and flush that urine away. Record the time.

- For the next 24 hours, save all your urine passed in the container provided.

- Store your urine container in the refrigerator or a cooler with ice.

- Return the sample container to your healthcare provider's office or the laboratory as instructed.

Will I Need to Do Anything to Prepare for the Test?

You don't need any special preparations for a crystals in urine test. Be sure to carefully follow all the instructions for providing a 24-hour urine sample.

Are There Any Risks to the Test?

There is no known risk to having a crystals in urine test.

What Do the Results Mean?

If a large number, large size, or certain types of crystal are found in your urine, it may mean you have a kidney stone that requires medical treatment, but it doesn't always mean you need treatment. Sometimes a small kidney stone can pass through your urine on its own, and cause little or no pain. Also, certain medicines, your diet, and other factors can affect your results. If you have questions about your urine crystal results, talk to your healthcare provider.

Is There Anything Else I Need to Know about a Crystals in Urine Test?

If a urinalysis is part of your regular checkup, your urine will be tested for a variety of substances in addition to crystals. These include red and white blood cells (WBCs), proteins, acid and sugar levels, cell fragments, bacteria, and yeast.

Section 19.7

Ketones in Urine

This section includes text excerpted from "Ketones in Urine," MedlinePlus, National Institutes of Health (NIH), September 22, 2017.

What Is a Ketones in Urine Test?

The test measures ketone levels in your urine. Normally, your body burns glucose (sugar) for energy. If your cells don't get enough glucose, your body burns fat for energy instead. This produces a substance called ketones, which can show up in your blood and urine. High ketone levels in urine may indicate diabetic ketoacidosis (DKA), a complication of diabetes that can lead to a coma or even death. A ketones in urine test can prompt you to get treatment before a medical emergency occurs.

Other names: ketones urine test, ketone test, urine ketones, ketone bodies

What Is It Used For?

The test is often used to help monitor people at a higher risk of developing elevated ketone levels. These include people with type 1 or type 2 diabetes. If you have diabetes, ketones in urine can mean that you are not getting enough insulin. If you don't have diabetes, you may still be at risk for developing ketones if you:

- Experience chronic vomiting and/or diarrhea
- Have a digestive disorder
- Participate in strenuous exercise
- Are on a very low-carbohydrate diet
- Have an eating disorder
- Are pregnant

Why Do I Need a Ketones in Urine Test?

Your healthcare provider may order a ketones in urine test if you have diabetes or other risk factors for developing ketones. You may also need this test if you have symptoms of ketoacidosis. These include:

- Nausea or vomiting
- Abdominal pain
- Confusion
- Trouble breathing
- Feeling extremely sleepy

People with type 1 diabetes are at a higher risk for ketoacidosis.

What Happens during a Ketones in Urine Test?

A ketones in urine test can be done in the home as well as in a lab. If in a lab, you will be given instructions to provide a "clean catch" sample. The clean catch method generally includes the following steps:

1. Wash your hands.

2. Clean your genital area with a cleansing pad. Men should wipe the tip of their penis. Women should open their labia and clean from front to back.

3. Start to urinate into the toilet.

4. Move the collection container under your urine stream.

5. Collect at least an ounce or two of urine into the container, which should have markings to indicate the amount.

6. Finish urinating into the toilet.

7. Return the sample container as instructed by your healthcare provider.

If you do the test at home, follow the instructions that are in your test kit. Your kit will include a package of strips for testing. You will either be instructed to provide a clean catch sample in a container as described above or to put the test strip directly in the stream of your urine. Talk to your healthcare provider about specific instructions.

Will I Need to Do Anything to Prepare for the Test?

You may have to fast (not eat or drink) for a certain period of time before taking a ketones in urine test. Ask your healthcare provider if you need to fast or do any other type of preparation before your test.

Are There Any Risks to the Test?

There is no known risk to having a ketones in urine test.

What Do the Results Mean?

Your test results may be a specific number or listed as a "small," "moderate," or "large" amount of ketones. Normal results can vary, depending on your on your diet, activity level, and other factors. Because high ketone levels can be dangerous, be sure to talk to your healthcare provider about what is normal for you and what your results mean.

Is There Anything Else I Need to Know about a Ketones in Urine Test?

Ketone test kits are available at most pharmacies without a prescription. If you are planning to test for ketones at home, ask your healthcare provider for recommendations on which kit would be best for you. At-home urine tests are easy to perform and can provide accurate results as long as you carefully follow all instructions.

Section 19.8

Nitrites in Urine

This section includes text excerpted from "Nitrites in Urine," MedlinePlus, National Institutes of Health (NIH), September 22, 2017.

How Do You Test for Nitrites in Urine?

A urinalysis, also called a urine test, can detect the presence of nitrites in the urine. Normal urine contains chemicals called nitrates. If bacteria enter the urinary tract, nitrates can turn into different, similarly named chemicals called nitrites. Nitrites in urine may be a sign of a urinary tract infection (UTI).

UTIs are one of the most common types of infections, especially in women. Fortunately, most UTIs are not serious and are usually treated with antibiotics. It's important to see your healthcare provider if you have symptoms of a UTI so you can start treatment right away.

Other names: urine test, urine analysis, microscopic urine analysis, microscopic examination of urine, UA

What Is It Used For?

A urinalysis, which includes a test for nitrites in urine, may be part of a regular exam. It may also be used to check for a UTI.

Why Do I Need a Nitrites in Urine Test?

Your healthcare provider may have ordered a urinalysis as part of a routine checkup or if you have symptoms of a UTI. Symptoms of a UTI may include:

- Frequent urge to urinate, but little urine comes out

- Painful urination

- Dark, cloudy, or reddish colored urine

- Bad smelling urine

- Weakness and fatigue, particularly in older women and men

- Fever

211

What Happens during a Nitrites in Urine Test?

Your healthcare provider will need to collect a sample of your urine. During your office visit, you will receive a container to collect the urine and special instructions to make sure that the sample is sterile. These instructions are often called the "clean catch method." The clean catch method includes the following steps:

1. Wash your hands.

2. Clean your genital area with a cleansing pad given to you by your provider. Men should wipe the tip of their penis. Women should open their labia and clean from front to back.

3. Start to urinate into the toilet.

4. Move the collection container under your urine stream.

5. Collect at least an ounce or two of urine into the container, which should have markings to indicate the amounts.

6. Finish urinating into the toilet.

7. Return the sample container as instructed by your healthcare provider

Will I Need to Do Anything to Prepare for the Test?

You don't need any special preparations to test for nitrites in urine. If your healthcare provider has ordered other urine or blood tests, you may need to fast (not eat or drink) for several hours before the test. Your healthcare provider will let you know if there are any special instructions to follow.

Are There Any Risks to the Test?

There is no known risk to having a urinalysis or a nitrites in urine test.

What Do the Results Mean?

If there are nitrites in your urine, it may mean that you have a UTI. However, even if no nitrites are found, you still may have an infection, because bacteria don't always change nitrates into nitrites. If you have symptoms of a UTI, your healthcare provider will also look at other results of your urinalysis, especially the white blood cell (WBC) count.

A high WBC count in urine is another possible sign of an infection. To learn what your results mean, talk to your healthcare provider.

Is There Anything Else I Need to Know about a Nitrites in Urine Test?

If a urinalysis is part of your regular checkup, your urine will be tested for a variety of substances along with nitrites. These include red and WBCs, proteins, acid and sugar levels, cell fragments, and crystals in your urine.

Section 19.9

Protein in Urine

This section includes text excerpted from "Protein in Urine," MedlinePlus, National Institutes of Health (NIH), September 22, 2017.

What Is a Protein in Urine Test?

A protein in urine test measures how much protein is in your urine. Proteins are substances that are essential for your body to function properly. Protein is normally found in the blood. If there is a problem with your kidneys, protein can leak into your urine. While a small amount is normal, a large amount of protein in urine may indicate kidney disease.

Other names: urine protein, 24-hour urine protein; urine total protein; ratio; reagent strip urinalysis

What Is It Used For?

A protein in urine test is often part of a urinalysis, a test that measures different cells, chemicals, and substances in your urine. Urinalysis is often included as part of a routine exam. This test may also be used to look for or to monitor kidney disease.

213

Why Do I Need a Protein in Urine Test?

Your healthcare provider may have ordered a protein test as part of your regular checkup, or if you have symptoms of kidney disease. These symptoms include:

- Difficulty urinating

- Frequent urination, especially at night

- Nausea and vomiting

- Loss of appetite

- Swelling in the hands and feet

- Fatigue

- Itching

What Happens during a Protein in Urine Test?

A protein in urine test can be done in the home as well as in a lab. If in a lab, you will receive instructions to provide a "clean catch" sample. The clean catch method includes the following steps:

1. Wash your hands.

2. Clean your genital area with a cleansing pad given to you by your provider. Men should wipe the tip of their penis. Women should open their labia and clean from front to back.

3. Start to urinate into the toilet.

4. Move the collection container under your urine stream.

5. Collect at least an ounce or two of urine into the container, which should have markings to indicate the amounts.

6. Finish urinating into the toilet.

7. Return the sample container as instructed by your healthcare provider.

If at home, you will use a test kit. The kit will include a package of strips for testing and instructions on how to provide a clean catch sample. Talk to your healthcare provider if you have any questions.

Your healthcare provider may also request you collect all your urine during a 24-hour period. This "24-hour urine sample test" is used because the amounts of substances in urine, including protein, can vary throughout the day. Collecting several samples in a day may provide a more accurate picture of your urine content.

Will I Need to Do Anything to Prepare for the Test?

You don't need any special preparations to test for protein in urine. If your healthcare provider has ordered a 24-hour urine sample, you will get specific instructions on how to provide and store your samples.

Are There Any Risks to the Test?

There is no known risk to having a urinalysis or a urine in protein test.

What Do the Results Mean?

If a large amount of protein is found in your urine sample, it doesn't necessarily mean that you have a medical problem needing treatment. Strenuous exercise, diet, stress, pregnancy, and other factors can cause a temporary rise in urine protein levels. Your healthcare provider may recommend additional urinalysis tests if a high level of protein is found This testing may include a 24-hour urine sample test.

If your urine protein levels are consistently high, it may indicate kidney damage or other medical condition. These include:

- Urinary tract infection (UTI)

- Lupus

- High blood pressure

- Preeclampsia, a serious complication of pregnancy, marked by high blood pressure. If it is not treated, preeclampsia can be life-threatening to the mother and baby.

- Diabetes

- Certain types of cancer

To learn what your results mean, talk to your healthcare provider.

Is There Anything Else I Need to Know about a Protein in Urine Test?

If you will be doing your urine test at home, ask your healthcare provider for recommendations on which test kit would be best for you.

At-home urine tests are easy to do and provide accurate results as long as you carefully follow all instructions.

Section 19.10

Urobilinogen in Urine

This section includes text excerpted from "Urobilinogen in Urine," MedlinePlus, National Institutes of Health (NIH), September 22, 2017.

What Is a Urobilinogen in Urine Test?

A urobilinogen in urine test measures the amount of urobilinogen in a urine sample. Urobilinogen is formed from the reduction of bilirubin. Bilirubin is a yellowish substance found in your liver that helps break down red blood cells (RBCs). Normal urine contains some urobilinogen. If there is little or no urobilinogen in urine, it can mean your liver isn't working correctly. Too much urobilinogen in urine can indicate a liver disease such as hepatitis or cirrhosis.

Other names: urine test; urine analysis; UA, chemical urinalysis

What Is It Used For?

A urobilinogen test may part of a urinalysis, a test that measures different cells, chemicals, and other substances in your urine. A urinalysis is often part of a routine exam.

Why Do I Need a Urobilinogen in Urine Test?

Your healthcare provider may have ordered this test as part of your regular checkup, to monitor an existing liver condition, or if you have symptoms of a liver disease. These include:

- Jaundice, a condition that causes your skin and eyes to turn yellow

- Nausea and/or vomiting

- Dark colored urine

- Pain and swelling in the abdomen

- Itchy skin

What Happens during a Urobilinogen in Urine Test?

Your healthcare provider will need to collect a sample of your urine. He or she will provide you with special instructions to ensure the sample is sterile. These instructions are often called as the "clean catch method." The clean catch method includes the following steps:

1. Wash your hands.

2. Clean your genital area with a cleansing pad given to you by your provider. Men should wipe the tip of their penis. Women should open their labia and clean from front to back.

3. Start to urinate into the toilet.

4. Move the collection container under your urine stream.

5. Collect at least an ounce or two of urine into the container, which should have markings to indicate the amounts.

6. Finish urinating into the toilet.

7. Return the sample container as instructed by your healthcare provider.

Will I Need to Do Anything to Prepare for the Test?

You don't need any special preparations. If your healthcare provider has ordered other urine or blood tests, you may need to fast (not eat or drink) for several hours before the test. Your healthcare provider will let you know if there are any special instructions to follow.

Are There Any Risks to the Test?

There is no known risk to having this test.

What Do the Results Mean?

If your test results show too little or no urobilinogen in your urine, it may indicate:

- A blockage in the structures that carry bile from your liver

- A blockage in the blood flow of the liver

- A problem with liver function

If your test results show a higher-than-normal level of urobilinogen, it may indicate:

- Hepatitis

- Cirrhosis

- Liver damage due to drugs

- Hemolytic anemia, a condition in which RBCs are destroyed before they can be replaced. This leaves the body without enough healthy RBCs

If your results are abnormal, it does not necessarily indicate you have a medical condition requiring treatment. Be sure to tell your healthcare provider about any medicines and supplements you are taking, as these can affect your results. If you are a woman, you should tell your healthcare provider if you are menstruating.

Is There Anything Else I Need to Know about a Urobilinogen in Urine Test?

This test is only one measure of liver function. If your healthcare provider thinks you might have a liver disease, additional urine and blood tests may be ordered.

Chapter 20

Yeast Infection Test

What Is a Yeast Test?

Yeast is a type of fungus that can live on the skin, mouth, digestive tract, and genitals. Some yeast in the body is normal, but if there is an overgrowth of yeast on your skin or other areas, it can cause an infection. A yeast test can help determine whether you have a yeast infection. Candidiasis is another name for a yeast infection.

Other names: potassium hydroxide (KOH) preparation, fungal culture; fungal antigen and antibody tests, calcofluor white stain, fungal smear.

What Is It Used For?

A yeast test is used to diagnose and detect yeast infections. There are different methods of yeast testing, depending on where you have symptoms.

Why Do I Need a Yeast Test?

Your healthcare provider may order a test if you have symptoms of a yeast infection. Your symptoms will vary, depending on where the infection is on your body. Yeast infections tend to happen in moist

---

This chapter includes text excerpted from "Yeast Infection Test," MedlinePlus, National Institutes of Health (NIH), September 22, 2017.

areas of the skin and mucous membranes. Below are symptoms of some common types of yeast infections. Your individual symptoms may vary.

Yeast infections on the folds of the skin include conditions such as athlete's foot and diaper rash. Symptoms include:

- Bright red rash, often redness or ulcers in the skin

- Itching

- Burning sensation

- Pimples

Yeast infections on the vagina are common. Nearly 75 percent of women will get at least one yeast infection in their lifetime. Symptoms include:

- Genital itching and/or burning

- A white, cottage cheese-like discharge

- Painful urination

- Redness in the vagina

Yeast infection of the penis may cause:

- Redness

- Scaling

- Rash

Yeast infection of the mouth is called thrush. It is common in young children. Thrush in adults may indicate a weakened immune system. Symptoms include:

- White patches on the tongue and inside of cheeks

- Soreness on the tongue and inside of cheeks

Yeast infection at the corners of the mouth may be caused by thumb sucking, ill-fitting dentures, or frequent licking of the lips. Symptoms include:

- Cracks and tiny cuts at the corners of the mouth

Yeast infection in the nail beds can happen in the fingers or toes, but are more common in toenails. Symptoms include:

- Pain and redness around the nail

- Discoloration of nail
- Cracks in the nail
- Swelling
- Pus
- White or yellow nail that separates from nail bed

What Happens during a Yeast Test?

The type of test depends on the location of your symptoms:

- **If a vaginal yeast infection is suspected,** your healthcare provider will perform a pelvic exam and take a sample of the discharge from your vagina.

- **If thrush is suspected,** your healthcare provider will look at the infected area in the mouth and may also take a small scraping to examine under the microscope.

- **If a yeast infection is suspected on the skin or nails,** your healthcare provider may use a blunt-edged instrument to scrape off a small bit of skin or part of a nail for examination. During this type of test, you may feel some pressure and a little discomfort.

Your healthcare provider may be able to tell if you have a yeast infection just by examining the infected area and looking at the cells under a microscope. If there are not enough cells to detect an infection, you may need a culture test. During a culture test, the cells in your sample will be put in a special environment in a lab to encourage cell growth. Results are often available within a few days. But some yeast infections grow slowly, and it may take weeks to get a result.

Will I Need to Do Anything to Prepare for the Test?

You don't need any special preparations for a yeast test.

Are There Any Risks to the Test?

There is no known risk to having a yeast test.

What Do the Results Mean?

If your results indicate a yeast infection, your healthcare provider may recommend an over-the-counter (OTC) antifungal medicine or prescribe an antifungal medicine. Depending on where your infection is, you may need a vaginal suppository, a medicine applied directly to the skin, or a pill. Your healthcare provider will tell you which treatment is best for you.

Is There Anything Else I Need to Know about a Yeast Test?

Certain antibiotics can also cause an overgrowth of yeast. Be sure to tell your healthcare provider about any medicines you are taking.

Yeast infections of the blood, heart, and brain are less common but more serious than yeast infections of the skin and genitals. Serious yeast infections occur more often in hospital patients and in people with weakened immune systems.

Part Three

Imaging Tests

Chapter 21

Medical Imaging Tests

Medical imaging tests are noninvasive procedures that allow doctors to diagnose diseases and injuries without being intrusive. Some of these tests involve exposure to ionizing radiation, which can present risks to patients. However, if patients understand the benefits and risks, they can make the best decisions about choosing a particular medical imaging procedure.

Medical Imaging Procedures

Most people have had one or more medical imaging tests. Imaging procedures are medical tests that allow doctors to see inside the body in order to diagnose, treat, and monitor health conditions. Doctors often use medical imaging procedures to determine the best treatment options for patients. The type of imaging procedure that your doctor may suggest will depend on your health concern and the part of the body that is being examined. Some common examples of imaging tests include:

- X-rays (including dental X-rays, chest X-rays, spine X-rays)

- Computed tomography (CT) or computed axial tomography (CAT) scans

- Fluoroscopy

This chapter includes text excerpted from "Radiation in Medicine: Medical Imaging Procedures," Centers for Disease Control and Prevention (CDC), May 30, 2017.

If your doctor suggests X-rays or other medical imaging tests, you should consider the following:

- medical imaging tests should be performed only when necessary
- the U.S. Food and Drug Administration (FDA) recommends discussing the benefits and risks of medical imaging procedures with your doctor

Benefits and Risks of Medical Imaging Procedures That Use Ionizing Radiation

Medical imaging tests can help doctors:

- obtain a better view of organs, blood vessels, tissues, and bones
- determine whether surgery is a good treatment option
- guide medical procedures involving placement of catheters, stents, or other devices inside the body; locate tumors for treatment and locate blood clots or other blockages
- guide joint replacement options and treatment of fractures

As in many areas of medicine, there are risks associated with the use of medical imaging which uses ionizing radiation to create images of the body. Risks from exposure to ionizing radiation include:

- a small increase in the likelihood that a person exposed to radiation will develop cancer later in life
- health effects that could occur after a large acute exposure to ionizing radiation such as skin reddening and hair loss
- possible allergic reactions associated with a contrast dye injected into the veins to better see body structures being examined

Reducing Your Exposure to Diagnostic Ionizing Radiation

In the case of X-rays or other tests involving exposure to ionizing radiation, doctors and radiation experts can help reduce your exposure to and risk of harm from diagnostic ionizing radiation by:

- checking to see if you have had a similar test done that can provide them with the background information they need

- checking to see if a test that does not use ionizing radiation can provide similar information

- making certain the least possible amount of radiation needed to obtain a good quality image is used for your procedure

- providing protective lead shielding to prevent exposing other areas of the body to radiation

Risks of Medical Imaging Procedures for Pregnant Women

Talk to your physician about the potential risks and benefits from the medical procedures. In many cases, the risk of an X-ray procedure to the mother and the unborn child is very small compared to the benefit of finding out about the medical condition of the mother or the child.

However, small risks should not be taken if they're unnecessary. You can reduce risks from medical imaging procedures by telling your doctor if you are, or think you might be, pregnant whenever an abdominal X-ray is suggested by your doctor. Other options suggested by the FDA that may be considered are as follows:

- If you are pregnant, the doctor may decide that it would be best to cancel the medical imaging procedure, to postpone it, or to modify it to reduce the amount of radiation.

- Depending on your medical needs, and realizing that the risk is very small, the doctor may feel that it is best to proceed with using a medical imaging procedure as planned.

In any case, you should feel free to discuss the decision with your doctor.

Special Considerations for Children

It is important that X-rays and other imaging procedures performed on children use the lowest exposure setting needed to obtain a good clinical image. The Image Gently Alliance (IGA), part of the Alliance for Radiation in Pediatric Imaging, suggests the following for imaging of children:

- Use imaging examinations when the medical benefit outweighs the risk.

- Use the most appropriate imaging techniques, matched to the size of the child.

- Use alternative imaging methods (such as ultrasound or magnetic resonance imaging (MRI)) when possible.

Chapter 22

Benefits and Risks of Medical Imaging

Benefits of Medical Imaging

The discovery of X-rays and the invention of computed tomography (CT) represented major advances in medicine. X-ray imaging exams are recognized as a valuable medical tool for a wide variety of examinations and procedures. They are used to:

- noninvasively and painlessly help to diagnose disease and monitor therapy;

- support medical and surgical treatment planning; and

- guide medical personnel as they insert catheters, stents, or other devices inside the body, treat tumors, or remove blood clots or other blockages.

Risks of Medical Imaging

As in many aspects of medicine, there are risks associated with the use of X-ray imaging, which uses ionizing radiation to generate images of the body. Ionizing radiation is a form of radiation that has enough

This chapter includes text excerpted from "Medical X-Ray Imaging," U.S. Food and Drug Administration (FDA), May 2, 2018.

energy to potentially cause damage to deoxyribonucleic acid (DNA). Risks from exposure to ionizing radiation include:

- a small increase in the possibility that a person exposed to X-rays will develop cancer later in life

- tissue effects such as cataracts, skin reddening, and hair loss, which occur at relatively high levels of radiation exposure and are rare for many types of imaging exams. For example, the typical use of a CT scanner or conventional radiography equipment should not result in tissue effects, but the dose to the skin from some long, complex interventional fluoroscopy procedures might, in some circumstances, be high enough to result in such effects.

Another risk of X-ray imaging is possible reactions associated with an intravenously injected contrast agent (or "dye") that is sometimes used to improve visualization.

The risk of developing cancer from medical imaging radiation exposure is generally very small, and it depends on:

- **Radiation dose.** The lifetime risk of cancer increases the larger the dose and the more X-ray exams a patient undergoes.

- **Patient's age.** The lifetime risk of cancer is larger for a patient who receives X-rays at a younger age than for one who receives them at an older age.

- **Patient's sex.** Women are at a somewhat higher lifetime risk than men for developing radiation-associated cancer after receiving the same exposures at the same ages.

- **Body region.** Some organs are more radiosensitive than others.

The above statements are generalizations based on scientific analyses of large population data sets, such as survivors exposed to radiation from the atomic bomb. One of the reports of such analyses is *Health Risks from Exposure to Low Levels of Ionizing Radiation: BEIR VII Phase 2* (Committee to Assess Health Risks from Exposure to Low Levels of Ionizing Radiation, National Research Council (NRC)). While specific individuals or cases may not fit into such generalizations, they are still useful in developing an overall approach to medical imaging radiation safety by identifying at-risk populations or higher-risk procedures.

Because radiation risks are dependent on exposure to radiation, an awareness of the typical radiation exposures involved in different imaging exams is useful for communication between the physician and patient.

The medical community has emphasized radiation dose reduction in CT because of the relatively high radiation dose for CT exams (as compared to radiography) and their increased use, as reported in the National Council on Radiation Protection and Measurements (NCRP) Report No. 160. Because tissue effects are extremely rare for typical use of many X-ray imaging devices (including CT), the primary radiation risk concern for most imaging studies is cancer; however, the long exposure times needed for complex interventional fluoroscopy exams and resulting high skin doses may result in tissue effects, even when the equipment is used appropriately.

Balancing Benefits and Risks

While the benefit of a clinically appropriate X-ray imaging exam generally far outweighs the risk, efforts should be made to minimize this risk by reducing unnecessary exposure to ionizing radiation. To help reduce risk to the patient, all exams using ionizing radiation should be performed only when necessary to answer a medical question, treat a disease, or guide a procedure. If there is a medical need for a particular imaging procedure and other exams using no or less radiation are less appropriate, then the benefits exceed the risks, and radiation risk considerations should not influence the physician's decision to perform the study or the patient's decision to have the procedure. However, the "As Low as Reasonably Achievable" (ALARA) principle should always be followed when choosing equipment settings to minimize radiation exposure to the patient.

Patient factors are important to consider in this balance of benefits and risks. For example:

- Because younger patients are more sensitive to radiation, special care should be taken in reducing radiation exposure to pediatric patients for all types of X-ray imaging exams.

- Special care should also be taken in imaging pregnant patients due to possible effects of radiation exposure to the developing fetus.

- The benefit of possible disease detection should be carefully balanced against the risks of an imaging screening study on healthy, asymptomatic patients.

Chapter 23

Medical X-Rays

Chapter Contents

Section 23.1

Medical X-Rays—Basics

This section includes text excerpted from "Reducing
Radiation from Medical X-Rays—Consumer Updates,"
U.S. Food and Drug Administration (FDA), November 15, 2017.

One of medicine's most remarkable achievements is the use of X-rays to see inside the body without having a surgeon wield a scalpel. Before medical X-ray machines were available, people who were in an accident and had serious injuries would often need exploratory surgery to find out what was wrong," says CAPT Thomas Ohlhaber, U.S. Public Health Service (PHS), a physicist and deputy director of the U.S. Food and Drug Administration's (FDA) Division of Mammography Quality and Radiation Programs (DMQRP).

"But today, if you're brought to the emergency room with severe injuries, within a few minutes you can be X-rayed, often with a sophisticated computed tomography, or 'CT,' unit, have your injuries assessed, and be treated quickly before you progress to a much more serious state," says Ohlhaber.

X-rays are used for much more than identifying injuries from accidents. They are used to screen for, diagnose, and treat various medical conditions. X-rays can be used on just about any part of the body—from the head down to the toes—to identify health problems ranging from a broken bone to pneumonia, heart disease, intestinal blockages, and kidney stones. And X-rays cannot only find cancerous tumors, but can often destroy them.

Along with their tremendous value, medical X-rays have a drawback: they expose people to radiation. The FDA regulates radiation-emitting products including X-ray machines. But everyone has a critical role in reducing radiation while still getting the maximum benefit from X-ray exams.

What Are X-Rays?

X-rays are a form of electromagnetic radiation that can penetrate clothing, body tissue, and internal organs. An X-ray machine sends this radiation through the body. Some of the radiation emerges on the other side of the body, where it exposes film or is absorbed by a digital detector to create an image. And some of it is absorbed in body tissues. It is the radiation absorbed by the body that contributes to the "radiation dose" a patient gets.

Because of their effectiveness in the early detection and treatment of diseases, and their ready access in doctor's offices, clinics, and hospitals, X-rays are used more today and on more people than in the past, according to the National Council on Radiation Protection and Measurements (NCRP).

- In the early 1980s, medical X-rays made up about 11 percent of all the radiation exposure to the U.S. population. Now the estimates attribute nearly 35 percent of all radiation exposure to medical X-rays. (Nuclear medicine procedures, which use radioactive material to create images of the body, account for about 12 percent of radiation exposure, and natural sources of radiation in the environment that we're exposed to all the time make up approximately 50 percent.)

- Radiation dose per person from medical X-rays has increased almost 500 percent since 1982.

- Nearly half of all medical X-ray exposures as of now come from CT equipment, and radiation doses from CT are higher than other X-ray studies.

Risks of X-Rays

The risks of medical X-rays include:

- A small increase in the chance of developing cancer later in life
- Developing cataracts and skin burns following exposure to very high levels of radiation

The small risk of cancer depends on several factors:

- The lifetime risk of cancer increases as a person undergoes more X-ray exams and the accumulated radiation dose gets higher.

- The lifetime risk is higher for a person who received X-rays at a younger age than for someone who receives them at an older age.

- Women are at a somewhat higher lifetime risk than men for developing cancer from radiation after receiving the same exposures at the same ages.

The risk of cataracts and skin burns are mainly associated with repeated or prolonged interventional fluoroscopy procedures. These types of procedures show a continuous X-ray image on a monitor (an X-ray "movie") to determine, for example, where to remove plaque from coronary arteries.

"The benefits of medical X-rays far outweigh their risks," says CDR Sean Boyd, PHS, an engineer and chief of the FDA's Diagnostic Devices Branch (DDB). "And everyone involved with medical X-rays can do their part to reduce radiation exposure—whether they're a consumer or patient, doctor, physicist, radiologist, technologist, manufacturer, or installer."

Steps for Consumers

Consumers have an important role in reducing radiation risks from medical X-rays. The FDA recommends these steps:

- **Ask your healthcare professional how an X-ray will help.** How will it help find out what's wrong or determine your treatment? Ask if there are other procedures that might be lower risk but still allow a good assessment or treatment for your medical situation.

- **Don't refuse an X-ray.** If your healthcare professional explains why it is medically needed, then don't refuse an X-ray. The risk of not having a needed X-ray is greater than the small risk from radiation.

- **Don't insist on an X-ray.** If your healthcare professional explains there is no need for an X-ray, then don't demand one.

- **If you are, or might be pregnant.** Tell the X-ray technologist in advance if you are, or might be, pregnant.

- **Ask if a protective shield can be used.** If you or your children are getting an X-ray, ask whether a lead apron or other shield should be used.

- **Ask your dentist if he/she uses the faster (E or F) speed film for X-rays.** It costs about the same as the conventional D speed film and offers similar benefits with a lower radiation dose. Using digital imaging detectors instead of film further reduces radiation dose.

- **Know your X-ray history.** "Just as you may keep a list of your medications with you when visiting the doctor, keep a list of your imaging records, including dental X-rays," says Ohlhaber. When an X-ray is taken, fill out the card with the date and type of exam, referring physician, and facility and address where the images are kept. Show the card to your healthcare professionals to avoid unnecessary duplication of X-rays of the same body part. Keep a record card for everyone in your family.

Section 23.2

Chest X-Ray

This section includes text excerpted from "Chest X-Ray," National Heart, Lung, and Blood Institute (NHLBI), December 10, 2016.

A chest X-ray is a fast and painless imaging test that uses certain electromagnetic waves to create pictures of the structures in and around your chest.

What a Chest X-Ray Shows

Chest X-rays show the structures in and around the chest. The test is used to look for and track conditions of the heart, lungs, bones, and chest cavity. For example, chest X-ray pictures may show signs of pneumonia, heart failure, lung cancer, lung tissue scarring, or sarcoidosis.

Chest X-rays do have limits. They only show conditions that change the size of tissues in the chest or how the tissues absorb radiation. Also, chest X-rays create two-dimensional pictures. This means that denser structures, like bone or the heart, may hide some signs of disease. Very small areas of cancer and blood clots in the lungs usually don't show up on chest X-rays.

For these reasons, your doctor may recommend other tests to confirm a diagnosis.

Who Needs a Chest X-Ray?

Doctors may recommend chest X-rays for people who have symptoms such as shortness of breath, chest pain, chronic cough (a cough that lasts a long time), or fever. The test can help find the cause of these symptoms.

Chest X-rays look for conditions such as pneumonia, heart failure, lung cancer, lung tissue scarring, or sarcoidosis. The test also is used to check how well treatments for certain conditions are working.

Chest X-rays also are used to evaluate people who test positive for tuberculosis (TB) exposure on skin tests. Sometimes, doctors recommend more chest X-rays within hours, days, or months of an earlier chest X-ray. This allows them to follow up on a condition.

People who are having certain types of surgery also may need chest X-rays. Doctors often use the test before surgery to look at the structures inside the chest.

What to Expect before a Chest X-Ray

You don't have to do anything special to prepare for a chest X-ray. However, you may want to wear a shirt that's easy to take off. Before the test, you'll be asked to undress from the waist up and wear a gown.

You also may want to avoid wearing jewelry and other metal objects. You'll be asked to take off any jewelry, eyeglasses, and metal objects that might interfere with the X-ray picture. Let the X-ray technician (a person specially trained to do X-ray tests) know if you have any body piercings on your chest.

Let your doctor know if you're pregnant or may be pregnant. In general, women should avoid all X-ray tests during pregnancy. Sometimes, though, having an X-ray is important to the health of the mother and fetus. If an X-ray is needed, the technician will take extra steps to protect the fetus from radiation.

What to Expect during a Chest X-Ray

Chest X-rays are done at doctors' offices, clinics, hospitals, and other healthcare facilities. The location depends on the situation. An X-ray technician oversees the test. This person is specially trained to do X-ray tests.

The entire test usually takes about 15 minutes.

During the Test

Depending on your doctor's request, you'll stand, sit, or lie for the chest X-ray. The technician will help position you correctly. He or she may cover you with a heavy lead apron to protect certain parts of your body from the radiation.

The X-ray equipment usually consists of two parts. One part, a box-like machine, holds the X-ray film or a special plate that records the picture digitally. You'll sit or stand next to this machine. The second part is the X-ray tube, which is located about 6 feet away.

Before the pictures are taken, the technician will walk behind a wall or into the next room to turn on the X-ray machine. This helps reduce his or her exposure to the radiation.

Usually, two views of the chest are taken. The first is a view from the back. The second is a view from the side. For a view from the back, you'll sit or stand so that your chest rests against the image plate. The X-ray tube will be behind you. For the side view, you'll turn to your side and raise your arms above your head.

If you need to lie down for the test, you'll lie on a table that contains the X-ray film or plate. The X-ray tube will be over the table. You'll need to hold very still while the pictures are taken. The technician may ask you to hold your breath for a few seconds. These steps help prevent a blurry picture.

Although the test is painless, you may feel some discomfort from the coolness of the exam room and the X-ray plate. If you have arthritis or injuries to the chest wall, shoulders, or arms, you may feel discomfort holding a position during the test. The technician may be able to help you find a more comfortable position.

When the test is done, you'll need to wait while the technician checks the quality of the X-ray pictures. He or she needs to make sure that the pictures are good enough for the doctor to use.

What to Expect after a Chest X-Ray

You usually can go back to your normal routine right after a chest X-ray. A radiologist will analyze, or "read," your X-ray images. This doctor is specially trained to supervise X-ray tests and look at the X-ray pictures. The radiologist will send a report to your doctor (who requested the X-ray test). Your doctor will discuss the results with you.

In an emergency, you'll get the X-ray results right away. Otherwise, it may take 24 hours or more. Talk with your doctor about when you should expect the results.

Risks of a Chest X-Ray

Chest X-rays have few risks. The amount of radiation used in a chest X-ray is very small. Talk to your doctor and the technicians performing the test about whether you are or could be pregnant. If the procedure is not urgent, they may have you wait to do the test until after your pregnancy. If it is urgent, the technicians will take extra steps to protect your baby during this test.

Section 23.3

Dental Imaging

"Dental Imaging" © 2017 Omnigraphics.
Reviewed July 2018.

What Is Dental Imaging?

Dental imaging refers to the practice of creating pictures of a person's mouth and teeth using X-rays. X-rays, also known as radiographs, are electromagnetic waves of energy that can pass through many materials including bones and teeth. Because different materials absorb X-rays to varying degrees, X-rays are used to show the internal composition of things that are not normally visible. X-rays provide dentists with a way to see inside a person's teeth and jawbone without surgery or other invasive procedures. X-rays are an important part of good dental care and are the most commonly used form of radiograph technology.

Dentists use X-rays to identify, diagnose, and monitor dental health issues for their patients. Dental X-rays allow dentists and other medical professionals to see details of teeth, bones, and mouth tissue. X-rays are used to examine the roots of teeth and their position within the jaw, locate cavities, diagnose dental diseases and other problems, and monitor the development of teeth.

Dental Imaging Procedures

Dental X-rays are classified in two groups: intraoral and extraoral. To create intraoral X-rays, technicians place X-ray film inside a person's mouth. Extraoral X-rays are created using film that is located outside the mouth.

Intraoral X-rays result in a highly detailed images and are the most common form of dental imaging. There are four main types of intraoral dental X-ray that are used to examine different aspects of the teeth and mouth. Intraoral X-ray procedures are painless and quick, usually taking only a few seconds to complete.

- **Bite-wing X-rays** are used to see examine the crowns of teeth in the back of the mouth, including the molars and bicuspids. To create bite-wing X-ray images, the technician asks the patient to bite down on a device that holds the X-ray film while the image is created.

- **Periapical X-rays** are used to examine one or two teeth in full, including the entire length of the tooth from crown to root. The procedure for periapical X-rays is similar to that of bite-wing X-rays.

- A **full-mouth radiographic survey**, or FMX, is a set of intraoral X-rays that includes images of every tooth from crown to root, including supporting tissue. An FMX survey is created using both bite-wing and periapical X-rays.

- **Occlusal X-rays** are used to produce images that are larger than other types of dental imaging, including the full arch of teeth in either the upper or lower jaw. Occlusal X-rays are most often used to monitor the dental health of children.

Extraoral X-rays provide fewer details than intraoral X-rays, and are generally used to create images that provide a broad view of a person's teeth, jaw, and skull. Dentists use extraoral X-rays to monitor the growth of teeth, the position of teeth in relation to the bones of the jaw and face, and the position of teeth relative to each other within the jaw bone. There are five main types of extraoral X-rays.

- **Panoramic X-rays** allow dentists and other medical professionals to create a single image of the entire mouth, including all the teeth and upper and lower jaws. Panoramic X-rays are created using a machine that directs X-rays forward from behind the head, while the film is gradually moved from one side of the face to the other. The panoramic X-ray machine holds a fixed position and the film moves on a fixed path. The procedure requires people to be positioned with attachments that hold the head and jaw in place for the duration of the X-ray. The procedure is safe, painless, and typically takes only a few minutes to complete.

- **Cephalometric projections** are extraoral X-rays that provide a view of the entire side of a person's head. These images are used to examine a person's profile and the location of their teeth in relation to the jaw. These X-rays are most often used by orthodontists in planning treatment strategies.

- **Cone-beam computed tomography (CT)** is a type of extraoral X-ray that is used to create three-dimensional images of a person's entire head. During this procedure, a person stands or sits without moving while the X-ray machine moves around their head. These images are most often used to determine treatment strategies for people who need dental implants.

- **Standard CT** is a type of dental imaging procedure that is usually conducted at a hospital or a radiologist's office. The procedure usually requires a person to lie down while the image is created. These images are similar to cone-beam computed tomography and are used for similar purposes.

Digital radiography is a type of dental imaging that replaces standard X-ray film with a tablet computer or other type of sensor. Digital X-ray images are created and stored as computer files. These images can then be viewed on screen or printed.

Radiation and Radiation Dose

X-ray images are created through the use of emitted radiation (electromagnetic energy waves). Radiation dose is the measurement of the amount of energy that is absorbed when a person is exposed to X-rays. Dental and medical X-rays emit extremely small doses of radiation. Excessive absorption of radiation can cause health problems, and people working with X-rays or those who are exposed to many X-rays over time should take precautions to protect themselves.

Modern X-ray machines are built to limit the amount of emitted radiation to the smallest possible effective dose. Dental X-ray machines generally emit radiation in a narrow beam that is less than three inches in diameter. Very little radiation is emitted outside of this beam. Modern X-ray film has also been engineered to produce images using the smallest possible amount of radiation. Film holders keep X-ray films in place without the need for people to directly handle the film. Digital radiography further reduces the emitted radiation dose by as much as 80 percent. X-ray procedures commonly include the use of lead shields or aprons that cover patients from the neck to the knees. A lead collar is also sometimes used for further protection of people with thyroid disease or other specific health concerns. Lead blocks emitted radiation and, therefore, protects the body from harm. To limit exposure to X-ray radiation over time, X-ray technicians typically leave the procedure room and operate X-ray machines remotely.

Dental Radiology and Pregnancy

Pregnant women and their fetuses are considered to be at a higher risk of physical damage from excessive radiation exposure over time. Although dental X-rays expose people to extremely small doses of radiation, it is common practice to protect pregnant women with lead aprons when creating dental X-rays.

References

1. "Radiation Protection of Patients: Dental Radiology—X Rays," International Atomic Energy Agency, 2013.

2. "Treatments and Procedures: Types of Dental X-Rays," Cleveland Clinic Foundation, 2015.

3. "Types of X-Rays," Aetna, 2013.

Section 23.4

Fluoroscopy

This section includes text excerpted from "Radiation in Medicine—Fluoroscopy," Centers for Disease Control and Prevention (CDC), November 8, 2016.

Fluoroscopy is a medical imaging test that uses an X-ray beam that passes continuously through the body to create an image. The image is projected on a monitor which allows doctors to see the movement of internal organs in real-time.

Medical imaging procedures such as fluoroscopy play a valuable role in preventing health problems and diagnosing diseases. During a hospital stay or outpatient procedures your doctor may request that you undergo fluoroscopy to determine treatment procedures for a particular health concern. Fluoroscopy procedures involve exposure to ionizing radiation, which can present risks. However, if patients understand the benefits and risks they can make the best decisions about their healthcare.

Before and during the Fluoroscopy Procedure

Before the Procedure

Ask your healthcare provider to explain the procedure and make sure you ask him/her if you still have additional questions. Some fluoroscopy procedures may use a "contrast dye" which allows doctors to see specific organ(s). The dye may be administered by swallowing, an intravenous (IV) line in your hand or arm, or an enema.

Make sure to let the doctor know if:

- you have ever had a reaction to any contrast dye

- you are pregnant or suspect that you may be pregnant

During the Procedure

- You will be asked to remove any clothing and jewelry that may interfere with the procedure.

- You will be positioned on the X-ray table, and depending on the type of procedure, you may be asked to do the following: assume different positions, move a specific body part, or hold your breath at intervals while the fluoroscopy is being performed.

- A special X-ray machine will produce fluoroscopic views of the body structure being examined or treated.

Benefits and Risks of Fluoroscopy

Medical imaging tests such as fluoroscopy are noninvasive procedures that allow doctors to diagnose diseases and injuries.

These tests can help doctors:

- Obtain a better view of organs, blood vessels, tissues and bones

- Determine whether surgery is a good treatment option

- Guide medical procedures involving placement of catheters, stents, or other devices inside the body, locate tumors for treatment and locate blood clots or other blockages

- Guide joint replacement options and treatment for fractures

As in many areas of medicine, there are risks associated with the use of fluoroscopy, which uses ionizing radiation to generate images of the body. Risks from exposure to ionizing radiation include:

- A small increase in the likelihood that a person exposed to radiation will develop cancer later in life.

- Health effects that could occur after a large exposure to ionizing radiation such as acute skin reddening, and hair loss.

- Possible allergic reactions associated with a contrast dye injected intravenously into the veins to better see body structures being examined.

While fluoroscopy itself is not painful, the particular procedure being performed may be painful, such as the injection into a joint or accessing of an artery or vein for angiography. In these cases, the radiologist will take all comfort measures possible, which could include local anesthesia, conscious sedation, or general anesthesia, depending on the particular procedure.

Section 23.5

Pediatric X-Ray Imaging

This section includes text excerpted from "Pediatric X-Ray Imaging," U.S. Food and Drug Administration (FDA), January 1, 2018.

X-Ray Imaging for Pediatrics

Medical X-ray imaging has led to improvements in the diagnosis and treatment of numerous medical conditions in pediatric patients. The Federal Food, Drug, and Cosmetic Act (FD&C Act) defines pediatric patients as persons aged 21 or younger at the time of their diagnosis or treatment. Typically these are broken down into different groups based on age ranges (neonates, infants, children, and adolescents). For medical X-ray imaging, the pediatric patient's size is even more important to consider than age, because patient size determines how much radiation is needed to produce a quality medical image.

The individual risk from X-ray imaging is small when compared to the benefits that it can provide through helping with accurate diagnosis. Still, efforts should be made to minimize risk by reducing unnecessary exposure to ionizing radiation. This is important because:

- Pediatric patients are more radiosensitive than adults (i.e., the cancer risk per unit dose of ionizing radiation is higher);

- Use of equipment and exposure settings designed for adults may result in excessive radiation exposure if used on smaller patients;

- Pediatric patients have a longer expected lifetime, putting them at higher risk of cancer from the effects of radiation exposure.

- The U.S. Food and Drug Administration (FDA) recommends that medical X-ray imaging exams, which include computed tomography (CT), fluoroscopy, and conventional X-rays, use the lowest radiation dose necessary, taking into account the size and age of the patient. Whether grouped by age or by size, an X-ray image should always be adjusted to meet the needs of the specific type of pediatric patient receiving the exam.

- X-ray exams should be performed for children only when the child's physician believes they are necessary to answer the clinical question or to guide treatment. Medical imaging professionals should use techniques that are adjusted to administer the lowest radiation dose that yields an image quality adequate for diagnosis or intervention (i.e., radiation doses should be "As Low as Reasonably Achievable"). The technique factors used should be chosen based on the clinical indication, patient size, and anatomical area scanned, and the equipment should be properly maintained and tested.

The FDA's Role in X-Ray Safety

The FDA collaborates with stakeholders across the imaging community to protect children's health by helping prevent unnecessary radiation exposure from X-ray exams, which includes:

- Encouraging manufacturers to address pediatric safety issues in current X-ray imaging devices and consider radiation safety of pediatric populations in the design of new X-ray imaging devices

- Publishing guidelines and other tools and resources to help enable imaging professionals to safely use imaging equipment on pediatric patients

- Fostering and strengthening relationships between manufacturers and healthcare professionals to improve device design and instructions for use

- Engaging in broad outreach efforts to incorporate radiation protection principles into facility quality assurance and personnel credentialing and training requirements

Examples of the FDA's medical radiation protection activities include:

- Publication of the *Pediatric Information for X-ray Imaging Device Premarket Notifications—Final Guidance* that encourages equipment design and instructions that help medical professionals more easily optimize equipment settings for patients of all sizes.

- The FDA's Center for Devices and Radiological Health (CDRH) and Critical Path Program funded two contracts awarded to the Image Gently Alliance. The contracts supported the development of educational tools for imaging practitioners to encourage reduction of radiation dose to pediatric patients.

- The FDA's Initiative to Reduce Unnecessary Ionizing Radiation Exposure from Medical Imaging has resulted in numerous dose reduction programs, national and international standards, and educational resources.

Section 23.6

Radiography

This section includes text excerpted from "Medical X-Ray
Imaging—Radiography," U.S. Food and Drug
Administration (FDA), May 2, 2018.

Medical radiography is a broad term that covers several types of studies that require the visualization of the internal parts of the body using X-ray techniques. Radiography is a technique for generating and recording an X-ray pattern for the purpose of providing the user with a static image(s) after termination of the exposure. It is different from fluoroscopy, mammography, and computed tomography (CT). Radiography may also be used during the planning of radiation therapy treatment. It is used to diagnose or treat patients by recording images of the internal structure of the body to assess the presence or absence of disease, foreign objects, and structural damage or anomaly.

During a radiographic procedure, an X-ray beam is passed through the body. A portion of the X-rays are absorbed or scattered by the internal structure and the remaining X-ray pattern is transmitted to a detector so that an image may be recorded for later evaluation. The recording of the pattern may occur on film or through electronic means.

Uses of Radiography

Radiography is used in many types of examinations and procedures where a record of a static image is desired. Some examples include:

- Dental examination

- Verification of correct placement of surgical markers prior to invasive procedure

- Mammography

- Orthopedic evaluations

- Spot film or static recording during fluoroscopy

- Chiropractic examinations

Risks and Benefits of Radiography

Radiography is a type of X-ray procedure, and it carries the same types of risks as other X-ray procedures. The radiation dose the patient receives varies depending on the individual procedure, but is generally less than that received during fluoroscopy and CT procedures.

The major risks associated with radiography are the small possibilities of:

- Developing a radiation-induced cancer or cataracts some time later in life, and

- Causing a disturbance in the growth or development of an embryo or fetus (teratogenic defect) when performed on a pregnant patient or one of childbearing age.

When an individual has a medical need, the benefit of radiography far exceeds the small cancer risk associated with the procedure. Even when radiography is medically necessary, it should use the lowest possible exposure and the minimum number of images. In most cases many of the possible risks can be reduced or eliminated with proper shielding.

Chapter 24

Contrast Radiography

Chapter Contents

Section 24.1

Coronary Angiography

This section includes text excerpted from "Coronary Angiography," National Heart, Lung, and Blood Institute (NHLBI), January 31, 2013. Reviewed July 2018.

Coronary angiography is a procedure that uses contrast dye, usually containing iodine, and X-ray pictures to detect blockages in the coronary arteries that are caused by plaque buildup.

Who Needs Coronary Angiography?

Your doctor may recommend coronary angiography if you have signs or symptoms of coronary heart disease (CHD). Signs and symptoms include:

- **Angina**. This is unexplained pain or pressure in your chest. You also may feel it in your shoulders, arms, neck, jaw, or back. The pain may even feel like indigestion. Angina may not only happen when you're active. Emotional stress also can trigger the pain associated with angina.

- **Sudden cardiac arrest (SCA).** This is a condition in which your heart suddenly and unexpectedly stops beating.

- **Abnormal results from tests** such as an EKG (electrocardiogram), exercise stress test, or other test

Coronary angiography also might be done on an emergency basis, such as during a heart attack. If angiography shows blockages in your coronary arteries, your doctor may do a procedure called percutaneous coronary intervention (PCI), also known as angioplasty. This procedure can open blocked heart arteries and prevent further heart damage.

Coronary angiography also can help your doctor plan treatment after you've had a heart attack, especially if you have major heart damage or if you're still having chest pain.

What to Expect before Coronary Angiography

Before having coronary angiography, talk with your doctor about:

- How the test is done and how to prepare for it

- Any medicines you're taking, and whether you should stop taking them before the test

- Whether you have diseases or conditions that may require taking extra steps during or after the test to avoid complications. Examples of such conditions include diabetes and kidney disease.

Your doctor will tell you exactly which procedures will be done. For example, your doctor may recommend PCI, also known as coronary angioplasty, if the angiography shows a blocked artery. You will have a chance to ask questions about the procedures. Also, you'll be asked to provide written informed consent to have the procedures.

It's not safe to drive after having cardiac catheterization, which is part of coronary angiography. You'll need to have someone drive you home after the procedure.

What to Expect during Coronary Angiography

During coronary angiography, you're kept on your back and awake. This allows you to follow your doctor's instructions during the test. You'll be given medicine to help you relax. The medicine might make you sleepy.

Your doctor will numb the area on the arm, groin (upper thigh), or neck where the catheter will enter your blood vessel. Then, he or she will use a needle to make a small hole in the blood vessel. The catheter will be inserted in the hole.

Next, your doctor will thread the catheter through the vessel and into the coronary arteries. Special X-ray movies are taken of the catheter as it's moved into the heart. The movies help your doctor see where to place the tip of the catheter.

Once the catheter is properly placed, your doctor will inject a special type of dye into the tube. The dye will flow through your coronary arteries, making them visible on an X-ray. This X-ray is called an angiogram.

If the angiogram reveals blocked arteries, your doctor may use PCI, commonly known as coronary angioplasty to restore blood flow to your heart.

After your doctor completes the procedure(s), he or she will remove the catheter from your body. The opening left in the blood vessel will then be closed up and bandaged. A small sandbag or other type of weight might be placed on the bandage to apply pressure. This will help prevent major bleeding from the site.

What to Expect after Coronary Angiography

After coronary angiography, your doctor will remove the catheter, possibly use a closure device to close the blood vessel, and close and bandage the opening on your arm, groin, or neck. You may develop a bruise and soreness where the catheter was inserted.

You will stay in the hospital for a few hours or overnight. During this time, your heart rate and blood pressure will be monitored. Your movement will be limited to prevent bleeding from the hole where the catheter was inserted. You will need a ride home after the procedure because of the medicines or anesthesia you received.

Risks of Coronary Angiography

Coronary angiography is a common procedure that rarely causes serious problems. Possible complications may include bleeding, allergic reactions to the contrast dye, infection, blood vessel damage, arrhythmias, blood clots that can trigger a heart attack or stroke, kidney damage, and fluid build up around the heart. The risk of complications is higher in people who are older or who have certain conditions such as chronic kidney disease or diabetes.

An imaging test called coronary computed tomography angiography, or coronary CTA, may be preferred over coronary angiography to detect blockages in the heart. Although coronary CTA still uses contrast dye, it does not require the invasive cardiac catheterization procedure that causes many of the complications of coronary angiography.

Section 24.2

Cystogram

What Is a Cystogram?

A cystogram is a study of the urinary tract, which is located in the pelvic region. Cystograms employ fluoroscopic imaging to show how the bladder fills up. This imaging allows the radiologist to monitor a patient's internal organs. A cystogram is used to diagnose a condition called urinary reflux, which causes urine to move back up the ureter from the bladder to the kidneys. Usually, a cystogram is performed when a patient has experienced pelvic injury or in case of a torn bladder. It is also used to detect polyps or tumors in the bladder.

Why Should I Have a Cystogram?

The cystogram helps your doctor diagnose a problem in the urinary tract. In the case of urinary tract infections or urinary incontinence, a follow-up examination detects any structural problems in the bladder. After the cystogram, further questions can be taken up with the doctor.

A cystogram helps determine the following conditions:

- Urinary reflux, when urine flows back into the ureter and, in some cases, to one or both kidneys

- Urinary tract infections that keep coming back

- Problems emptying your bladder, a bladder tear, or trauma to the bladder

- Problems with nerve supply

- Blood clots in the bladder

- Blockages in the ureters

- Urinary incontinence

- Foreign bodies

- Bladder fistulae

- Tumors

What are the Risk Factors?

It is important to consider the following risk factors before a cystogram:

- Radiation exposure might lead to birth defects during pregnancy.

- Check with your doctor if you are allergic or sensitive to medicines, contrast dyes, local anesthesia, iodine, or latex, or you have kidney failure or other kidney problems.

You are at risk in the case of bleeding or hematuria. It is important to consider the following conditions in case the test results are less accurate. These include:

- if you have gas or stool in your intestines
- if you have had a barium enema

You may not be able to have a cystogram if you:

- are allergic to contrast dyes
- are pregnant
- had recent bladder surgery
- have a blocked or damaged urethra
- have a urinary tract infection

In the case of a specific health condition, be sure to talk with your health provider about any concerns you have before the procedure.

What Happens before a Cystogram?

A cystogram examination does not require any specific preparation. Your physician will ask you to take your medicines promptly and to follow up on appointments. The physician will also make sure to keep you involved in decisions concerning your care and treatment. With your consent, the physician will proceed with the treatment. It is important to consider the following before proceeding with a cystogram:

- Ask your healthcare provider if you have any concerns about the procedure and read the instructions in the consent form before proceeding with the treatment.
- Your healthcare provider will give you specific instructions regarding your dietary plan before the procedure.
- Tell your provider if you are pregnant or think you may be pregnant.
- If you have had a reaction to any contrast dye, it is important to keep your healthcare provider informed.
- If you are allergic to any medicines, latex, tape, or anesthetic medicines, inform your health provider prior to any procedures or treatment.

- If you have a bleeding disorder or if you are taking blood-thinning medicines (anticoagulants), aspirin, or other medicines that affect blood clotting, your physician might ask you to stop these medicines before the test.

- The physician will give you an enema or medicine to make you have a bowel movement before the test.

What Happens during a Cystogram?

- The physician will ask you to remove your clothing and put on a gown.

- You will be asked to empty your bladder before the test.

- After placing a thin tube (catheter) into your bladder, the physician will inject the contrast dye.

- The physician will take an X-ray of your kidneys, ureters, and bladder (KUB) to make sure that he or she can monitor the urinary tract system.

- After injecting the contrast dye into your bladder through the catheter, the physician will clamp the catheter tubing to keep the dye from draining out of your bladder.

- Your healthcare provider will take X-rays while the dye is in your bladder.

What Happens after a Cystogram?

The radiologist will monitor the radiographs before handing over the report to your physician. After discussing the results and further courses of action with you, the physician will ask you to resume your normal diet (unless your healthcare provider informs you differently). It is important to drink additional fluids for the next few days. This will help to prevent any bladder infection. It is important to keep your healthcare provider informed if you observe any of the following conditions:

- Pain when you urinate that gets worse or lasts more than two days

- Less urine than usual

- Pain in your belly

- Fever or chills

- Blood in your urine

When Will I Get the Results?

The cystogram report is studied by the radiologist and sent to a physician. The referred physician will discuss the results with you. Follow-up on the treatment by visiting your physician.

References

1. "What You Need to Know about Cystogram," American Society of Radiologic Technologists (ASRT), 2009.

2. "Cystogram," Guy's and St. Thomas' NHS Foundation Trust, April 2017.

3. "Cystogram," University of Washington Medicine, 2018.

4. "Cystography," Johns Hopkins Medicine (JHM), May 5, 2016.

Section 24.3

Upper Gastrointestinal (GI) Series

This section includes text excerpted from "Upper GI Series,"
National Institute of Diabetes and Digestive and Kidney
Diseases (NIDDK), August 2016.

An upper gastrointestinal (GI) series is a procedure in which a doctor uses X-rays, fluoroscopy, and a chalky liquid called barium to view your upper GI tract. The barium will make your upper GI tract more visible on an X-ray.

The two types of upper GI series are:

• A standard barium upper GI series, which uses only barium

• A double-contrast upper GI series, which uses both air and barium for a clearer view of your stomach lining

Purpose of Upper Gastrointestinal (GI) Series

An upper GI series can help a doctor find the cause of:

• Nausea and vomiting

- Pain in the abdomen
- Problems swallowing
- Unexplained weight loss

An upper GI series can also show:

- Abnormal growths such as cancer
- Esophageal varices
- Gastroesophageal reflux
- A hiatal hernia
- Scars or strictures
- Ulcers

What to Expect before Performing an Upper GI Series

To prepare for an upper GI series, don't eat, drink, smoke, or chew gum. You also will need to talk with your doctor.

Don't Eat, Drink, Smoke, or Chew Gum

In order to see your upper GI tract clearly, your doctor will most likely ask you not to eat, drink, smoke, or chew gum during the 8 hours before the upper GI series.

Talk with Your Doctor

You should talk with your doctor about any medical conditions you have and all prescribed and over-the-counter (OTC) medicines, vitamins, and supplements you take.

Doctors don't recommend X-rays for pregnant women because X-rays may harm the fetus. Tell your doctor if you are, or may be, pregnant. Your doctor may suggest a different procedure.

A doctor may recommend an upper GI series for your child when the benefits of the procedure outweigh the relatively small risk of X-rays. Talk with your child's doctor about safety measures used to lower your child's exposure to X-rays during the procedure.

What to Expect during an Upper GI Series

An X-ray technician and a radiologist perform an upper GI series at a hospital or an outpatient center. You do not need anesthesia. The procedure usually takes about 2 hours. The procedure can take up to 5 hours if the barium moves slowly through your small intestine.

For the procedure, you'll be asked to stand or sit in front of an X-ray machine and drink barium, which coats the lining of your upper GI tract. You will then lie on the X-ray table, and the radiologist will watch the barium move through your GI tract on the X-ray and fluoroscopy. The technician may press on your abdomen or ask you to change position several times to evenly coat your upper GI tract with the barium.

If you are having a double-contrast study, you will swallow gas-forming crystals that mix with the barium coating your stomach. Gas forms when the crystals and barium mix. The gas expands your stomach, which lets the radiologist see more details of your upper GI tract lining. The technician will then take additional X-rays.

What to Expect after an Upper GI series

After an upper GI series, you can expect the following:

- You may have cramping in your abdomen and bloating during the first hour after the procedure.

- You may resume most normal activities after leaving the hospital or outpatient center.

- For several days, your stools may be white or light colored from the barium in your GI tract.

- A healthcare professional will give you instructions on how to care for yourself after the procedure. The instructions will explain how to flush the remaining barium from your GI tract. You should follow all instructions.

A specialist will read the X-rays and send a report of the findings to your doctor.

Risks of an Upper GI Series

The risks of an upper GI series include:

- Constipation from the barium—the most common complication of an upper GI series

- An allergic reaction to the barium or flavoring in the barium

- Intestinal obstruction

Seek Care Right Away

If you have any of the following symptoms after an upper GI series, seek medical attention right away:

- Fever

- No bowel movement within two days after the procedure

- Inability to pass gas

- Severe pain in your abdomen

Section 24.4

Lower Gastrointestinal (GI) Series (Barium Enema)

This section includes text excerpted from "Lower GI Series," National Institute of Diabetes and Digestive and Kidney Diseases (NIDDK), June 2016.

A lower gastrointestinal (GI) series is a procedure in which a doctor uses X-rays and a chalky liquid called barium to view your large intestine. The barium will make your large intestine more visible on an X-ray.

The two types of lower GI series are:

- A single-contrast lower GI series, which uses only barium

- A double-contrast or air-contrast lower GI series, which uses both barium and air for a clearer view of your large intestine

A lower GI series is also called a barium enema.

Purpose of Lower Gastrointestinal (GI) Series

A lower GI series can help a doctor find the cause of:

- Bleeding from your anus

- Changes in your bowel activity

- Chronic diarrhea

- Pain in your abdomen

- Unexplained weight loss

A lower GI series can also show:

- Cancerous growths

- Diverticula

- A fistula

- Polyps

- Ulcers

Prepare for a Lower GI Series

To prepare for a lower GI series, you will need to talk with your doctor, change your diet, and clean out your bowel.

Talk with Your Doctor

You should talk with your doctor about any medical conditions you have and all prescribed and over-the-counter (OTC) medicines, vitamins, and supplements you take. Also tell your doctor whether you've had a colonoscopy with a biopsy or polyp removal in the last 4 weeks.

Doctors don't recommend X-rays for pregnant women because X-rays may harm the fetus. Tell your doctor if you are, or may be, pregnant. Your doctor may suggest a different procedure.

Change Your Diet and Clean Out Your Bowel

A healthcare professional will give you written bowel prep instructions to follow at home before the procedure. A healthcare professional orders a bowel prep so that little to no stool is present in your intestine. A complete bowel prep lets you pass stool that is clear and liquid. Stool inside your colon can prevent the X-ray machine from taking clear images of your intestine.

You may need to follow a clear liquid diet for 1–3 days before the procedure. The instructions will provide specific direction about when to start and stop the clear liquid diet. In most cases, you may drink or eat the following:

- Fat-free bouillon or broth

- Gelatin in flavors such as lemon, lime, or orange

- Plain coffee or tea, without cream or milk

- Sports drinks in flavors such as lemon, lime, or orange

- Strained fruit juice, such as apple or white grape—doctors recommend avoiding orange juice

- Water

Your doctor will tell you how long before the procedure you should have nothing by mouth.

A healthcare professional will ask you to follow the directions for a bowel prep before the procedure. The bowel prep will cause diarrhea, so you should stay close to a bathroom.

Different bowel preps may contain different combinations of laxatives—pills that you swallow or powders that you dissolve in water and other clear liquids—and enemas. Some people will need to drink a large amount, often a gallon, of liquid laxative during a scheduled amount of time—most often the night before the procedure.

You may find this part of the bowel prep difficult; however, completing the prep is very important. Your doctor will not be able to see your large intestine clearly if the prep is incomplete.

Call a healthcare professional if you have side effects that prevent you from finishing the prep.

How Doctors Perform a Lower GI Series

An X-ray technician and a radiologist perform a lower GI series at a hospital or an outpatient center. You do not need anesthesia. The procedure usually takes 30–60 minutes.

For the procedure, you'll be asked to lie on a table while the radiologist inserts a flexible tube into your anus and fills your large intestine with barium. The radiologist prevents barium from leaking from your anus by inflating a balloon on the end of the tube. You may be asked to change position several times to evenly coat the large intestine with the barium. If you are having a double-contrast lower GI series, the radiologist will inject air through the tube to inflate the large intestine.

During the procedure, you may have some discomfort and feel the urge to have a bowel movement. You will need to hold still in various positions while the radiologist and technician take X-ray images and possibly an X-ray video, called fluoroscopy.

The radiologist or technician will deflate the balloon on the tube when the imaging is complete. Most of the barium will drain through the tube. You will push out the remaining barium into a bedpan or nearby toilet. A healthcare professional may give you an enema to flush out the rest of the barium.

After a Lower GI Series

After a lower GI series, you can expect the following:

- You may have cramping in your abdomen and bloating during the first hour after the procedure.

- You may resume most normal activities after leaving the hospital or outpatient center.

- For several days, your stools may be white or light colored from the barium in your large intestine.

- A healthcare professional will give you instructions on how to care for yourself after the procedure. The instructions will explain how to flush the remaining barium from your large intestine. You should follow all instructions.

The radiologist will read the X-rays and send a report of the findings to your doctor.

Risks of a Lower GI Series

The risks of a lower GI series include:

- Constipation from the barium enema—the most common complication of a lower GI series
- An allergic reaction to the barium
- Intestinal obstruction
- Leakage of barium into your abdomen through a tear or hole in the lining of the large intestine

Seek Care Right Away

If you have any of the following symptoms after a lower GI series, seek medical care right away:

- Bloody bowel movements or bleeding from your anus

- Fever

- Inability to pass gas

- Severe constipation

- Severe pain in your abdomen

Section 24.5

Lung Ventilation/Perfusion Scan

This section includes text excerpted from "Lung VQ Scan,"
National Heart, Lung, and Blood Institute (NHLBI),
December 10, 2016.

A lung pulmonary ventilation and perfusion (VQ) scan is an imaging test that uses a ventilation scan to measure airflow in your lungs and a perfusion scan to see where blood flows in your lungs. This scan is also known as lung or pulmonary ventilation and perfusion scans.

Lung Ventilation/Perfusion (VQ) Scan—Who Needs

You may need a lung VQ scan if you have signs or symptoms of a pulmonary embolism (PE). A PE is a sudden blockage in a lung artery. A blood clot usually causes the blockage.

Signs and symptoms of a PE include chest pain, trouble breathing, rapid breathing, coughing, and coughing up blood. An irregular heartbeat called an arrhythmia also may suggest a PE.

Some blood clots that can cause a PE travel to the lungs from veins deep in the legs. This can cause pain and swelling in the affected limb.

Doctors use VQ scans to help find out whether a PE is causing these signs and symptoms. A VQ scan alone, however, won't confirm whether you have a PE. Your doctor also will consider other factors when making a diagnosis.

Doctors also use VQ scans to detect poor blood flow in the lungs' blood vessels, air trapping or uneven air distribution, and to examine the lungs before some types of surgery.

What to Expect before a Lung VQ Scan

A lung VQ scan may be done during an emergency to help diagnose or rule out a pulmonary embolism (PE). A PE is a sudden blockage in a lung artery. This serious condition can cause low blood oxygen levels, damage to the lungs, or even death.

If your VQ scan isn't done during an emergency, your doctor will tell you how to prepare for the test. Most people don't need to take any special steps to prepare for a VQ scan.

Your doctor may ask you to wear clothing that has no metal hooks or snaps. These materials can block the scanner's view. Or, you may be asked to wear a hospital gown for the test.

Tell your doctor whether you're pregnant or may be pregnant. If possible, you should avoid radiation exposure during pregnancy, as it may harm the fetus.

You and your doctor will decide whether the benefits of a VQ scan outweigh the small risk to the fetus, or whether another test might be better.

If you're breastfeeding, ask your doctor how long you should wait after the test before you breastfeed. The radioisotopes used for VQ scans can pass through your breast milk to your baby.

You may want to prepare for the scan by pumping and saving milk for 24–48 hours in advance. You can bottle-feed your baby in the hours after the VQ scan.

What to Expect during a Lung VQ Scan

Lung VQ scans are done at radiology clinics or hospitals.

For the test, you lie on a table for about 1 hour and have two types of scans: ventilation and perfusion. The ventilation scan shows the pattern of airflow in your lungs. The perfusion scan shows the pattern of blood flow in your lungs.

You must lie very still during the tests or the pictures may blur. If you're having trouble staying still, your doctor may give you medicine to help you relax.

Both scans use radioisotopes (a low-risk radioactive substance). This substance releases energy inside your body. Special scanners outside of your body use the energy to create images of air and blood flow in your lungs.

The radioisotopes used in VQ scans can cause an allergic reaction, including itching and hives. Medicines can relieve these symptoms.

Ventilation

For this scan, you lie on a table that moves under the arm of the scanner. You wear a breathing mask over your nose and mouth and inhale a small amount of radioisotope gas mixed with oxygen.

As you breathe, the scanner takes pictures that show air going into your lungs. You'll need to hold your breath for a few seconds at the start of each picture.

The scan is painless, and each picture takes only a few minutes. However, wearing the mask can make some people feel anxious. If this happens, your doctor may give you medicine to help you relax.

Perfusion

For this scan, a small amount of radioisotope is injected into a vein in your arm. The scanner then takes pictures of blood flow through your lungs.

The scan itself doesn't hurt, but you may feel some discomfort from the radioisotope injection.

What to Expect after a Lung VQ Scan

Most people can return to their normal activities right after a lung VQ scan.

If you got medicine to help you relax during the scan, your doctor will tell you when you can return to your normal activities. The medicine may make you tired, so you'll need someone to drive you home.

You may have a bruise on your arm where the radioisotopes were injected. You'll need to drink plenty of fluids to flush the radioisotopes out of your body. Your doctor can advise you about how much fluid to drink.

If you're breastfeeding, ask your doctor how long you should wait after the test before you breastfeed. The radioisotopes used for VQ scans can pass through your breast milk to your baby.

You may want to prepare for the scan by pumping and saving milk for 24–48 in advance. You can bottle-feed your baby in the hours after the VQ scan.

Risk Factors

Lung VQ scans involve little risk for most people. The radioisotopes used for both tests expose you to a small amount of radiation. The amount of radiation in the gas and injection together are about the same as the amount a person is naturally exposed to in 1 year.

Although rare, the radioisotopes may cause an allergic reaction.

Radiation

The radiation from a VQ scan leaves your body after a few days. Exposure to radiation is associated with a risk of cancer. However, it's not known whether the amount of radiation from a VQ scan increases your risk for cancer.

You and your doctor will decide whether the benefits of a VQ scan outweigh the possible risks. Your doctor also will try to avoid ordering multiple VQ scans for you over a short period.

If you're pregnant or breastfeeding, talk with your doctor about the risk of radiation to your baby. He or she will consider whether another test can be used instead.

Allergic Reaction

Very rarely, the radioisotopes used in VQ scans can cause an allergic reaction. Hives or a rash may result. Medicines can relieve this reaction.

Chapter 25

Ultrasound (Sonography) Exams

Chapter Contents

Section 25.1

Ultrasound Overview

This section includes text excerpted from "Ultrasound,"
National Institute of Biomedical Imaging and
Bioengineering (NIBIB), July 2016.

What Is Medical Ultrasound?

Medical ultrasound falls into two distinct categories: diagnostic and therapeutic.

Diagnostic ultrasound is a noninvasive diagnostic technique used to image inside the body. Ultrasound probes, called transducers, produce sound waves that have frequencies above the threshold of human hearing (above 20KHz), but most transducers at present use operate at much higher frequencies (in the megahertz (MHz) range). Most diagnostic ultrasound probes are placed on the skin. However, to optimize image quality, probes may be placed inside the body via the gastrointestinal tract, vagina, or blood vessels. In addition, ultrasound is sometimes used during surgery by placing a sterile probe into the area being operated on.

Diagnostic ultrasound can be further subdivided into anatomical and functional ultrasound. Anatomical ultrasound produces images of internal organs or other structures. Functional ultrasound combines information such as the movement and velocity of tissue or blood, softness or hardness of tissue, and other physical characteristics, with anatomical images to create "information maps." These maps help doctors visualize changes/differences in function within a structure or organ.

Therapeutic ultrasound also uses sound waves above the range of human hearing but does not produce images. Its purpose is to interact with tissues in the body such that they are either modified or destroyed. Among the modifications possible are: moving or pushing tissue, heating tissue, dissolving blood clots, or delivering drugs to specific locations in the body. These destructive, or ablative, functions are made possible by use of very high-intensity beams that can destroy diseased or abnormal tissues such as tumors. The advantage of using ultrasound therapies is that, in most cases, they are noninvasive. No incisions or cuts need to be made to the skin, leaving no wounds or scars.

How Does It Work?

Ultrasound waves are produced by a transducer, which can both emit ultrasound waves, as well as detect the ultrasound echoes reflected back. In most cases, the active elements in ultrasound transducers are made of special ceramic crystal materials called piezoelectrics. These materials are able to produce sound waves when an electric field is applied to them, but can also work in reverse, producing an electric field when a sound wave hits them. When used in an ultrasound scanner, the transducer sends out a beam of sound waves into the body. The sound waves are reflected back to the transducer by boundaries between tissues in the path of the beam (e.g., the boundary between fluid and soft tissue or tissue and bone). When these echoes hit the transducer, they generate electrical signals that are sent to the ultrasound scanner. Using the speed of sound and the time of each echo's return, the scanner calculates the distance from the transducer to the tissue boundary. These distances are then used to generate two-dimensional images of tissues and organs.

During an ultrasound exam, the technician will apply a gel to the skin. This keeps air pockets from forming between the transducer and the skin, which can block ultrasound waves from passing into the body.

What Is Ultrasound Used For?

Diagnostic ultrasound. Diagnostic ultrasound is able to noninvasively image internal organs within the body. However, it is not good for imaging bones or any tissues that contain air, like the lungs. Under some conditions, ultrasound can image bones (such as in a fetus or in small babies) or the lungs and lining around the lungs, when they are filled or partially filled with fluid. One of the most common uses of ultrasound is during pregnancy, to monitor the growth and development of the fetus, but there are many other uses, including imaging the heart, blood vessels, eyes, thyroid, brain, breast, abdominal organs, skin, and muscles. Ultrasound images are displayed in either 2D, 3D, or 4D (which is 3D in motion).

Functional ultrasound. Functional ultrasound applications include Doppler and color Doppler ultrasound for measuring and visualizing blood flow in vessels within the body or in the heart. It can also measure the speed of the blood flow and direction of movement. This is done using color-coded maps called color Doppler imaging. Doppler ultrasound is commonly used to determine whether plaque build up inside the carotid arteries is blocking blood flow to the brain.

Another functional form of ultrasound is elastography, a method for measuring and displaying the relative stiffness of tissues, which can be used to differentiate tumors from healthy tissue. This information can be displayed as either color-coded maps of the relative stiffness; black-and white maps that display high-contrast images of tumors compared with anatomical images; or color-coded maps that are overlaid on the anatomical image. Elastography can be used to test for liver fibrosis, a condition in which excessive scar tissue builds up in the liver due to inflammation.

Ultrasound is also an important method for imaging interventions in the body. For example, ultrasound-guided needle biopsy helps physicians see the position of a needle while it is being guided to a selected target, such as a mass or a tumor in the breast. Also, ultrasound is used for real-time imaging of the location of the tip of a catheter as it is inserted in a blood vessel and guided along the length of the vessel. It can also be used for minimally invasive surgery to guide the surgeon with real-time images of the inside of the body.

Therapeutic or interventional ultrasound. Therapeutic ultrasound produces high levels of acoustic output that can be focused on specific targets for the purpose of heating, ablating, or breaking up tissue. One type of therapeutic ultrasound uses high-intensity beams of sound that are highly targeted, and is called high-intensity focused ultrasound (HIFU). HIFU is being investigated as a method for modifying or destroying diseased or abnormal tissues inside the body (e.g., tumors) without having to open or tear the skin or cause damage to the surrounding tissue. Either ultrasound or magnetic resonance imaging (MRI) is used to identify and target the tissue to be treated, guide and control the treatment in real time, and confirm the effectiveness of the treatment. HIFU is U.S. Food and Drug Administration (FDA) approved for the treatment of uterine fibroids, to alleviate pain from bone metastases, and for the ablation of prostate tissue. HIFU is also being investigated as a way to close wounds and stop bleeding, to break up clots in blood vessels, and to temporarily open the blood brain barrier so that medications can pass through.

Are There Risks?

Diagnostic ultrasound is generally regarded as safe and does not produce ionizing radiation like that produced by X-rays. Still, ultrasound is capable of producing some biological effects in the body under specific settings and conditions. For this reason, the FDA requires that diagnostic ultrasound devices operate within acceptable limits. The FDA, as well as many professional societies, discourage the casual use of ultrasound (e.g., for keepsake videos) and recommend that it be used only when there is a true medical need.

Section 25.2

Carotid Ultrasound

This section includes text excerpted from "Carotid Ultrasound,"
National Heart, Lung, and Blood Institute (NHLBI),
November 5, 2011. Reviewed July 2018.

Carotid ultrasound is a painless imaging test that uses high-frequency sound waves to create pictures of the inside of your carotid arteries. It is also known as carotid duplex.

Who Needs Carotid Ultrasound?

A carotid ultrasound shows whether you have plaque buildup in your carotid arteries. Over time, plaque can harden or rupture (break open). This can reduce or block the flow of oxygen-rich blood to your brain and cause a stroke.

Your doctor may recommend a carotid ultrasound if you:

- **Had a stroke or mini-stroke recently.** During a mini-stroke, you may have some or all of the symptoms of a stroke. However, the symptoms usually go away on their own within 24 hours.

- **Have an abnormal sound called a carotid bruit in one of your carotid arteries.** Your doctor can hear a carotid bruit using a stethoscope. A bruit might suggest a partial blockage in your carotid artery, which could lead to a stroke.

Your doctor also may recommend a carotid ultrasound if he or she thinks you have:

- Blood clots in one of your carotid arteries

- A split between the layers of your carotid artery wall. The split can weaken the wall or reduce blood flow to your brain.

A carotid ultrasound also might be done to see whether carotid artery surgery, also called carotid endarterectomy, has restored normal blood flow through a carotid artery.

If you had a procedure called carotid stenting, your doctor might use carotid ultrasound afterward to check the position of the stent in your carotid artery. (The stent, a small mesh tube, supports the inner artery wall.)

Carotid ultrasound sometimes is used as a preventive screening test in people at increased risk of stroke, such as those who have high blood pressure and diabetes.

What to Expect during Carotid Ultrasound

Carotid ultrasound usually is done in a doctor's office or hospital. The test is painless and often doesn't take more than 30 minutes. The ultrasound machine includes a computer, a screen, and a transducer. The transducer is a hand-held device that sends and receives ultrasound waves.

You will lie on your back on an exam table for the test. Your technician or doctor will put gel on your neck where your carotid arteries are located. The gel helps the ultrasound waves reach the arteries. Your technician or doctor will put the transducer against different spots on your neck and move it back and forth. The transducer gives off ultrasound waves and detects their echoes as they bounce off the artery walls and blood cells. Ultrasound waves can't be heard by the human ear. The computer uses the echoes to create and record pictures of the insides of the carotid arteries. These pictures usually appear in black and white. The screen displays these live images for your doctor to review.

Your carotid ultrasound test might include a Doppler ultrasound. Doppler ultrasound is a special test that shows the movement of blood through your arteries. Blood flow through the arteries usually appears in color on the ultrasound pictures.

What to Expect after Carotid Ultrasound

You usually can return to your normal activities as soon as the carotid ultrasound is over. Your doctor will likely be able to tell you the results of the carotid ultrasound when it occurs or soon afterward.

Risks of Carotid Ultrasound

Carotid ultrasound has no risks because the test uses harmless sound waves. They are the same type of sound waves that doctors use to record pictures of fetuses in pregnant women.

Section 25.3

Echocardiography (Heart)

This section includes text excerpted from
"Echocardiography," National Heart, Lung, and Blood
Institute (NHLBI), December 12, 2017.

What Is Echocardiography (Echo)?

Echocardiography, or echo, is a painless test that uses sound waves to create moving pictures of your heart. The pictures show the size and shape of your heart. They also show how well your heart's chambers and valves are working.

Echo also can pinpoint areas of heart muscle that aren't contracting well because of poor blood flow or injury from a previous heart attack. A type of echo called Doppler ultrasound shows how well blood flows through your heart's chambers and valves.

Echo can detect possible blood clots inside the heart, fluid buildup in the pericardium (the sac around the heart), and problems with the aorta. The aorta is the main artery that carries oxygen-rich blood from your heart to your body.

Doctors also use echo to detect heart problems in infants and children.

Who Needs Echo?

Your doctor may recommend echo if you have signs or symptoms of heart problems. For example, shortness of breath and swelling in the legs are possible signs of heart failure. Heart failure is a condition in which your heart can't pump enough oxygen-rich blood to meet your body's needs. Echo can show how well your heart is pumping blood.

Echo also can help your doctor find the cause of abnormal heart sounds, such as heart murmurs. Heart murmurs are extra or unusual sounds heard during the heartbeat. Some heart murmurs are harmless, while others are signs of heart problems.

Your doctor also may use echo to learn about:

- **The size of your heart.** An enlarged heart might be the result of high blood pressure, leaky heart valves, or heart failure. Echo also can detect increased thickness of the ventricles (the heart's lower chambers). Increased thickness may be due to high blood pressure, heart valve disease, or congenital heart defects.

- **Heart muscles that are weak and aren't pumping well.** Damage from a heart attack may cause weak areas of heart muscle. Weakening also might mean that the area isn't getting enough blood supply, a sign of coronary heart disease.

- **Heart valve problems.** Echo can show whether any of your heart valves don't open normally or close tightly.

- **Problems with your heart's structure.** Echo can detect congenital heart defects, such as holes in the heart. Congenital heart defects are structural problems present at birth. Infants and children may have echo to detect these heart defects.

- **Blood clots or tumors.** If you've had a stroke, you may have echo to check for blood clots or tumors that could have caused the stroke.

Your doctor also might recommend echo to see how well your heart responds to certain heart treatments, such as those used for heart failure.

Types of Echo

There are several types of echo—all use sound waves to create moving pictures of your heart. This is the same technology that allows doctors to see an unborn baby inside a pregnant woman.

Unlike X-rays and some other tests, echo doesn't involve radiation.

Transthoracic Echo

Transthoracic echo is the most common type of echocardiogram test. It's painless and noninvasive. "Noninvasive" means that no surgery is done and no instruments are inserted into your body.

This type of echo involves placing a device called a transducer on your chest. The device sends special sound waves, called ultrasound, through your chest wall to your heart. The human ear can't hear ultrasound waves. As the ultrasound waves bounce off the structures of your heart, a computer in the echo machine converts them into pictures on a screen.

Stress Echo

Stress echo is done as part of a stress test. During a stress test, you exercise or take medicine (given by your doctor) to make your heart work hard and beat fast. A technician will use echo to create pictures of your heart before you exercise and as soon as you finish.

Some heart problems, such as coronary heart disease, are easier to diagnose when the heart is working hard and beating fast.

Transesophageal Echo (TEE)

Your doctor may have a hard time seeing the aorta and other parts of your heart using a standard transthoracic echo. Thus, he or she may recommend transesophageal echo, or TEE. During this test, the transducer is attached to the end of a flexible tube. The tube is guided down your throat and into your esophagus (the passage leading from your mouth to your stomach). This allows your doctor to get more detailed pictures of your heart.

Fetal Echo

Fetal echo is used to look at an unborn baby's heart. A doctor may recommend this test to check a baby for heart problems. When recommended, the test is commonly done at about 18–22 weeks of pregnancy. For this test, the transducer is moved over the pregnant woman's belly.

Three-Dimensional Echo

A three-dimensional (3D) echo creates 3D images of your heart. These detailed images show how your heart looks and works. During transthoracic echo or TEE, 3D images can be taken as part of the process used to do these types of echo. Doctors may use 3D echo to diagnose heart problems in children. They also may use 3D echo for planning and overseeing heart valve surgery.

Researchers continue to study other ways to use 3D echo.

What to Expect before Echo

Echo is done in a doctor's office or a hospital. No special preparations are needed for most types of echo. You usually can eat, drink, and take any medicines as you normally would.

The exception is if you're having a transesophageal echo. This test usually requires that you don't eat or drink for 8 hours prior to the test.

If you're having a stress echo, you may need to take steps to prepare for the stress test. Your doctor will let you know what steps you need to take.

What to Expect during Echo

Echo is painless; the test usually takes less than an hour to do. For some types of echo, your doctor will need to inject saline or a special dye into one of your veins. The substance makes your heart show up more clearly on the echo pictures.

The dye used for echo is different from the dye used during angiography (a test used to examine the body's blood vessels). For most types of echo, you will remove your clothing from the waist up. Women will be given a gown to wear during the test. You'll lie on your back

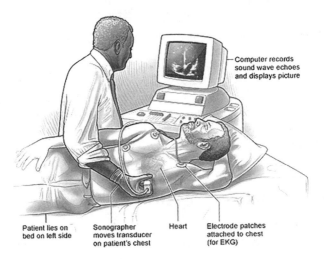

Computer records sound wave echoes and displays picture

Patient lies on bed on left side | Sonographer moves transducer on patient's chest | Heart | Electrode patches attached to chest (for EKG)

Figure 25.1. *Echocardiography*

The illustration shows a patient having echocardiography. The patient lies on his left side. A sonographer moves the transducer on the patient's chest, while viewing the echo pictures on a computer.

278

or left side on an exam table or stretcher. Soft, sticky patches called electrodes will be attached to your chest to allow an EKG (electrocardiogram) to be done. An EKG is a test that records the heart's electrical activity.

A doctor or sonographer (a person specially trained to do ultrasounds) will apply gel to your chest. The gel helps the sound waves reach your heart. A wand-like device called a transducer will then be moved around on your chest.

The transducer transmits ultrasound waves into your chest. A computer will convert echoes from the sound waves into pictures of your heart on a screen. During the test, the lights in the room will be dimmed so the computer screen is easier to see.

The sonographer will record pictures of various parts of your heart. He or she will put the recordings on a computer disc for a cardiologist (heart specialist) to review. During the test, you may be asked to change positions or hold your breath for a short time. This allows the sonographer to get better pictures of your heart.

At times, the sonographer may apply a bit of pressure to your chest with the transducer. You may find this pressure a little uncomfortable, but it helps get the best picture of your heart. You should let the sonographer know if you feel too uncomfortable. The process described above is similar to the process for fetal echo. For that test, however, the transducer is placed over the pregnant woman's belly at the location of the baby's heart.

Transesophageal Echo (TEE)

Transesophageal echo (TEE) is used if your doctor needs a more detailed view of your heart. For example, your doctor may use TEE to look for blood clots in your heart. A doctor, not a sonographer, will perform this type of echo. TEE uses the same technology as transthoracic echo, but the transducer is attached to the end of a flexible tube.

Your doctor will guide the tube down your throat and into your esophagus (the passage leading from your mouth to your stomach). From this angle, your doctor can get a more detailed image of the heart and major blood vessels leading to and from the heart.

For TEE, you'll likely be given medicine to help you relax during the test. The medicine will be injected into one of your veins.

Your blood pressure, the oxygen content of your blood, and other vital signs will be checked during the test. You'll be given oxygen through a tube in your nose. If you wear dentures or partials, you'll have to remove them.

The back of your mouth will be numbed with gel or spray. Your doctor will gently place the tube with the transducer in your throat and guide it down until it's in place behind your heart.

The pictures of your heart are then recorded as your doctor moves the transducer around in your esophagus and stomach. You shouldn't feel any discomfort as this happens.

Although the imaging usually takes less than an hour, you may be watched for a few hours at the doctor's office or hospital after the test.

Stress Echo

Stress echo is a transthoracic echo combined with either an exercise or pharmacological stress test. For an exercise stress test, you'll walk or run on a treadmill or pedal a stationary bike to make your heart work hard and beat fast. For a pharmacological stress test, you'll be given medicine to increase your heart rate. A technician will take pictures of your heart using echo before you exercise and as soon as you finish.

What You May See and Hear during Echo

As the doctor or sonographer moves the transducer around, you will see different views of your heart on the screen of the echo machine. The structures of your heart will appear as white objects, while any fluid or blood will appear black on the screen.

Doppler ultrasound often is used during echo tests. Doppler ultrasound is a special ultrasound that shows how blood is flowing through the blood vessels.

This test allows the sonographer to see blood flowing at different speeds and in different directions. The speed and direction of blood flow appear as different colors moving within the black and white images.

The human ear is unable to hear the sound waves used in echo. If you have a Doppler ultrasound, you may be able to hear "whooshing" sounds. Your doctor can use these sounds to learn about blood flow through your heart.

What to Expect after Echo

You usually can go back to your normal activities right after having echo. If you have a TEE, you may be watched for a few hours at the doctor's office or hospital after the test. Your throat might be sore for a few hours after the test. You also may not be able to drive for a short time after having TEE. Your doctor will let you know whether you need to arrange for a ride home.

What Does Echo Show?

Echo shows the size, structure, and movement of various parts of your heart. These parts include the heart valves, the septum (the wall separating the right and left heart chambers), and the walls of the heart chambers. Doppler ultrasound shows the movement of blood through your heart.

Your doctor may use echo to:

- Diagnose heart problems

- Guide or determine next steps for treatment

- Monitor changes and improvement

- Determine the need for more tests

Echo can detect many heart problems. Some might be minor and pose no risk to you. Others can be signs of serious heart disease or other heart conditions. Your doctor may use echo to learn about:

- **The size of your heart.** An enlarged heart might be the result of high blood pressure, leaky heart valves, or heart failure. Echo also can detect increased thickness of the ventricles (the heart's lower chambers). Increased thickness may be due to high blood pressure, heart valve disease, or congenital heart defects.

- **Heart muscles that are weak and aren't pumping well.** Damage from a heart attack may cause weak areas of heart muscle. Weakening also might mean that the area isn't getting enough blood supply, a sign of coronary heart disease.

- **Heart valve problems.** Echo can show whether any of your heart valves don't open normally or close tightly.

- **Problems with your heart's structure.** Echo can detect congenital heart defects, such as holes in the heart. Congenital heart defects are structural problems present at birth. Infants and children may have echo to detect these heart defects.

- **Blood clots or tumors.** If you've had a stroke, you may have echo to check for blood clots or tumors that could have caused the stroke.

281

What Are the Risks of Echo?

Transthoracic and fetal echo have no risks. These tests are safe for adults, children, and infants.

If you have a TEE, some risks are associated with the medicine given to help you relax. For example, you may have a bad reaction to the medicine, problems breathing, and nausea (feeling sick to your stomach).

Your throat also might be sore for a few hours after the test. Rarely, the tube used during TEE causes minor throat injuries. Stress echo has some risks, but they're related to the exercise or medicine used to raise your heart rate, not the echo. Serious complications from stress tests are very uncommon.

Section 25.4

Pelvic Ultrasound

"Pelvic Ultrasound," © 2018 Omnigraphics.
Reviewed July 2018.

What Is a Pelvic Ultrasound?

A pelvic ultrasound is a diagnostic procedure that uses ultrasound waves to generate images of the pelvic organs, including the uterus, cervix, vagina, fallopian tubes, and the ovaries. A transducer sends out ultrasound waves at a high frequency when placed over the skin. The sound waves reflected by the transducer are converted into images on the computer screen. The transducer translates the different types of tissues encountered in the process, depending on the speed of the sound waves. The pelvic ultrasound can be done either as a transabdominal ultrasound or transvaginal ultrasound. Other procedures related to problems of the pelvis include hysteroscopy, colposcopy, and laparoscopy.

Why Is a Pelvic Ultrasound Performed?

The pelvic ultrasound procedure may not offer all the answers to pelvic problems but it is important for diagnosis and treatment.

A pelvic ultrasound is used for the treatment of the following conditions:

- Postmenopausal bleeding
- Monitoring fetal development during pregnancy
- Abnormalities in the uterine structure, including endometrial conditions
- Fibroid tumors, pelvic masses, ovarian cysts, and other types of tumors in the pelvic region
- Pelvic inflammatory disease (PID) and other types of inflammation
- Ectopic pregnancy (pregnancy occurring outside of the uterus, usually in the fallopian tube)
- Aspiration of follicle fluid and eggs from ovaries for *in vitro* fertilization

Certain factors in a pelvic ultrasound may interfere with the results of the test, such as:

- Intestinal gas, barium in the intestines
- Severe obesity
- Inadequate filling of the bladder
- Keep your doctor informed if any concern arises during the procedure.

How Do I Prepare for a Pelvic Ultrasound?

- It is important to ask for instructions from your doctor to help you prepare for a pelvic ultrasound.
- No fasting is required for a pelvic ultrasound unless the procedure requires the use of general anesthesia.
- Drink at least three cups (24 ounces) of clear fluid an hour before the procedure; but don't empty your bladder. A full bladder helps the physician look at the pelvic organs clearly.
- You will be asked to empty your bladder before a transvaginal procedure.

Your doctor will explain the procedure to you if any other preparation is required because of your medical condition.

The Procedure

The procedure of a pelvic ultrasound may differ based on hospital practices and is usually carried out either in the doctor's office or at an outpatient clinic.

For a Transabdominal Ultrasound

The transabdominal ultrasound procedure is as follows:

- You will be given a gown to wear during the examination.

- You will be asked to lie down on the examination table, and then a gel-like substance will be applied to your abdomen.

- The transducer will be pressed against the skin of your abdomen and moved around over the area being studied.

- When blood flow is being assessed, you may hear a "whoosh, whoosh" sound if a Doppler probe is being used.

- Images of structures will be displayed on the computer screen for the doctor to analyze or detect any abnormalities.

- Once the procedure is completed, you can empty your bladder.

For a Transvaginal Ultrasound

The transvaginal ultrasound is as follows:

- You will be given a gown to wear during the examination.

- After your legs are placed into position for a pelvic examination, a transvaginal transducer will be lubricated and inserted into the vagina. Make sure to inform your doctor if you experience any discomfort during this procedure.

- The transducer will be angled and gently turned to bring the area of study into focus. You might feel some pressure when the transducer is being moved.

- Images of the organs and structures will be displayed on the computer screen for the doctor to analyze or detect any abnormalities.

- Once the procedure is completed, the transducer will be removed.

- Most pelvic ultrasounds are performed using both the transabdominal and transvaginal approaches.

Results

A normal result indicates that there is no problem with the pelvic organs or structures. However, an abnormal result may be due to the following conditions:

- Adenomyosis (benign infiltration of the endometrium into the surrounding uterine muscle)
- Growths in or around the uterus and ovaries (such as cysts or fibroids, or benign muscular growths)
- Endometrial polyps as a result of abnormal vaginal bleeding
- Abscess in the ovaries, fallopian tubes, or pelvis
- Ectopic pregnancy and appendicitis
- Blockages in the fallopian tube
- Cancers of the bladder, cervix, uterus, ovaries, vagina, and other pelvic structures

References

1. "Pelvic/Gynaecologic Ultrasound," Advanced Women's Imaging, May 19, 2010.

2. "Pelvic Ultrasound—Abdominal," MedlinePlus, National Institutes of Health (NIH), April 30, 2018.

3. "Pelvic Ultrasound," Johns Hopkins Medicine (JHM), n.d.

Chapter 26

Computed Tomography (CT)

Chapter Contents

Section 26.1

Introduction to Computed Tomography (CT)

This section includes text excerpted from "Computed Tomography (CT)," National Institute of Biomedical Imaging and Bioengineering (NIBIB), December 9, 2016.

What Is a Computed Tomography (CT) Scan?

The term "computed tomography," or CT, refers to a computerized X-ray imaging procedure in which a narrow beam of X-rays is aimed at a patient and quickly rotated around the body, producing signals that are processed by the machine's computer to generate cross-sectional images—or "slices"—of the body. These slices are called tomographic images and contain more detailed information than conventional X-rays. Once a number of successive slices are collected by the machine's computer, they can be digitally "stacked" together to form a three-dimensional (3D) image of the patient that allows for easier identification and location of basic structures as well as possible tumors or abnormalities.

How Does CT Work?

Unlike a conventional X-ray—which uses a fixed X-ray tube—a CT scanner uses a motorized X-ray source that rotates around the circular opening of a donut-shaped structure called a gantry. During a CT scan, the patient lies on a bed that slowly moves through the gantry while the X-ray tube rotates around the patient, shooting narrow beams of X-rays through the body. Instead of film, CT scanners use special digital X-ray detectors, which are located directly opposite the X-ray source. As the X-rays leave the patient, they are picked up by the detectors and transmitted to a computer.

Each time the X-ray source completes one full rotation, the CT computer uses sophisticated mathematical techniques to construct a 2D image slice of the patient. The thickness of the tissue represented in each image slice can vary depending on the CT machine used, but usually ranges from 1–10 millimeters. When a full slice is completed, the image is stored and the motorized bed is moved forward incrementally into the gantry. The X-ray scanning process is then repeated to produce another image slice. This process continues until the desired number of slices is collected.

Image slices can either be displayed individually or stacked together by the computer to generate a 3D image of the patient that shows the skeleton, organs, and tissues as well as any abnormalities the physician is trying to identify. This method has many advantages including the ability to rotate the 3D image in space or to view slices in succession, making it easier to find the exact place where a problem may be located.

When Would I Get a CT Scan?

CT scans can be used to identify disease or injury within various regions of the body. For example, CT has become a useful screening tool for detecting possible tumors or lesions within the abdomen. A CT scan of the heart may be ordered when various types of heart disease or abnormalities are suspected. CT can also be used to image the head in order to locate injuries, tumors, clots leading to stroke, hemorrhage, and other conditions. It can image the lungs in order to reveal the presence of tumors, pulmonary embolisms (blood clots), excess fluid, and other conditions such as emphysema or pneumonia. A CT scan is particularly useful when imaging complex bone fractures, severely eroded joints, or bone tumors since it usually produces more detail than would be possible with a conventional X-ray.

What Is a CT Contrast Agent?

As with all X-rays, dense structures within the body—such as bone—are easily imaged, whereas soft tissues vary in their ability to stop X-rays and, thus, may be faint or difficult to see. For this reason, intravenous (IV) contrast agents have been developed that are highly visible in an X-ray or CT scan and are safe to use in patients. Contrast agents contain substances that are better at stopping X-rays and, thus, are more visible on an X-ray image. For example, to examine the circulatory system, a contrast agent based on iodine is injected into the bloodstream to help illuminate blood vessels. This type of test is used to look for possible obstructions in blood vessels, including those in the heart. Oral contrast agents, such as barium-based compounds, are used for imaging the digestive system, including the esophagus, stomach, and gastrointestinal (GI) tract.

Are There Risks?

CT scans can diagnose possibly life-threatening conditions such as hemorrhage, blood clots, or cancer. An early diagnosis of these conditions could potentially be life-saving. However, CT scans use X-rays, and all X-rays produce ionizing radiation. Ionizing radiation has the potential to cause biological effects in living tissue. This is a risk that increases with the number of exposures added up over the life of an individual. However, the risk of developing cancer from radiation exposure is generally small.

A CT scan in a pregnant woman poses no known risks to the baby if the area of the body being imaged isn't the abdomen or pelvis. In general, if imaging of the abdomen and pelvis is needed, doctors prefer to use exams that do not use radiation, such as magnetic resonance imaging (MRI) or ultrasound. However, if neither of those can provide the answers needed, or there is an emergency or other time constraint, CT may be an acceptable alternative imaging option.

In some patients, contrast agents may cause allergic reactions, or in rare cases, temporary kidney failure. IV contrast agents should not be administered to patients with abnormal kidney function since they may induce a further reduction of kidney function, which may sometimes become permanent.

Children are more sensitive to ionizing radiation and have a longer life expectancy and, thus, a higher relative risk for developing cancer than adults. Parents may want to ask the technologist or doctor if their machine settings have been adjusted for children.

Section 26.2

Chest CT Scan

This section includes text excerpted from "Chest CT Scan,"
National Heart, Lung, and Blood Institute (NHLBI),
July 25, 2012. Reviewed July 2018.

A chest computerized tomography (CT) scan is a more detailed type of chest X-ray that takes many detailed pictures of your lungs and the inside of your chest. It is also known as chest CT, X-ray computed tomography (X-ray CT), computed axial tomography (CAT) scan.

What Does a Chest Computerized Tomography (CT) Scan Show?

A chest CT scan provides detailed pictures of the size, shape, and position of your lungs and other structures in your chest. Doctors use this test to:

- Follow up on abnormal results from standard chest X-rays

- Find the cause of lung symptoms, such as shortness of breath or chest pain

- Find out whether you have a lung problem, such as a tumor, excess fluid around the lungs, or a pulmonary embolism (a blood clot in the lungs). The test also is used to check for other conditions, such as tuberculosis (TB), emphysema, and pneumonia.

Who Needs a Chest CT Scan?

Your doctor may recommend a chest CT scan if you have symptoms of lung problems, such as chest pain or trouble breathing. The scan can help find the cause of the symptoms.

A chest CT scan looks for problems such as tumors, excess fluid around the lungs, and pulmonary embolism (a blood clot in the lungs). The scan also checks for other conditions, such as TB, emphysema, and pneumonia.

Your doctor may recommend a chest CT scan if a standard chest X-ray doesn't help diagnose the problem. The chest CT scan can:

- Provide more detailed pictures of your lungs and other chest structures than a standard chest X-ray

- Find the exact location of a tumor or other problem

- Show something that isn't visible on a chest X-ray

What to Expect during a Chest CT Scan

A chest CT scan takes about 30 minutes, which includes preparation time. The actual scanning time is much shorter, only a few minutes or less. The CT scanner is a large, tunnel-like machine that has a hole in the middle. You'll lie on a narrow table that moves through the hole. While you're inside the scanner, an X-ray tube moves around your body. You'll hear soft buzzing, clicking, or whirring noises as the scanner takes pictures.

The CT scan technician who controls the machine will be in the next room. He or she can see you through a glass window and talk to you through a speaker.

Moving your body can cause the pictures to blur. The technician will ask you to lie still and hold your breath for short periods. This will help make the pictures as clear as possible.

The scan itself doesn't hurt, but you may feel anxious if you get nervous in tight or closed spaces. Your doctor may give you medicine to help you relax.

What to Expect after a Chest CT Scan

You usually can return to your normal routine right after a chest CT scan.

If you got medicine to help you relax during the CT scan, your doctor will tell you when you can return to your normal routine. The medicine may make you sleepy, so you'll need someone to drive you home.

If contrast dye was used during the test, you may have a bruise where the needle was inserted. Your doctor may give you special instructions, such as drinking plenty of liquids to flush out the contrast dye.

If you're breastfeeding, the contrast dye can be passed to your baby through your breast milk. Ask your doctor how long you should wait after the test before you breastfeed.

You may want to prepare for the test by pumping and saving milk for 24–48 hours in advance. You can bottle-feed your baby in the hours after the CT scan.

What Are the Risks of a Chest CT Scan?

Chest CT scans have some risks. In rare instances, some people have an allergic reaction to the contrast dye. There is a slight risk of cancer, particularly in growing children, because the test uses radiation. Although the amount of radiation from one test is usually less than the amount of radiation you are naturally exposed to over three years, patients should not receive more CT scans than the number that clinical guidelines recommend.

Another risk is that chest CT scans may detect an incidental finding, which is something that doesn't cause symptoms but now may require more tests after being found.

Talk to your doctor and the technicians performing the test about whether you are or could be pregnant. If the test is not urgent, they may have you wait to do the test until after your pregnancy. If it is urgent, the technicians will take extra steps to protect your baby during this test.

Let your doctor know if you are breastfeeding because contrast dye can pass into your breast milk. If you must have contrast dye injected, you may want to pump and save enough breast milk for one to two days after your test or you may bottle-feed your baby for that time.

Section 26.3

Coronary Calcium Scan

This section includes text excerpted from "Coronary Calcium Scan," National Heart, Lung, and Blood Institute (NHLBI), June 11, 2014. Reviewed July 2018.

What Is a Coronary Calcium Scan?

A coronary calcium scan is a test that looks for specks of calcium in the walls of the coronary (heart) arteries. These specks of calcium are called calcifications. Calcifications in the coronary arteries are an early sign of coronary heart disease (CHD). CHD is a disease in which a waxy substance called plaque builds up in the coronary arteries.

Over time, plaque can harden or rupture (break open). Hardened plaque narrows the coronary arteries and reduces the flow of oxygen-rich blood to the heart. This can cause chest pain or discomfort called angina.

If the plaque ruptures, a blood clot can form on its surface. A large blood clot can mostly or completely block blood flow through a coronary artery. This is the most common cause of a heart attack. Over time, ruptured plaque also hardens and narrows the coronary arteries.

CHD also can lead to heart failure and arrhythmias. Heart failure is a condition in which your heart can't pump enough blood to meet your body's needs. Arrhythmias are problems with the rate or rhythm of your heartbeat.

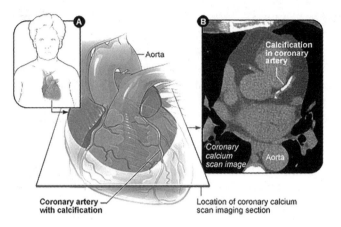

Figure 26.1. *Coronary Calcium Scan*

Figure A shows the position of the heart in the body and the location and angle of the coronary calcium scan image. Figure B is a coronary calcium scan image showing calcifications in a coronary artery.

What to Expect before a Coronary Calcium Scan

You don't need to take any special steps before having a coronary calcium scan. However, your doctor may ask you to avoid caffeine and smoking for 4 hours before the test.

For the scan, you'll remove your clothes above the waist and wear a hospital gown. You also will remove any jewelry from around your neck or chest.

What to Expect during a Coronary Calcium Scan

A coronary calcium scan is done in a hospital or outpatient office. The X-ray machine that's used for the scan is called a computed tomography (CT) scanner. The technician who runs the scanner will clean areas of your chest and apply sticky patches with sensors called electrodes. The patches are connected to an EKG (electrocardiogram) machine.

The EKG will record your heart's electrical activity during the scan. This makes it possible to take pictures of your heart when it's relaxed between beats. The CT scanner is a large machine that has a hollow, circular tube in the center. You'll lie on your back on a sliding table. The table can move up and down, and it goes inside the tunnel-like machine.

The table will slowly slide into the opening in the machine. Inside the scanner, an X-ray tube will move around your body to take pictures of your heart. The technician will control the CT scanner from the next room. He or she will be able to see you through a glass window and talk to you through a speaker.

The technician will ask you to lie still and hold your breath for short periods while each picture is taken. You may be given medicine to slow your heart rate. This helps the machine take clearer pictures of your heart. The medicine will be given by mouth or injected into a vein.

The coronary calcium scan will take about 10–15 minutes, although the actual scanning will take only a few seconds. During the test, the machine will make clicking and whirring sounds as it takes pictures. The scan causes no discomfort, but the exam room might be chilly to keep the machine working properly. If you get nervous in enclosed or tight spaces, you might receive medicine to help you stay calm. Your head will remain outside the opening in the machine during the test.

What to Expect after a Coronary Calcium Scan

You'll be able to return to your normal activities after the coronary calcium scan is done. Your doctor will discuss the results of the test with you.

What Does a Coronary Calcium Scan Show?

After a coronary calcium scan, you'll get a calcium score called an Agatston score. The score is based on the amount of calcium found in your coronary (heart) arteries. You may get an Agatston score for each major artery and a total score.

The test is negative if no calcifications are found in your arteries. This means your chance of having a heart attack in the next 2–5 years is low. The test is positive if calcifications are found in your arteries. Calcifications are a sign of atherosclerosis and CHD. (Atherosclerosis is a condition in which plaque builds up in the arteries.) The higher your Agatston score is, the more severe the atherosclerosis.

The National Heart, Lung, and Blood Institute (NHLBI) has a calculator you can use to see how your Agatston score compares with scores of people your age and of the same ethnic background. An Agatston score of 0 is normal. In general, the higher your score, the more likely you are to have CHD. If your score is high, your doctor may recommend more tests.

What Are the Risks of a Coronary Calcium Scan?

Coronary calcium scans have very few risks. The test isn't invasive, which means that no surgery is done and no instruments are inserted into your body. Unlike some CT scans, coronary calcium scans don't require an injection of contrast dye to make your heart or arteries visible on X-ray images.

Coronary calcium scans involve radiation, although the amount used is considered small. Electron beam computed tomography (EBCT) uses less radiation than multidetector computed tomography (MDCT).

In either case, the amount of radiation is about equal to the amount of radiation you're naturally exposed to in a single year.

Section 26.4

Virtual Colonoscopy

This section includes text excerpted from "Virtual Colonoscopy," National Institute of Diabetes and Digestive and Kidney Diseases (NIDDK), August 2016.

What Is Virtual Colonoscopy?

Virtual colonoscopy is a procedure in which a radiologist uses X-rays and a computer to create images of your rectum and colon from outside the body. Virtual colonoscopy can show ulcers, polyps, and cancer. Virtual colonoscopy is also called computerized tomography (CT) colonography.

How Virtual Colonoscopy Differs from Colonoscopy

Colonoscopy and virtual colonoscopy are different in several ways. Colonoscopy is a procedure in which a trained specialist uses a long, flexible, narrow tube with a light and tiny camera on one end, called a colonoscope or scope, to look inside your rectum and colon. Virtual colonoscopy is an X-ray test, takes less time, and does not require a doctor to insert a scope into the entire length of your colon. Unlike colonoscopy, virtual colonoscopy does not require sedation or anesthesia.

However, virtual colonoscopy may not be as effective as colonoscopy at finding certain polyps. Also, doctors cannot remove polyps or treat certain other problems during virtual colonoscopy, as they can during colonoscopy. Your health insurance coverage for virtual colonoscopy and colonoscopy also may be different.

Why Do Doctors Use Virtual Colonoscopy?

Doctors mainly use virtual colonoscopy to screen for polyps or cancer. Screening may find diseases at an early stage, when a doctor has a better chance of curing the disease. Occasionally, doctors may use virtual colonoscopy when colonoscopy is incomplete or not possible due to other medical reasons.

Screening for Colon and Rectal Cancer

Your doctor will recommend screening for colon and rectal cancer at age 50 if you don't have health problems or other factors that make you more likely to develop colon cancer.

Factors that make you more likely to develop colorectal cancer include:

- Someone in your family has had polyps or cancer of the colon or rectum

- A personal history of inflammatory bowel disease (IBD), such as ulcerative colitis (UC) or Crohn's disease

- Other factors, such as if you weigh too much or smoke cigarettes

If you are more likely to develop colorectal cancer, your doctor may recommend screening at a younger age, and you may need to be tested more often.

If you are older than age 75, talk with your doctor about whether you should be screened.

Government health insurance plans, such as Medicare, and private health insurance plans sometimes change whether and how often they pay for cancer screening tests. Check with your insurance plan to find out if and how often your insurance will cover a screening virtual colonoscopy.

How Do I Prepare for a Virtual Colonoscopy?

To prepare for a virtual colonoscopy, you will need to talk with your doctor, change your diet, clean out your bowel, and drink a special liquid called contrast medium. The contrast medium makes your rectum and colon easier to see in the X-rays.

Talk with Your Doctor

You should talk with your doctor about any medical conditions you have and all prescribed and over-the-counter (OTC) medicines, vitamins, and supplements you take, including:

- Arthritis medicines

- Aspirin or medicines that contain aspirin

- Blood thinners

- Diabetes medicines

- Nonsteroidal anti-inflammatory drugs (NSAIDs), such as ibuprofen or naproxen vitamins that contain iron or iron supplements

X-rays may interfere with personal medical devices. Tell your doctor if you have any implanted medical devices, such as a pacemaker. Doctors don't recommend X-rays for pregnant women because X-rays may harm the fetus. Tell your doctor if you are, or may be, pregnant. Your doctor may suggest a different procedure, such as a colonoscopy.

Change Your Diet and Clean Out Your Bowel

As in colonoscopy, a healthcare professional will give you written bowel prep instructions to follow at home before the procedure. A healthcare professional orders a bowel prep so that little or no stool is present in your intestine. A complete bowel prep lets you pass stool that is clear and liquid. Stool inside your colon can prevent the X-ray machine from taking clear images of the lining of your intestine.

You may need to follow a clear liquid diet the day before the procedure. The instructions will provide specific direction about when to start and stop the clear liquid diet. In most cases, you may drink or eat the following:

- Fat-free bouillon or broth

- Gelatin in flavors such as lemon, lime, or orange

- Plain coffee or tea, without cream or milk

- Sports drinks in such flavors as lemon, lime, or orange

- Strained fruit juice, such as apple or white grape—doctors recommend avoiding orange juice and red or purple beverages

- Water

Your doctor will tell you how long before the procedure you should have nothing by mouth.

A healthcare professional will ask you to follow the directions for a bowel prep before the procedure. The bowel prep will cause diarrhea, so you should stay close to a bathroom.

Different bowel preps may contain different combinations of laxatives—pills that you swallow or powders that you dissolve in water and other clear liquids, and enemas. Some people will need to drink a large amount, often a gallon, of liquid laxative over a scheduled amount of time—most often the night before the procedure.

You may find this part of the bowel prep difficult; however, completing the prep is very important. The images will not be clear if the prep is incomplete.

Drink Contrast Medium

The night before the procedure, you will drink a contrast medium. Contrast medium is visible on X-rays and can help your doctor tell the difference between stool and polyps.

How Do Healthcare Professionals Perform a Virtual Colonoscopy?

A specially trained X-ray technician performs a virtual colonoscopy at an outpatient center or a hospital. You do not need anesthesia.

For the procedure, you will lie on a table while the technician inserts a thin tube through your anus and into your rectum. The tube inflates your large intestine with air for a better view. The table slides into a tunnel-shaped device where the technician takes the X-ray images. The technician may ask you to hold your breath several times during the procedure to steady the images. The technician will ask you to turn over on your side or stomach so he or she can take different images of the large intestine. The procedure lasts about 10–15 minutes.

What Should I Expect after a Virtual Colonoscopy?

After a virtual colonoscopy, you can expect to:

- Feel cramping or bloating during the first hour after the test

- Resume your regular activities right after the test

- Return to a normal diet

After the test, a radiologist looks at the images to find any problems and sends a report to your doctor. If the radiologist finds problems, your doctor may perform a colonoscopy the same day or at a later time.

What Are the Risks of a Virtual Colonoscopy?

Inflating the colon with air has a small risk of perforating the lining of the large intestine. The doctor may need to treat perforation with surgery.

Seek Care Right Away

If you have any of the following symptoms after a virtual colonoscopy, you should seek medical attention right away:

- Severe pain in your abdomen

- Fever

- Bloody bowel movements or bleeding from your anus

- Dizziness

- Weakness

Section 26.5

Full Body CT Scans—What You Need to Know

This section includes text excerpted from "Full-Body CT
Scans—What You Need to Know," U.S. Food and Drug
Administration (FDA), December 5, 2017.

Using a technology that "takes a look" at people's insides and promises early warnings of cancer, cardiac disease, and other abnormalities, clinics and medical imaging facilities nationwide are touting a novel service for health-conscious people: "Whole-body computed tomography (CT) screening." This typically involves scanning the body from the chin to below the hips with a form of X-ray imaging that produces cross-sectional images.

The technology used is called "X-ray computed tomography" (CT), sometimes referred to as "computerized axial tomography" (CAT). A number of different types of X-ray CT systems are being promoted for various types of screening. For example, "multi-slice" CT (MSCT) and "electron beam" CT (EBCT)—also called "electron beam tomography" (EBT)—are X-ray CT systems that produce images rapidly and are often promoted for screening the buildup of calcium in arteries of the heart.

CT, MSCT, and EBCT all use X-rays to produce images representing "slices" of the body—like the slices of a loaf of bread. Each image slice corresponds to a wafer-thin section which can be viewed to reveal body structures in great detail.

CT is recognized as an invaluable medical tool for the diagnosis of disease, trauma, or abnormality in patients with signs or symptoms of disease. It's also used for planning, guiding, and monitoring therapy. CT is being marketed as a preventive or proactive healthcare measure to healthy individuals who have no symptoms of disease.

No Proven Benefits for Healthy People

Taking preventive action, finding unsuspected disease, uncovering problems while they are treatable, these all sound great, almost too good to be true! In fact, at this time the U.S. Food and Drug Administration (FDA) knows of no scientific evidence demonstrating that whole-body scanning of individuals without symptoms provides more benefit than harm to people being screened. The FDA is responsible for assuring the safety and effectiveness of such medical devices, and it prohibits manufacturers of CT systems to promote their use for whole-body screening of asymptomatic people. The FDA, however, does not regulate practitioners and they may choose to use a device for any use they deem appropriate.

Compared to most other diagnostic X-ray procedures, CT scans result in relatively high radiation exposure. The risks associated with such exposure are greatly outweighed by the benefits of diagnostic and therapeutic CT. However, for whole-body CT screening of asymptomatic people, the benefits are questionable:

- Can it effectively differentiate between healthy people and those who have a hidden disease?

301

- Do suspicious findings lead to additional invasive testing or treatments that produce additional risk with little benefit?

- Does a "normal" finding guarantee good health?

Many people don't realize that getting a whole body CT screening exam won't necessarily give them the "peace of mind" they are hoping for, or the information that would allow them to prevent a health problem. An abnormal finding, for example, may not be a serious one, and a normal finding may be inaccurate. CT scans, like other medical procedures, will miss some conditions, and "false" leads can prompt further, unnecessary testing.

Chapter 27

Magnetic Resonance Imaging (MRI)

Chapter Contents

Section 27.1

Introduction to MRI

This section includes text excerpted from "MRI (Magnetic Resonance Imaging)," U.S. Food and Drug Administration (FDA), March 27, 2018.

Magnetic resonance imaging (MRI) is a medical imaging procedure for making images of the internal structures of the body. MRI scanners use strong magnetic fields and radio waves (radiofrequency energy) to make images. The signal in an MR image comes mainly from the protons in fat and water molecules in the body.

During an MRI exam, an electric current is passed through coiled wires to create a temporary magnetic field in a patient's body. Radio waves are sent from and received by a transmitter/receiver in the machine, and these signals are used to make digital images of the scanned area of the body. A typical MRI scan last from 20–90 minutes, depending on the part of the body being imaged.

For some MRI exams, intravenous (IV) drugs, such as gadolinium-based contrast agents (GBCAs) are used to change the contrast of the MR image. Gadolinium-based contrast agents are rare earth metals that are usually given through an IV in the arm.

Uses of Magnetic Resonance Imaging (MRI)

MRI gives healthcare providers useful information about a variety of conditions and diagnostic procedures including:

- Abnormalities of the brain and spinal cord

- Abnormalities in various parts of the body such as breast, prostate, and liver

- Injuries or abnormalities of the joints

- The structure and function of the heart (cardiac imaging)

- Areas of activation within the brain (functional MRI or fMRI)

- Blood flow through blood vessels and arteries (angiography)

- The chemical composition of tissues (spectroscopy)

In addition to these diagnostic uses, MRI may also be used to guide certain interventional procedures.

Benefits and Risks of MRI

Benefits

An MRI scanner can be used to take images of any part of the body (e.g., head, joints, abdomen, legs, etc.), in any imaging direction. MRI provides better soft tissue contrast than CT and can differentiate better between fat, water, muscle, and other soft tissue than CT. (CT is usually better at imaging bones). These images provide information to physicians and can be useful in diagnosing a wide variety of diseases and conditions.

Risks

MR images are made without using any ionizing radiation, so patients are not exposed to the harmful effects of ionizing radiation. But while there are no known health hazards from temporary exposure to the MR environment, the MR environment involves a strong, static magnetic field, a magnetic field that changes with time (pulsed gradient field), and radiofrequency energy, each of which carry specific safety concerns:

- The strong, static magnetic field will attract magnetic objects (from small items such as keys and cell phones, to large, heavy items such as oxygen tanks and floor buffers) and may cause damage to the scanner or injury to the patient or medical professionals if those objects become projectiles. Careful screening of people and objects entering the MR environment is critical to ensure nothing enters the magnet area that may become a projectile.

- The magnetic fields that change with time create loud knocking noises which may harm hearing if adequate ear protection is not used. They may also cause peripheral muscle or nerve stimulation that may feel like a twitching sensation.

- The radiofrequency energy used during the MRI scan could lead to heating of the body. The potential for heating is greater during long MRI examinations.

The use of gadolinium-based contrast agents (GBCAs) also carries some risk, including side effects such as allergic reactions to the contrast agent.

Some patients find the inside of the MRI scanner to be uncomfortably small and may experience claustrophobia. Imaging in an open

MRI scanner may be an option for some patients, but not all MRI systems can perform all examinations, so you should discuss these options with your doctor. Your doctor may also be able to prescribe medication to make the experience easier for you.

To produce good quality images, patients must generally remain very still throughout the entire MRI procedure. Infants, small children, and other patients who are unable to lay still may need to be sedated or anesthetized for the procedure. Sedation and anesthesia carry risks not specific to the MRI procedure, such as slowed or difficult breathing, and low blood pressure.

Patients with Implants, External and Accessory Devices

The MR environment presents unique safety hazards for patients with implants, external devices and accessory medical devices. Examples of implanted devices include artificial joints, stents, cochlear implants, and pacemakers. An external device is a device that may touch the patient like an external insulin pump, a leg brace, or a wound dressing. An accessory device is a nonimplanted medical device (such as a ventilator, patient monitor) that is used to monitor or support the patient.

- The strong, static magnetic field of the MRI scanner will pull on magnetic materials and may cause unwanted movement of the medical device.

- The radiofrequency energy and magnetic fields that change with time may cause heating of the implanted medical device and the surrounding tissue, which could lead to burns.

- The magnetic fields and radiofrequency energy produced by an MRI scanner may also cause electrically active medical devices to malfunction, which can result in a failure of the device to deliver the intended therapy.

- The presence of the medical device will degrade the quality of the MR image, which may make the MRI scan uninformative or may lead to an inaccurate clinical diagnosis, potentially resulting in inappropriate medical treatment.

Therefore, patients with implanted medical devices should not receive an MRI exam unless the implanted medical device has been positively identified as MR Safe or MR Conditional. An MR Safe device is nonmagnetic, contains no metal, does not conduct electricity and poses no known hazards in all MR environments. An MR Conditional device may be used safely only within an MR environment that matches its conditions of safe use. Any device with an unknown MRI safety status should be assumed to be MR Unsafe.

Adverse Events

Adverse events for MRI scans are very rare. Millions of MRI scans are performed in the United States every year, and the U.S. Food and Drug Administration (FDA) receives around 300 adverse event reports for MRI scanners and coils each year from manufacturers, distributors, user facilities, and patients. The majority of these reports describe heating and/or burns (thermal injuries). Second degree burns are the most commonly reported patient problem. Other reported problems include injuries from projectile events (objects being drawn toward the MRI scanner), crushed and pinched fingers from the patient table, patient falls, and hearing loss or a ringing in the ear (tinnitus). The FDA has also received reports concerning the inadequate display or quality of the MR images.

What Patients Should Know before Having an MRI Exam

Before your MRI exam, you will likely be asked to fill out a screening questionnaire. For your safety, answering the questionnaire accurately is extremely important. In particular, make sure you notify the MRI technologist or radiologist if you have any implanted medical devices, such as stents, knee or hip replacements, pacemakers, or drug pumps. Also be sure to tell the technologist if you have any tattoos or drug patches as these can cause skin irritation or burns during the exam. The medical team will need to make sure that these devices can safely enter the MR environment.

Some devices are MR Safe or MR Conditional, meaning that they can be safely used in the MR environment under specific conditions. If you have an implant card for your device, bring it with you to your MRI exam so that you can help the doctor or the MRI technologist identify what type of device you have.

The space where you will lay in an MRI scanner to have your images taken can be a tight fit for some people, especially larger individuals. If you believe that you will feel claustrophobic, tell the MRI technologist or your doctor.

The MRI scanner will make a lot of noise as it takes images. This is normal. You should be offered earplugs and/or headphones to make the noise sound less loud. You may also be able to listen to music through the headphones to make the MRI exam more enjoyable.

If your exam includes a contrast agent, the MRI technologist will place a small IV line in one of your arms. You may feel some coldness when the contrast agent is injected. Be sure to notify the technologist if you feel any pain or discomfort.

Remember, your doctor has referred you to have an MRI because he or she believes the scan will provide useful information. If you have any questions about your procedure, don't be afraid to ask.

Questions to Ask Your Doctor

- What information will the MRI scan provide? How might this change my treatment options?

- Is there any reason why I shouldn't have an MRI scan? (If you have any implanted devices (such as a pacemaker, stents, an insulin pump, or an artificial joint), be sure your doctor knows about them.)

- Will my exam involve contrast agent? What additional information will using the contrast agent provide?

Questions to Ask the MRI Technologist

- How long can I expect my scan to last?

- Can I listen to music during my MRI scan? Can I choose the music?

- Where is the call button I can use to let you know if there is a problem?

Section 27.2

Cardiac MRI

This section includes text excerpted from "Cardiac MRI,"
National Heart, Lung, and Blood Institute (NHLBI),
April 26, 2013. Reviewed July 2018.

A cardiac magnetic resonance imaging (MRI) is a painless imaging test that uses radio waves, magnets, and a computer to create detailed pictures of your heart.

What Does a Cardiac Magnetic Resonance Imaging (MRI) Show?

The doctor supervising your scan will provide your doctor with the results of your cardiac MRI. Your doctor will discuss the findings with you.

Cardiac MRI can reveal various heart diseases and conditions, such as:

- Coronary heart disease (CHD)

- Damage caused by a heart attack

- Heart failure

- Heart valve problems

- Congenital heart defects (heart defects present at birth)

- Pericarditis (a condition in which the membrane, or sac, around your heart is inflamed)

- Cardiac tumors

Cardiac MRI is a fast, accurate tool that can help diagnose a heart attack. The test does this by detecting areas of the heart that don't move normally, have poor blood supply, or are scarred.

Cardiac MRI also can show whether any of the coronary arteries are blocked. A blockage prevents your heart muscle from getting enough oxygen-rich blood, which can lead to a heart attack.

Coronary angiography is the most common procedure for looking at blockages in the coronary arteries. Coronary angiography is an invasive procedure that uses X-rays and iodine-based dye.

Researchers have found that cardiac MRI can sometimes replace coronary angiography, avoiding the need to use X-ray radiation and iodine-based dye. This use of MRI is called MR angiography (MRA).

Echocardiography (echo) is the main test for diagnosing heart valve disease. However, your doctor also might recommend cardiac MRI to assess the severity of valve disease.

A cardiac MRI can confirm information about valve defects or provide more detailed information about heart valve disease. This information can help your doctor plan your treatment. An MRI also might be done before heart valve surgery to help your surgeon plan for the surgery.

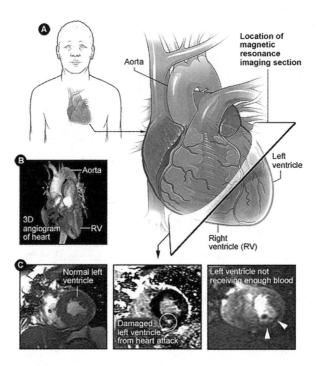

Figure 27.1. *Cardiac MRI*

Figure A shows the heart's position in the body and the location and angle of the MRI pictures shown in figure C. Figure B is a magnetic resonance angiogram, which sometimes is used instead of a standard angiogram. Figure C shows MRI pictures of a normal left ventricle (left image), a left ventricle damaged by a heart attack (middle image), and a left ventricle that isn't getting enough blood from the coronary arteries (right image).

What to Expect during Cardiac MRI

Cardiac MRI takes place in a hospital or medical imaging facility. A radiologist or other doctor who has special training in medical imaging oversees MRI testing.

Cardiac MRI usually takes 30–90 minutes, depending on how many pictures are needed. The test may take less time with some MRI machines.

The MRI machine will be located in a special room that prevents radio waves from disrupting the machine. It also prevents the MRI machines' strong magnetic fields from disrupting other equipment.

Traditional MRI machines look like long, narrow tunnels. The MRI machines (called short-bore systems) of present days are shorter, wider, and don't completely surround you. Some machines are open on all sides. Your doctor will help decide which type of machine is best for you.

Cardiac MRI is painless and harmless. You'll lie on your back on a sliding table that goes inside the tunnel-like machine. The MRI technician will control the machine from the next room. He or she will be able to see you through a glass window and talk to you through a speaker. Tell the technician if you have a hearing problem.

The MRI machine makes loud humming, tapping, and buzzing noises. Some facilities let you wear earplugs or listen to music during the test. You will need to remain very still during the MRI. Any movement can blur the pictures. If you're unable to lie still, you may be given medicine to help you relax.

The technician might ask you to hold your breath for 10–15 seconds at a time while he or she takes pictures of your heart. Researchers are studying ways that will allow someone having a cardiac MRI to breathe freely during the exam, while achieving the same image quality.

A contrast agent, such as gadolinium, might be used to highlight your blood vessels or heart in the pictures. The substance usually is injected into a vein in your arm using a needle.

You may feel a cool sensation during the injection and discomfort when the needle is inserted. Gadolinium doesn't contain iodine, so it won't cause problems for people who are allergic to iodine.

Your cardiac MRI might include a stress test to detect blockages in your coronary arteries. If so, you'll get other medicines to increase the blood flow in your heart or to increase your heart rate.

What to Expect after Cardiac MRI

You'll be able to return to your normal routine once the cardiac MRI is done. If you took medicine to help you relax during the test, your doctor will tell you when you can return to your normal routine. The medicine will make you sleepy, so you'll need someone to drive you home.

What Are the Risks of Cardiac MRI?

The magnetic fields and radio waves used in cardiac MRI have no side effects. This method of taking pictures of organs and tissues doesn't carry a risk of causing cancer or birth defects.

Serious reactions to the contrast agent used during some MRI tests are very rare. However, side effects are possible and include the following:

- Headache

- Nausea (feeling sick to your stomach)

- Dizziness

- Changes in taste

- Allergic reactions

Rarely, the contrast agent can harm people who have severe kidney or liver disease. The substance may cause a disease called nephrogenic systemic fibrosis (NSF). If your cardiac MRI includes a stress test, more medicines will be used during the test. These medicines may have other side effects that aren't expected during a regular MRI scan, such as:

- Arrhythmias, or irregular heartbeats

- Chest pain

- Shortness of breath

- Palpitations (feelings that your heart is skipping a beat, fluttering, or beating too hard or fast)

Section 27.3

Chest MRI

This section includes text excerpted from "Chest MRI,"
National Heart, Lung, and Blood Institute (NHLBI),
December 9, 2016.

A chest magnetic resonance imaging (MRI) is a painless imaging test that uses radio waves, magnets, and a computer to create detailed pictures of the structures in your chest, including your chest wall, heart, and blood vessels.

What Does a Chest Magnetic Resonance Imaging (MRI) Show?

Chest MRI can provide detailed information to help your doctor diagnose lung problems such as a tumor or pleural disorder, blood vessel problems, or abnormal lymph nodes. Chest MRI can help explain the results of other imaging tests such as chest X-rays and chest computerized tomography (CT) scans.

What to Expect during a Chest MRI

Chest MRI may be done in a medical imaging facility or hospital. Before your test, a technician may inject a contrast dye into a vein in your arm to highlight your heart and blood vessels. You may feel some discomfort from the needle or have a cool feeling as the contrast dye is injected. The MRI machine is a large, tunnel-like machine that has a table. You will lie still on the table, and the table will slide into the machine. You will hear loud humming, tapping, and buzzing sounds when you are inside the machine as pictures of your chest are being taken. You will be able to hear from and talk to the technician performing the test while you are inside the machine. The technician may ask you to hold your breath for a few seconds during the test.

What Are the Risks of a Chest MRI?

Chest MRI has few risks. In rare instances, the contrast dye may harm people who have kidney disease, or it may cause an allergic reaction. Researchers are studying whether multiple contrast dye

313

injections, defined as four or more, may cause other adverse effects. Talk to your doctor and the technicians performing the test about whether you are or could be pregnant. Let your doctor know if you are breastfeeding because the contrast dye can pass into your breast milk. If you must have the contrast dye injected, you may want to pump and save enough breast milk for one to two days after your test or you may bottle-feed your baby for that time. Tell your doctor if you have:

- A pacemaker or other implanted device because the MRI machine can damage these devices

- Metal inside your body from previous surgeries because it can interfere with the MRI machine

- Metal on your body from piercings, jewelry, or some transdermal skin patches because they can interfere with the MRI machine or cause skin burns. Tattoos may cause a problem because older tattoo inks may contain small amounts of metal.

Section 27.4

MRI of the Spine

"Magnetic Resonance Imaging (MRI) of the Spine," © 2018 Omnigraphics. Reviewed July 2018.

What Is Magnetic Resonance Imaging of the Spine?

Magnetic resonance imaging (MRI) is a medical test that helps physicians diagnose the medical condition of the body using a large magnet, radio frequencies, and a computer to produce images of organs and structures within the body. The anatomy of the vertebrae, the ligaments, disks, spinal cord, and the spaces between the vertebrae can be examined in an MRI scan. MRI machines usually look like narrow tunnels, although some are more spacious or wider. Typically, an MRI scan can last from 30 minutes to two hours.

What are Some Common Uses of MRI Scan?

- Explore the causes of back pain, compression fracture or bone swelling, such as edema

- Detect congenital anomalies of the vertebrae or the spinal cord

- Assess spinal anatomy, alignment, compression, and inflammation of spinal cord and nerves

- Help plan spinal surgical procedures, decompression of a pinched nerve, spinal fusion, or injection of steroids to relieve spinal pain

- Monitor changes after spinal surgery

How Does an MRI Scan Work?

The MRI scan utilizes radio frequencies to realign hydrogen atoms in your body without causing any chemical change in the tissues. When the hydrogen atoms return to their usual alignment, energy is emitted from different tissues of the body, which is captured by the MRI scanner. A radiologist interprets the signals processed by the computer. The MRI scan also helps differentiate between abnormal and normal tissue and is better than viewing the images by X-ray, computed tomography (CT), or ultrasound.

What Are the Risk Factors of MRI Scan?

The following risk factors may prohibit some patients from having an MRI scan:

- Cochlear implants or pacemakers

- Internal metal objects such as clips, plates, screws, or wire mesh

- Claustrophobic patients, or those taking anti-anxiety medications

- Patients allergic or sensitive to contrast dye or iodine

- Pregnant patients

The Procedure

- An MRI scan is usually painless. However, patients who experience anxiety or feel claustrophobic may opt to be sedated.

Make sure to inform the radiologist of any concerns. It is normal for the body to feel warm during an MRI scan, and important that a patient remain still while the images are being obtained. Each MRI scan usually takes a few seconds to a few minutes and the radiologist informs the patient before the scan begins and when it ends.

- Occasionally a contrast dye is administered intravenously in order to obtain certain images. On such occasions, you may experience irritation at the injection site or a metallic taste in your mouth after the contrast injection is administered. Some patients may experience allergic reactions to the contrast dye. It is important to keep the radiologist or the physician informed on such occasions.

- After an MRI scan, you may be required to rest for a period of time if you have been sedated. You will be under supervision for a period of time if a contrast dye was used as well. Inform your physician immediately if side effects such as itching, swelling, rashes, or breathing difficulties develop. Before leaving the medical center, the physician may give you additional instructions depending on your situation.

Who Interprets the Results and How Do I Get Them?

The radiologist will analyze the images, sign the report, and refer you to your physician. The physician will evaluate the results, explain your results, and prescribe medications as required. In case of any abnormalities, a follow-up exam may be recommended. Sometimes, follow-up examinations are the best way to determine if a treatment is working or discover any changes that have occurred as a result of your treatment.

References

1. "Magnetic Resonance Imaging (MRI)—Spine," Radiological Society of North America (RSNA), July 28, 2015.

2. "Magnetic Resonance Imaging (MRI) of the Spine and Brain," Johns Hopkins Medicine (JHM), August 23, 2015.

Chapter 28

Nuclear Imaging

Chapter Contents

Section 28.1

Molecular Imaging and Nuclear Imaging (PET and SPECT)

This section includes text excerpted from "Molecular and Nuclear Imaging (PET and SPECT)," Cancer Imaging Program (CIP), National Cancer Institute (NCI), December 22, 2016.

Molecular and Nuclear imaging use low doses of radioactive substances linked to compounds used by the body's cells or compounds that attach to tumor cells. Using special detection equipment, the radioactive substances can be traced in the body to see where and when they concentrate.

Positron Emission Tomography (PET) Scan

The positron emission tomography (PET) scan creates computerized images of chemical changes, such as sugar metabolism, that take place in tissue. Typically, the patient is given an injection of a substance that consists of a combination of a sugar and a small amount of radioactively labeled sugar. The radioactive sugar can help in locating a tumor, because cancer cells take up or absorb sugar more avidly than other tissues in the body.

After receiving the radioactive sugar, the patient lies still for about 60 minutes while the radioactively labeled sugar circulates throughout the body. If a tumor is present, the radioactive sugar will accumulate in the tumor. The patient then lies on a table, which gradually moves through the PET scanner incrementally several times during a 15–60-minute period. The PET scanner is used to detect the distribution of the sugar in the tumor and in the body. By the combined matching of a computerized tomography (CT) scan with PET images, there is an improved capacity to discriminate normal from abnormal tissues. A computer translates this information into the images that are interpreted by a radiologist.

PET scans may play a role in determining whether a mass is cancerous. However, PET scans are more accurate in detecting larger and more aggressive tumors than they are in locating tumors that are smaller than 8 mm a pinky nail (or half of a thumbnail) and/or less aggressive cancers. The size of smallest tumor mass that can be found at PET is constantly improving. They may also detect cancer when other imaging techniques show normal results. PET scans may be helpful in evaluating and staging recurrent disease (cancer that has come back). PET scans are beginning to be also commonly used to check if a treatment is working—if a tumor cells are dying and thus using less sugar.

Single Photon Emission Computed Tomography (SPECT) Scan

Similar to PET, single photon emission computed tomography (SPECT) uses radioactive tracers and a scanner to record data that a computer constructs into two- or three-dimensional (2D/3D) images. A small amount of a radioactive drug is injected into a vein and a scanner is used to make detailed images of areas inside the body where the radioactive material is taken up by the cells. SPECT can give information about blood flow to tissues and chemical reactions (metabolism) in the body.

In this procedure, antibodies (proteins that recognize and stick to tumor cells) can be linked to a radioactive substance. If a tumor is present, the antibodies will stick to it. Then a SPECT scan can be done to detect the radioactive substance and reveal where the tumor is located.

Section 28.2

Nuclear Heart Scan

This section includes text excerpted from "Nuclear Heart Scan," National Heart, Lung, and Blood Institute (NHLBI), December 10, 2016.

A nuclear heart scan is an imaging test that uses special cameras and a radioactive substance called a tracer to create pictures of your heart. It is also known as nuclear stress test and radionuclide scan.

What Does a Nuclear Heart Scan Show?

The results from a nuclear heart scan can help doctors:

- Diagnose heart conditions, such as coronary heart disease (CHD), and decide the best course of treatment

- Manage certain heart diseases, such as CHD and heart failure, and predict short- or long-term survival

- Determine your risk for a heart attack

- Decide whether other heart tests or procedures will help you. Examples of these tests and procedures include coronary angiography and cardiac catheterization.

- Decide whether procedures that increase blood flow to the coronary arteries will help you

Examples of these procedures include percutaneous coronary intervention, also known as coronary angioplasty, and coronary artery bypass grafting (CABG).

Monitor procedures or surgeries that have been done, such as CABG or a heart transplant.

What to Expect before a Nuclear Heart Scan

A nuclear heart scan can take a lot of time. Most scans take between 2–5 hours, especially if your doctor needs two sets of pictures.

Discuss with your doctor how a nuclear heart scan is done. Talk with him or her about your overall health, including health problems such as asthma, COPD (chronic obstructive pulmonary disease), diabetes, and kidney disease.

If you have lung disease or diabetes, your doctor will give you special instructions before the nuclear heart scan. If you're having a stress test as part of your nuclear heart scan, wear comfortable walking shoes and loose-fitting clothes for the test. You may be asked to wear a hospital gown during the test.

Let your doctor know about any medicines you take, including prescription and over-the-counter (OTC) medicines, vitamins, minerals, and other supplements. Some medicines and supplements can interfere with the medicines that might be used during the stress test to raise your heart rate.

What to Expect during a Nuclear Heart Scan

Many nuclear medicine centers are located in hospitals. A doctor who has special training in nuclear heart scans—a cardiologist or radiologist—will oversee the test. Cardiologists are doctors who specialize in diagnosing and treating heart problems. Radiologists are doctors who have special training in medical imaging techniques.

Before the test begins, the doctor or a technician will use a needle to insert an intravenous (IV) line into a vein in your arm. Through this IV line, he or she will put radioactive tracer into your bloodstream at the right time.

You also will have EKG (electrocardiogram) patches attached to your body to check your heart rate during the test. (An EKG is a simple test that detects and records the heart's electrical activity.)

During the Stress Test

If you're having an exercise stress test as part of your nuclear scan, you'll walk on a treadmill or pedal a stationary bike. During this time, you'll be attached to EKG and blood pressure monitors.

Your doctor will ask you to exercise until you're too tired to continue, short of breath, or having chest or leg pain. You can expect that your heart will beat faster, you'll breathe faster, your blood pressure will increase, and you'll sweat.

Tell your doctor if you have any chest, arm, or jaw pain or discomfort. Also, report any dizziness, light-headedness, or other unusual symptoms.

If you're unable to exercise, your doctor may give you medicine to increase your heart rate. This is called a pharmacological stress test. The medicine might make you feel anxious, sick, dizzy, or shaky for a short time. If the side effects are severe, your doctor may give you other medicine to relieve the symptoms. Before the exercise or pharmacological stress test ends, the tracer is injected through the IV line.

During the Nuclear Heart Scan

The nuclear heart scan will start shortly after the stress test. You'll lie very still on a padded table. The nuclear heart scan camera, called a gamma camera, is enclosed in metal housing. The camera can be put in several positions around your body as you lie on the padded table.

For some nuclear heart scans, the metal housing is shaped like a doughnut (with a hole in the middle). You lie on a table that slowly moves through the hole. A computer nearby or in another room collects pictures of your heart.

Usually, two sets of pictures are taken. One will be taken right after the stress test and the other will be taken after a period of rest. The pictures might be taken all in 1 day or over 2 days. Each set of pictures takes about 15–30 minutes.

Some people find it hard to stay in one position during the test. Others may feel anxious while lying in the doughnut-shaped scanner. The table may feel hard, and the room may feel chilly because of the air conditioning needed to maintain the machines.

Let your doctor or technician know how you're feeling during the test so he or she can respond as needed.

What to Expect after a Nuclear Heart Scan

Your doctor may ask you to return to the nuclear medicine center on a second day for more pictures. Outpatients will be allowed to go home after the scan or leave the nuclear medicine center between the two scans.

Most people can go back to their daily routines after a nuclear heart scan. The radioactivity will naturally leave your body in your urine or stool. It's helpful to drink plenty of fluids after the test, as your doctor advises.

The cardiologist or radiologist will read and interpret the results of your test. He or she will report the results to your doctor, who will contact you to discuss them. Or, the cardiologist or radiologist may contact you directly to discuss the results.

What Are the Risks of Nuclear Heart Scan

Nuclear heart scans have few risks. The amount of radiation in this test is small. In rare instances, some people have a treatable allergic reaction to the tracer. If you have CHD, you may have chest pain during the stress test. Medicine can help relieve your chest pain. Talk to your doctor and the technicians performing the test about whether you are or could be pregnant. If the test is not urgent, they may have you wait to do the test until after your pregnancy. Let your doctor know if you are breastfeeding because radiation can pass into your breast milk. If the test is urgent, you may want to pump and save enough breast milk for one to two days after your test, or you may bottle-feed your baby for that time.

Chapter 29

Mammograms

What Is a Mammogram?[1]

A mammogram is a low-dose X-ray exam of the breasts to look for changes that are not normal. The results are recorded on X-ray film or directly into a computer for a doctor called a radiologist to examine.

A mammogram allows the doctor to have a closer look for changes in breast tissue that cannot be felt during a breast exam. It is used for women who have no breast complaints and for women who have breast symptoms, such as a change in the shape or size of a breast, a lump, nipple discharge, or pain. Breast changes occur in almost all women. In fact, most of these changes are not cancer and are called "benign," but only a doctor can know for sure. Breast changes can also happen monthly, due to your menstrual period.

What Is the Best Method of Detecting Breast Cancer as Early as Possible?[1]

A high-quality mammogram plus a clinical breast exam, an exam done by your doctor, is the most effective way to detect breast cancer

This chapter includes text excerpted from documents published by two public domain sources. Text under the headings marked 1 are excerpted from "Mammograms," Office on Women's Health (OWH), U.S. Department of Health and Human Services (HHS), March 2, 2018; Text under the headings marked 2 are excerpted from "Frequently Asked Questions about Digital Mammography," U.S. Food and Drug Agency (FDA), November 14, 2017.

early. Finding breast cancer early greatly improves a woman's chances for successful treatment.

Like any test, mammograms have both benefits and limitations. For example, some cancers can't be found by a mammogram, but they may be found in a clinical breast exam.

Checking your own breasts for lumps or other changes is called a breast self-exam (BSE). Studies so far have not shown that BSE alone helps reduce the number of deaths from breast cancer. BSE should not take the place of routine clinical breast exams and mammograms.

If you choose to do BSE, remember that breast changes can occur because of pregnancy, aging, menopause, menstrual cycles, or from taking birth control pills or other hormones. It is normal for breasts to feel a little lumpy and uneven. Also, it is common for breasts to be swollen and tender right before or during a menstrual period. If you notice any unusual changes in your breasts, contact your doctor.

How Is a Mammogram Done?[1]

You stand in front of a special X-ray machine. The person who takes the X-rays, called a radiologic technician, places your breasts, one at a time, between an X-ray plate and a plastic plate. These plates are attached to the X-ray machine and compress the breasts to flatten them. This spreads the breast tissue out to obtain a clearer picture. You will feel pressure on your breast for a few seconds. It may cause you some discomfort; you might feel squeezed or pinched. This feeling only lasts for a few seconds, and the flatter your breast, the better the picture. Most often, two pictures are taken of each breast—one from the side and one from above. A screening mammogram takes about 20 minutes from start to finish.

Are There Different Types of Mammograms?[1]

- **Screening mammograms** are done for women who have no symptoms of breast cancer. It usually involves two X-rays of each breast. Screening mammograms can detect lumps or tumors that cannot be felt. They can also find microcalcifications or tiny deposits of calcium in the breast, which sometimes mean that breast cancer is present.

- **Diagnostic mammograms** are used to check for breast cancer after a lump or other symptom or sign of breast cancer has been found. Signs of breast cancer may include pain, thickened skin on the breast, nipple discharge, or a change in breast size or shape. This type of mammogram also can be used to find out more about breast changes found on a screening mammogram, or to view breast tissue that is hard to see on a screening mammogram. A diagnostic mammogram takes longer than a screening mammogram because it involves more X-rays in order to obtain views of the breast from several angles. The technician can magnify a problem area to make a more detailed picture, which helps the doctor make a correct diagnosis.

A digital mammogram also uses X-rays to produce an image of the breast, but instead of storing the image directly on film, the image is stored directly on a computer. This allows the recorded image to be magnified for the doctor to take a closer look. Current research has not shown that digital images are better at showing cancer than X-ray film images in general. But, women with dense breasts who are pre- or perimenopausal, or who are younger than age 50, may benefit from having a digital rather than a film mammogram. Digital mammography may offer these benefits:

- Long-distance consultations with other doctors may be easier because the images can be shared by computer.

- Slight differences between normal and abnormal tissues may be more easily noted.

- The number of follow-up tests needed may be fewer.

- Fewer repeat images may be needed, reducing exposure to radiation.

What Is Digital Mammography?[2]

Full field digital mammography (FFDM, also known simply as "digital mammography") is a mammography system where the X-ray film used in screen-film mammography is replaced by solid-state detectors, similar to those found in digital cameras, which convert X-rays into electrical signals. The electrical signals are used to produce images of the breast that can be seen on a computer screen, or printed on special films to look like screen-film mammograms. Types of digital mammography include direct radiography (the most common type, which captures the image directly onto a flat-panel detector), computed radiography (which involves the use of a cassette that contains an imaging plate), or digital breast tomosynthesis (DBT).

What Is Digital Breast Tomosynthesis?[2]

Digital breast tomosynthesis is a relatively new technology. In DBT, the X-ray tube moves in an arc around the breast and takes multiple images from different angles. Similar to computed tomography (CT scan), these images are then reconstructed into parallel "slices" through the breast. This allows interpreting physicians to see through layers of overlapping tissue.

How Often Should I Get a Mammogram?[1]

The U.S. Preventive Services Task Force (USPSTF) recommends:

- Women ages 50–74 years should get a mammogram every 2 years.

- Women younger than age 50 should talk to a doctor about when to start and how often to have a mammogram.

What Can Mammograms Show?[1]

The radiologist will look at your X-rays for breast changes that do not look normal and for differences in each breast. He or she will compare your past mammograms with your most recent one to check for changes. The doctor will also look for lumps and calcifications.

- **Lump or mass.** The size, shape, and edges of a lump sometimes can give doctors information about whether or not it may be cancer. On a mammogram, a growth that is benign often looks smooth and round with a clear, defined edge. Breast cancer often has a jagged outline and an irregular shape.

- **Calcification**. A calcification is a deposit of the mineral calcium in the breast tissue. Calcifications appear as small white spots on a mammogram. There are two types:

  - *Macrocalcifications* are large calcium deposits often caused by aging. These usually are not a sign of cancer.

  - *Microcalcifications* are tiny specks of calcium that may be found in an area of rapidly dividing cells.

If calcifications are grouped together in a certain way, it may be a sign of cancer. Depending on how many calcium specks you have, how big they are, and what they look like, your doctor may suggest that you have other tests. Calcium in the diet does not create calcium deposits, or calcifications, in the breast.

What If My Screening Mammogram Shows a Problem?[1]

If you have a screening test result that suggests cancer, your doctor must find out whether it is due to cancer or to some other cause. Your doctor may ask about your personal and family medical history. You may have a physical exam. Your doctor also may order some of these tests:

- **Diagnostic mammogram**, to focus on a specific area of the breast

- **Ultrasound**, an imaging test that uses sound waves to create a picture of your breast. The pictures may show whether a lump is solid or filled with fluid. A cyst is a fluid-filled sac. Cysts are not cancer. But a solid mass may be cancer. After the test, your doctor can store the pictures on video or print them out. This exam may be used along with a mammogram.

- **Magnetic resonance imaging (MRI)**, which uses a powerful magnet linked to a computer. MRI makes detailed pictures of breast tissue. Your doctor can view these pictures on a monitor or print them on film. MRI may be used along with a mammogram.

- Biopsy, a test in which fluid or tissue is removed from your breast to help find out if there is cancer. Your doctor may refer you to a surgeon or to a doctor who is an expert in breast disease for a biopsy.

Where Can I Get a High-Quality Mammogram?[1]

Women can get high-quality mammograms in breast clinics, hospital radiology departments, mobile vans, private radiology offices, and doctors' offices. The U.S. Food and Drug Administration (FDA) certifies mammography facilities that meet strict quality standards for their X-ray machines and staff and are inspected every year. You can ask your doctor or the staff at the mammography center about FDA certification before making your appointment.

Your doctor, local medical clinic, or local or state health department can tell you where to get no-cost or low-cost mammograms. You can also call the National Cancer Institute's (NCI) Cancer Information Service (CIS) toll-free at 800-422-6237.

What If I Have Breast Implants?[1]

Women with breast implants should also have mammograms. A woman who had an implant after breast cancer surgery in which the entire breast was removed (mastectomy) should ask her doctor whether she needs a mammogram of the reconstructed breast.

If you have breast implants, be sure to tell your mammography facility that you have them when you make your appointment. The technician and radiologist must be experienced in X-raying patients with breast implants. Implants can hide some breast tissue, making it harder for the radiologist to see a problem when looking at your mammogram. To see as much breast tissue as possible, the X-ray technician will gently lift the breast tissue slightly away from the implant and take extra pictures of the breasts.

How Do I Get Ready for My Mammogram?[1]

First, check with the place you are having the mammogram for any special instructions you may need to follow before you go. Here are some general guidelines to follow:

- If you are still having menstrual periods, try to avoid making your mammogram appointment during the week before your period. Your breasts will be less tender and swollen. The mammogram will hurt less and the picture will be better.

- If you have breast implants, be sure to tell your mammography facility that you have them when you make your appointment.

- Wear a shirt with shorts, pants, or a skirt. This way, you can undress from the waist up and leave your shorts, pants, or skirt on when you get your mammogram.

- Don't wear any deodorant, perfume, lotion, or powder under your arms or on your breasts on the day of your mammogram appointment. These things can make shadows show up on your mammogram.

- If you have had mammograms at another facility, have those X-ray films sent to the new facility so that they can be compared to the new films.

Are There Any Problems with Mammograms?[1]

Although they are not perfect, mammograms are the best method to find breast changes that cannot be felt. If your mammogram shows a breast change, sometimes other tests are needed to better understand it. Even if the doctor sees something on the mammogram, it does not mean it is cancer.

As with any medical test, mammograms have limits. These limits include:

They are only part of a complete breast exam. Your doctor also should do a clinical breast exam. If your mammogram finds something abnormal, your doctor will order other tests.

Finding cancer does not always mean saving lives. Even though mammography can detect tumors that cannot be felt, finding a small tumor does not always mean that a woman's life will be saved. Mammography may not help a woman with a fast growing cancer that has already spread to other parts of her body before being found.

False negatives can happen. This means everything may look normal, but cancer is actually present. False negatives don't happen often. Younger women are more likely to have a false negative mammogram than are older women. The dense breasts of younger women make breast cancers harder to find in mammograms.

False positives can happen. This is when the mammogram results look like cancer is present, even though it is not. False positives are more common in younger women, women who have had breast biopsies, women with a family history of breast cancer, and women who are taking estrogen, such as menopausal hormone therapy.

Mammograms (as well as dental X-rays and other routine X-rays) use very small doses of radiation. The risk of any harm is very slight, but repeated X-rays could cause cancer. The benefits nearly always outweigh the risk. Talk to your doctor about the need for each X-ray. Ask about shielding to protect parts of the body that are not in the picture. You should always let your doctor and the technician know if there is any chance that you are pregnant.

Chapter 30

Neurological Imaging

Neurological Imaging in the Past

- Neurologists and neurosurgeons made clinical decisions based on first generation computed tomography (CT) scans. This was a quantum advance over the insensitive plain film X-ray techniques of previous generations.

- Early positron emission tomography (PET) and single photon emission computed tomography (SPECT) techniques utilized first generation radiographic tracers (or tags) to map brain function.

- Functional magnetic resonance imaging (fMRI) allowed researchers to measure blood oxygen level dependent (BOLD) changes in the brain of humans for the first time. fMRI enabled the noninvasive study of everything from finger movements to thoughts and emotions.

Neurological Imaging Today

- Advanced magnetic resonance imaging (MRI) is revolutionizing the care of patients with neurologic disorders, as well as research in understanding the brain. Magnetic resonance

This chapter includes text excerpted from "Neurological Imaging," National Institutes of Health (NIH), March 29, 2013. Reviewed July 2018.

(MR) spectroscopy allows measurement of brain chemicals in living patients. PET imaging using compounds that bind to brain receptors now allows the study of molecular details not previously visualized.

- The resolution of brain and spinal cord imaging has increased tremendously. For example, modern techniques allow the neuroimaging of subtle abnormalities of neurological development that give rise to seizures and enable many more persons to benefit from a surgical treatment of epilepsy. MRI can now identify spinal vascular malformations that are amenable to treatment. Many of these went undiagnosed 30 years ago.

- Functional MRI BOLD imaging enables researchers not only to localize and measure important brain functions, but also to assess functional changes in the brain resulting from disease processes, injury, or response to treatment. fMRI is also being used to guide operative strategy in neurosurgery.

- Diffusion tensor imaging, a technique that allows for the visualization and characterization of white matter tracts in the human brain, is allowing researchers to assess changes in the brain's maturation from childhood to adulthood, as well as to detect differences in white matter integrity between healthy and diseased populations.

- Advanced diagnostics in many neurological diseases/disorders now are increasingly used as a means to monitor the progression of disease and response to treatment. For example, the development of Pittsburgh Compound B now permits the molecular imaging of the amyloid beta protein in patients with Alzheimer disease. In addition, MRI has become invaluable in the diagnosis of patients with multiple sclerosis and spinal cord disorders.

- Advanced image processing allows clinicians and researchers to measure the subtle shrinkage of brain regions over time (from chronic disease progression) and use this information to test new therapies. Furthermore, neuroimaging has made it possible to detect, characterize, and monitor objective brain changes after insults such as traumatic brain injury.

- Neuroimaging has played a crucial role in advancing understanding and treatment of stroke, and is now recommended by national guidelines for acute assessment and treatment decisions and for secondary prevention. Ongoing studies are using different forms of imaging at different time points after stroke to help hospitals better identify patients who could benefit from treatment beyond the current window.

Future of Neurological Imaging

- Advanced neuroimaging techniques will allow researchers to understand all of the structural and functional pathways in the entire, living human brain. This groundbreaking advance could lead to more accurate diagnosis and treatment of a variety of neurological and mental disorders. The NIH has launched the Human Connectome Project (www.humanconnectomeproject. org), a $30 million multi-site project that aims to understand genetic and environmental influences on brain connectivity, as well as how dysfunction in connectivity can contribute to neurological and mental conditions.

- Scientists will be able to use imaging to understand cognitive impairment in neurodegenerative diseases such as Alzheimer disease. The ongoing Alzheimer's Disease Neuroimaging Initiative (ADNI) (adni.loni.usc.edu), a multi-site, longitudinal, prospective study of normal cognitive aging, mild cognitive impairment (MCI), and early Alzheimer disease, will enable researchers to define rates of impairment, design improved methods for clinical trials, and develop more effective techniques to treat and prevent Alzheimer disease.

- In the future, scientists will be able to use neuroimaging to determine consciousness states of individuals. A series of intriguing studies has improved the clinical assessment of states such as coma, vegetative state, minimally conscious state, and locked in syndrome, providing new information about evaluation of brain function, formation of diagnoses, and estimation of prognosis.

Chapter 31

Optical Imaging

Optical imaging is a technique for noninvasively looking inside the body, as is done with X-rays. Unlike X-rays, which use ionizing radiation, optical imaging uses visible light and the special properties of photons to obtain detailed images of organs and tissues as well as smaller structures including cells and even molecules. These images are used by scientists for research and by clinicians for disease diagnosis and treatment.

What Are the Advantages of Optical Imaging?

- Optical imaging significantly reduces patient exposure to harmful radiation by using nonionizing radiation, which includes visible, ultraviolet, and infrared light. These types of light generate images by exciting electrons without causing the damage that can occur with ionizing radiation used in some other imaging techniques. Because it is much safer for patients, and significantly faster, optical imaging can be used for lengthy and repeated procedures over time to monitor the progression of disease or the results of treatment.

- Optical imaging is particularly useful for visualizing soft tissues. Soft tissues can be easily distinguished from one another due

---

This chapter includes text excerpted from "Optical Imaging," National Institute of Biomedical Imaging and Bioengineering (NIBIB), May 2016.

to the wide variety of ways different tissues absorb and scatter light. Because it can obtain images of structures across a wide range of sizes and types, optical imaging can be combined with other imaging techniques, such as MRI or X-rays, to provide enhanced information for doctors monitoring complex diseases or researchers working on intricate experiments.

- Optical imaging takes advantage of the various colors of light in order to see and measure many different properties of an organ or tissue at the same time. Other imaging techniques are limited to just one or two measurements.

What Types of Optical Imaging Are There and What Are They Used For?

- **Endoscopy:** The simplest and most widely recognized type of optical imaging is endoscopy. An endoscope consists of a flexible tube with a system to deliver light to illuminate an organ or tissue. For example, a physician can insert an endoscope through a patient's mouth to see the digestive cavity to find the cause of symptoms such as abdominal pain, difficulty swallowing, or gastrointestinal bleeding. Endoscopes are also used for minimally invasive robotic surgery to allow a surgeon to see inside the patient's body while remotely manipulating the thin robotic arms that perform the procedure.

- **Optical Coherence Tomography (OCT):** Optical coherence tomography is a technique for obtaining subsurface images such as diseased tissue just below the skin. OCT is a well-developed technology with commercially available systems now in use in a variety of applications, including art conservation and diagnostic medicine. For example, ophthalmologists use OCT to obtain detailed images from within the retina. Cardiologists also use it to help diagnose coronary artery disease.

- **Photoacoustic Imaging:** During photoacoustic imaging, laser pulses are delivered to a patient's tissues; the pulses generate heat, expanding the tissues and enabling their structure to be imaged. The technique can be used for a number of clinical applications including monitoring blood vessel growth in tumors, detecting skin melanomas, and tracking blood oxygenation in tissues.

- **Diffuse Optical Tomography (DOT):** DOT can be used to obtain information about brain activity. A laser that uses near-infrared light is positioned on the scalp. The light goes through the scalp and harmlessly traverses the brain. The absorption of light reveals information about chemical concentrations in the brain. The scattering of the light reflects physiological characteristics such as the swelling of a neuron upon activation to pass on a neural signal.

- **Raman Spectroscopy:** This technique relies on what is known as Raman scattering of visible, near-infrared, or near-ultraviolet light that is delivered by a laser. The laser light interacts with molecular vibrations in the material being examined, and shifts in energy are measured that reveal information about the properties of the material. The technique has a wide variety of applications including identifying chemical compounds and characterizing the structure of materials and crystals. In medicine, Raman gas analyzers are used to monitor anesthetic gas mixtures during surgery.

- **Super-resolution Microscopy:** This form of light microscopy encompasses a number of techniques used in research to obtain very high-resolution images of individual cells, at a level of detail not feasible using normal microscopy. One example is a technique called photoactivated localization microscopy (PALM), which uses fluorescent markers to pinpoint single molecules. PALM can be performed sequentially to create a super-resolution image from the series of molecules isolated in the sample tissue.

- **Terahertz Tomography:** This relatively new, experimental technique involves sectional imaging using terahertz radiation. Terahertz radiation consists of electromagnetic waves, which are found on the spectrum between microwaves and infrared light waves. They are of great interest to scientists because terahertz radiation can "see" what visible and infrared light cannot, and holds great promise for detecting unique information unavailable via other optical imaging methods.

What Are NIBIB-Funded Researchers Developing in the Area of Optical Imaging to Improve Biomedical Research and Medical Care?

Scanning laser microscope to identify cancer of the epithelium without painful biopsies: Scientists are building a miniature scanning laser microscope that can identify skin cancer cells and can also be attached to an endoscope (a thin illuminated tube) to examine cells on the epithelium of the oral cavity, GI tract and elsewhere. The device combines high-resolution images showing cellular detail, with wide-field color video images of the surrounding tissue. The two views will allow the clinician to see the exact position in the tissue where the microscopic images are being taken, which is essential for accurately identifying and sampling the cells most likely to be cancerous. The instrument will improve early cancer diagnosis leading to higher survival rates at lower healthcare costs.

Near-infrared brain imaging for guiding treatment in children with cerebral palsy: Cerebral palsy affects a child's ability to develop typical motor skills and to engage fully in play, and routine daily activities. Currently, treatments are tried blindly and as a result, many pediatric patients undergo futile, prolonged and taxing treatments that have no benefit. This project uses functional near infrared (fNIR) imaging to detect brain activation patterns in the cortex, located at the top of the skull. The images will allow researchers to identify strong cortical activation patterns, which indicate a positive response to therapies. Ultimately, the scientists hope to refine the system so that physicians can readily use it to assess the initial severity of cerebral palsy and help them decide which specific treatment is likely to have a positive outcome for each individual patient.

Digital holograms to test response to therapies for ovarian cancer: Ovarian cancer is often not detected until late stages when it is difficult to treat and can be fatal. Scientists are using a new technique called tissue dynamics imaging (TDI) to measure the sensitivity of ovarian tumors to chemotherapy and biological treatments. TDI constructs 3D holograms inside ovarian cancer tissue samples that measure cellular function and growth of tumors in response to drug treatments. The method predicts the clinical outcome expected following each round of treatment and determines the best subsequent treatment. The approach of analyzing the changing cellular properties of ovarian tumor tissue is designed to determine the optimal therapy for each patient. The ultimate goal is to establish TDI as a novel drug-response monitoring system that could transform personalized ovarian cancer care.

Optical imaging includes a variety of techniques that use light to obtain images from inside the body, tissues or cells.

Part Four

Catheterization, Endoscopic, and Electrical Tests and Assessments

Chapter 32

Cardiac Catheterization

What Is Cardiac Catheterization?

Cardiac catheterization is a medical procedure used to diagnose and treat some heart conditions.

A long, thin, flexible tube called a catheter is put into a blood vessel in your arm, groin (upper thigh), or neck and threaded to your heart. Through the catheter, your doctor can do diagnostic tests and treatments on your heart.

For example, your doctor may put a special type of dye into the catheter. The dye will flow through your bloodstream to your heart. Then, your doctor will take X-ray pictures of your heart. The dye will make your coronary (heart) arteries visible on the pictures. This test is called coronary angiography.

The dye can show whether a waxy substance called plaque has built up inside your coronary arteries. Plaque can narrow or block the arteries and restrict blood flow to your heart.

The buildup of plaque in the coronary arteries is called coronary heart disease (CHD) or coronary artery disease (CAD).

Doctors also can use ultrasound during cardiac catheterization to see blockages in the coronary arteries. Ultrasound uses sound waves to create detailed pictures of the heart's blood vessels.

Doctors may take samples of blood and heart muscle during cardiac catheterization or do minor heart surgery.

This chapter includes text excerpted from "Cardiac Catheterization," National Heart, Lung, and Blood Institute (NHLBI), April 26, 2013. Reviewed July 2018.

Cardiologists (heart specialists) usually do cardiac catheterization in a hospital. You're awake during the procedure, and it causes little or no pain. However, you may feel some soreness in the blood vessel where the catheter was inserted.

Cardiac catheterization rarely causes serious complications.

Who Needs Cardiac Catheterization?

Doctors may recommend cardiac catheterization for various reasons. The most common reason is to evaluate chest pain.

Chest pain might be a symptom of CHD. Cardiac catheterization can show whether plaque is narrowing or blocking your coronary arteries.

Doctors also can treat CHD during cardiac catheterization using a procedure called percutaneous coronary intervention (PCI), also known as coronary angioplasty.

During PCI, a catheter with a balloon at its tip is threaded to the blocked coronary artery. Once in place, the balloon is inflated, pushing the plaque against the artery wall. This creates a wider path for blood to flow to the heart.

Sometimes a stent is placed in the artery during PCI. A stent is a small mesh tube that supports the inner artery wall.

Most people who have heart attacks have narrow or blocked coronary arteries. Thus, cardiac catheterization might be used as an emergency procedure to treat a heart attack. When used with PCI, the procedure allows your doctor to open up blocked arteries and prevent further heart damage.

Cardiac catheterization also can help your doctor figure out the best treatment plan for you if:

- You recently recovered from a heart attack, but are having chest pain

- You had a heart attack that caused major heart damage

- You had an EKG (electrocardiogram), stress test, or other tests with results that suggested heart disease

Cardiac catheterization also might be used if your doctor thinks you have a heart defect or if you're about to have heart surgery. The procedure shows the overall shape of your heart and the four large spaces (heart chambers) inside it. This inside view of the heart will show certain heart defects and help your doctor plan your heart surgery.

Sometimes doctors use cardiac catheterization to see how well the heart valves work. Valves control blood flow in your heart. They open and shut to allow blood to flow between your heart chambers and into your arteries.

Your doctor can use cardiac catheterization to measure blood flow and oxygen levels in different parts of your heart. He or she also can check how well a human-made heart valve is working and how well your heart is pumping blood.

If your doctor thinks you have a heart infection or tumor, he or she may take samples of your heart muscle through the catheter. With the help of cardiac catheterization, doctors can even do minor heart surgery, such as repair certain heart defects.

What to Expect before Cardiac Catheterization

Before having cardiac catheterization, discuss with your doctor:

- How to prepare for the procedure

- Any medicines you're taking, and whether you should stop taking them before the procedure

- Whether you have any conditions (such as diabetes or kidney disease) that may require taking extra steps during or after the procedure to avoid problems

Your doctor will let you know whether you need to arrange for a ride home after the procedure.

What to Expect during Cardiac Catheterization

Cardiac catheterization is done in a hospital. During the procedure, you'll be kept on your back and awake. This allows you to follow your doctor's instructions during the procedure. You'll be given medicine to help you relax, which might make you sleepy.

Your doctor will numb the area on the arm, groin (upper thigh), or neck where the catheter will enter your blood vessel. Then, a needle will be used to make a small hole in the blood vessel. Your doctor will put a tapered tube called a sheath through the hole.

Next, your doctor will put a thin, flexible guide wire through the sheath and into your blood vessel. He or she will thread the wire through your blood vessel to your heart.

Your doctor will use the guide wire to correctly place the catheter. He or she will put the catheter through the sheath and slide it over the guide wire and into the coronary arteries.

343

Special X-ray movies will be taken off the guide wire and the catheter as they're moved into the heart. The movies will help your doctor see where to put the tip of the catheter.

When the catheter reaches the right spot, your doctor will use it to do tests or treatments on your heart. For example, your doctor may perform a PCI, also known as coronary angioplasty, and stenting.

During the procedure, your doctor may put a special type of dye into the catheter. The dye will flow through your bloodstream to your heart. Then, your doctor will take X-ray pictures of your heart. The dye will make your coronary (heart) arteries visible on the pictures. This test is called coronary angiography.

Coronary angiography can show how well the heart's lower chambers, called the ventricles, are pumping blood.

When the catheter is inside your heart, your doctor may use it to take blood and tissue samples or do minor heart surgery.

To get a more detailed view of a blocked coronary artery, your doctor may do an intracoronary ultrasound. For this test, your doctor will thread a tiny ultrasound device through the catheter and into the artery. This device gives off sound waves that bounce off the artery wall (and its blockage). The sound waves create a picture of the inside of the artery.

If the angiogram or intracoronary ultrasound shows blockages in the coronary arteries, your doctor may use PCI to treat the blocked arteries.

After your doctor does all of the needed tests or treatments, he or she will pull back the catheter and take it out along with the sheath. The opening left in the blood vessel will be closed up and bandaged.

A small weight might be put on top of the bandage for a few hours to apply more pressure. This will help prevent major bleeding from the site.

What to Expect after Cardiac Catheterization

After cardiac catheterization, you will be moved to a special care area. You will rest there for several hours or overnight. During that time, you'll have to limit your movement to avoid bleeding from the site where the catheter was inserted.

While you recover in this area, nurses will check your heart rate and blood pressure regularly. They also will check for bleeding from the catheter insertion site.

A small bruise might form at the catheter insertion site, and the area may feel sore or tender for about a week. Let your doctor know if you have problems such as:

- A constant or large amount of bleeding at the insertion site that can't be stopped with a small bandage

- Unusual pain, swelling, redness, or other signs of infection at or near the insertion site

Talk to your doctor about whether you should avoid certain activities, such as heavy lifting, for a short time after the procedure.

What Are the Risks of Cardiac Catheterization?

Cardiac catheterization is a common medical procedure. It rarely causes serious problems. However, complications can include:

- Bleeding, infection, and pain at the catheter insertion site

- Damage to blood vessels. Rarely, the catheter may scrape or poke a hole in a blood vessel as it's threaded to the heart.

- An allergic reaction to the dye that's used during coronary angiography

Other, less common complications include:

- Arrhythmias (irregular heartbeats). These irregular heartbeats often go away on their own. However, your doctor may recommend treatment if they persist.

- Kidney damage caused by the dye used during coronary angiography

- Blood clots that can trigger a stroke, heart attack, or other serious problems

- Low blood pressure

- A buildup of blood or fluid in the sac that surrounds the heart. This fluid can prevent the heart from beating properly.

As with any procedure involving the heart, complications sometimes can be fatal. However, this is rare with cardiac catheterization.

The risks of cardiac catheterization are higher in people who are older and in those who have certain diseases or conditions (such as chronic kidney disease (CKD) and diabetes).

Chapter 33

Endoscopy

Chapter Contents

Section 33.1

Endoscopy Overview

This section includes text excerpted from "Endoscopy,"
National Cancer Institute (NCI), December 3, 2016.

An endoscopic exam involves using an instrument, inserted into natural openings or man-made openings, to examine internal passages or the inside of hollow organs or viscera. This can be effective in the nasopharynx, larynx, esophagus, stomach, large bowel, bladder and parts of the lungs. The common endoscopic procedures used in diagnosis are listed in the table below.

Table 33.1. Common Endoscopic Examinations

Examination	Site Examined
bronchoscopy	bronchi
colonoscopy	colon and rectum
cystoscopy	urinary bladder
esophagoscopy	esophagus
gastroscopy	stomach
laryngoscopy	larynx
nasopharyngoscopy	nasopharynx, pharynx
ophthalmoscopy	interior of the eye
panendoscopy	urinary bladder and urethra
proctoscopy	rectum
sigmoidoscopy	colon up to sigmoid flexure

A bronchoscopy is the examination of the bronchi in the lungs. The scope can be inserted through the oral or nasal cavity. The pharynx, larynx, and trachea can be seen as the bronchoscope goes through to the bronchi. Using the flexible bronchoscope, the interior segmental and subsegmental bronchi can be visualized. The endoscopist looks for irregular bronchial folds, mucosal thickening, stenosis, friable tissue, and many other abnormalities such a tumor mass. Normally, biopsies bronchial washings are obtained during a bronchoscopic exam. A proctoscopy is often done using a rigid scope.

A sigmoidoscope is more flexible and can be used to observe the colon, up into the descending colon at greater than 30 cm. In the past, rigid sigmoidoscopes were often used but they have been replaced with flexible sigmoidoscopes. Flexible scopes allow greater visualization of the sigmoid colon. A fiberoptic colonoscope is a flexible instrument that examines the colon to the cecum. Often, the physician will photograph and biopsy any abnormalities or suspicious areas seen during colonoscopy.

A cystoscope is used to examine the interior of the bladder. It is inserted through the urethra, so the urethra can also be examined. Abnormalities can be surgically removed or electrocauterized during the cystoscopic procedure.

The entire endoscopic procedure report must be read to obtain pertinent information. Endoscopic reports define certain observations, tumor location, pertinent findings, diagnosis, or the impressions of the condition. For example, colonoscopy reports should state the distance of the abnormality from the anal verge. Esophagoscopy reports should state the distance of the abnormality from the incisors to help determine the exact location of the tumor. Any biopsies or washings sent for microscopic examination should be noted. It is important to locate copies of the pathology and cytology reports to confirm the diagnosis of the disease.

Some endoscopic procedures can be accomplished through natural openings in the body. Others must be performed through incisions into the body. For example, thoracoscopy is used to examine the pleural cavity. The instrument is inserted through an intercostal space. Mediastinoscopy is performed through an incision in the neck and allows visualization of the area between the lungs.

Laparoscopy, performed through an incision in the abdominal wall, allows the visualization of intra-abdominal structures. Laparoscopy is useful in gastrointestinal and gynecologic malignancies to diagnose both the primary organ and metastatic involvement. Needle biopsies of the liver are often done under the direct visualization of the laparoscope. Some surgeries can be completed as laparoscopic or laparoscope-aided procedures.

Section 33.2

Bronchoscopy

This section includes text excerpted from "Bronchoscopy,"
National Heart, Lung, and Blood Institute (NHLBI),
December 10, 2016.

Bronchoscopy is a procedure that looks inside the lung airways. It involves inserting a bronchoscope tube, with its light and small camera, through your nose or mouth, down your throat into your trachea, or windpipe, and to the bronchi and bronchioles of your lungs.

What Does Bronchoscopy Show?

Bronchoscopy may show a tumor, signs of an infection, excess mucus in the airways, the site of bleeding, or something blocking your airway. Your doctor will use the procedure results to decide how to treat any lung problems that were found. Other tests may be needed.

Who Needs Bronchoscopy?

The most common reason why your doctor may decide to do a bronchoscopy is if you have an abnormal chest X-ray or chest computed tomography (CT) scan. These tests may show a tumor, a pneumothorax (collapsed lung), or signs of an infection.

A chest X-ray takes a picture of your heart and lungs. A chest CT scan uses special X-rays to take pictures of the inside of your body. Other reasons for bronchoscopy include if you're coughing up blood or if you have a cough that has lasted more than a few weeks.

The procedure also can be done to remove something that's stuck in an airway (like a piece of food), to place medicine in a lung to treat a lung problem, or to insert a stent (small tube) in an airway to hold it open when a tumor or other condition causes a blockage.

Bronchoscopy also can be used to check for swelling in the upper airways and vocal cords of people who were burned around the throat area or who inhaled smoke from a fire. In children, the procedure most often is used to remove something blocking an airway. In some cases, it's used to find out what's causing a cough that has lasted for at least a few weeks.

350

What to Expect before Bronchoscopy?

Your doctor will do the bronchoscopy in a special clinic or in a hospital. To prepare for the procedure, tell your doctor:

- What medicines you're taking, including prescription and over-the-counter (OTC) medicines. It's helpful to give your doctor a list of the medicines you take.

- About any previous bleeding problems

- About any allergies to medicines or latex

The medicine you'll get before the procedure will make you sleepy, so you should arrange for a ride home from the clinic or hospital. Avoid eating or drinking for 4–8 hours before the procedure. Your doctor will let you know the right amount of time.

What to Expect during Bronchoscopy?

Your doctor will do the bronchoscopy in an exam room at a special clinic or in a hospital. The bronchoscopy itself usually lasts about 30 minutes. But the entire procedure, including preparation and recovery time, takes about 4 hours.

Your doctor will give you medicine through an intravenous (IV) line in your bloodstream or by mouth to make you sleepy and relaxed. Your doctor also will squirt or spray a liquid medicine into your nose and throat to make them numb. This helps prevent coughing and gagging when the bronchoscope (long, thin tube) is inserted.

Then, your doctor will insert the bronchoscope through your nose or mouth and into your airways. As the tube enters your mouth, you may gag a little. Once it enters your throat, that feeling will go away.

Your doctor will look at your vocal cords and airways through the bronchoscope (which has a light and a small camera). The doctor inserts a bronchoscope into a patient's nose and passes it down into the airways. This allows the doctor to look inside the airways. During the procedure, your doctor may take a sample of lung fluid or tissue for further testing. Samples can be taken using:

- **Bronchoalveolar lavage.** For this method, your doctor passes a small amount of salt water (a saline solution) through the bronchoscope and into part of your lung. He or she then suctions the salt water back out. The fluid picks up cells and bacteria from the airway, which your doctor can study.

- **Transbronchial lung biopsy.** For this method, your doctor inserts forceps into the bronchoscope and takes a small sample of tissue from inside the lung.

- **Transbronchial needle aspiration.** For this method, your doctor inserts a needle into the bronchoscope and removes cells from the lymph nodes in your lungs. These nodes are small, bean-shaped masses. They trap bacteria and cancer cells and help fight infection.

You may feel short of breath during bronchoscopy, but enough air is getting to your lungs. Your doctor will check your oxygen level. If the level drops, you'll be given oxygen.

If you have a lot of bleeding in your lungs or a large object stuck in your throat, your doctor may use a bronchoscope with a rigid tube. The rigid tube, which is passed through the mouth, is wider. This allows your doctor to see inside it more easily, treat bleeding, and remove stuck objects.

A rigid bronchoscopy usually is done in a hospital operating room using general anesthesia. The term "anesthesia" refers to a loss of feeling and awareness. General anesthesia temporarily puts you to sleep.

After the procedure is done, your doctor will remove the bronchoscope.

What to Expect after Bronchoscopy?

After bronchoscopy, you'll need to stay at the clinic or hospital for up to a few hours. If your doctor uses a bronchoscope with a rigid tube, the recovery time is longer. While you're at the clinic or hospital:

- You may have a chest X-ray if your doctor took a sample of lung tissue. This test will check for a pneumothorax and bleeding. A pneumothorax is a condition in which air or gas collects in the space around the lungs. This can cause one or both lungs to collapse. Usually, this condition is easily treated.

- A nurse will check your breathing and blood pressure

- You can't eat or drink until the numbness in your throat wears off. This takes 1–2 hours.

After recovery, you'll need to have someone take you home. You'll be too sleepy to drive.

If samples of tissue or fluid were taken during the procedure, they'll be tested in a lab. Talk to your doctor about when you'll get the lab results.

Recovery and Recuperation

Your doctor will let you know when you can return to your normal activities, such as driving, working, and physical activity. For the first few days, you may have a sore throat, cough, and hoarseness. Call your doctor right away if you:

- Develop a fever

- Have chest pain

- Have trouble breathing

- Cough up more than a few tablespoons of blood

What Are the Risks of Bronchoscopy?

Bronchoscopy usually is a safe procedure. However, there's a small risk for problems, such as:

- A drop in your oxygen level during the procedure. Your doctor will give you oxygen if this happens.

- Minor bleeding and developing a fever or pneumonia

A rare, but more serious side effect is a pneumothorax. A pneumothorax is a condition in which air or gas collects in the space around the lungs. This can cause one or both lungs to collapse.

Usually, this condition is easily treated or may go away on its own. If it interferes with breathing, a tube may need to be placed in the space around the lungs to remove the air.

A chest X-ray may be done after bronchoscopy to check for problems.

Section 33.3

Capsule Endoscopy

"Capsule Endoscopy," © 2018 Omnigraphics.
Reviewed July 2018.

What Is Capsule Endoscopy?

Capsule endoscopy is a tested method for screening polyps. The procedure allows physicians to examine a patient's gastrointestinal (GI) tract through the use of a wireless, pill-sized camera, also known as capsule enteroscopy. The camera has a light source of its own and captures images of the intestines, which are then passed to a small recording device attached to your waist.

Why Is Capsule Endoscopy Done?

Capsule endoscopy is recommended by your doctor in the following cases:

- Follow-up testing after X-rays or other imaging tests
- Gastrointestinal bleeding
- Ulcers
- Screening for polyps
- Inflammatory bowel disease, such as Crohn's disease
- Celiac disease
- Tumors or cancer

Risk Factors for Capsule Endoscopy

Capsule endoscopy is considered a safe procedure although complications are possible:

- If the capsule gets stuck in the digestive tract
- In the case of Crohn's disease or a previous surgery in the digestive tract
- If the following problems arise after swallowing the capsule, call your health provider immediately:
  - Chest pain, cramping, or abdominal pain

- Trouble swallowing

- Vomiting or indigestion

- Fever

How to Prepare for a Capsule Endoscopy?

Your doctor will give you specific instructions on how to prepare for a capsule endoscopy:

- **Avoid consumption of food or beverages for 12 hours before the procedure.** This will ensure quality images of your digestive tract.

- **Stop taking certain medications.** Your doctor may instruct you to specifically stop taking certain medicines that may interfere with the procedure.

- **Plan to take it easy for the day.** In most cases, you will be allowed to resume regular activities after you've swallowed the camera capsule. However, heavy lifting and strenuous exercises must be avoided.

The Procedure

The pill-sized capsule is about an inch long and less than half inch wide. The capsule has a slippery coating that makes it easier to swallow. A recorder is placed on your waist or shoulder and adhesive patches are attached to your abdomen. Each patch has an antenna that receives signals from the capsule and connects to the recorder. The recorder collects and stores the images that a physician uses later to examine your GI tract.

Generally, a physician will permit you to drink fluids after two hours and to consume food after four hours. The procedure is, however, completed only after eight hours when the physician removes the patches and the recorder from your body. The capsule will leave your body later during a bowel movement; however, it is important to inform your physician if this has not happened within two weeks.

Following the procedure, your doctor will give you specific instructions (such as avoiding strenuous physical activities). In most cases, the results of the test will be given to you a week after the procedure, although some tests may take a little longer.

Results

The images saved on the recorder are transferred to your physician via software and made available to your physician as individual images and as images that have been strung together to create a video. Your physician may take a week or more to analyze these results, and will share them with you once analysis is complete.

Normal Result

If no problems were revealed during your test, then your result is normal.

Abnormal Result

If a problem with your digestive tract was discovered during the test, then your physician will discuss this result and further courses of treatment with you.

References

1. "Capsule Endoscopy," Mayo Clinic, January 10, 2018.

2. "Understanding Capsule Endoscopy," American Society for Gastrointestinal Endoscopy (ASGE), February 9, 2017.

3. "Capsule Endoscopy," MedlinePlus, National Institutes of Health (NIH), April 30, 2018.

Section 33.4

Colonoscopy

This section includes text excerpted from "Colonoscopy,"
National Institute of Diabetes and Digestive and Kidney
Diseases (NIDDK), July 2017.

What Is Colonoscopy?

Colonoscopy is a procedure in which a doctor uses a colonoscope or scope, to look inside your rectum and colon. Colonoscopy can show irritated and swollen tissue, ulcers, polyps, and cancer.

How Is Virtual Colonoscopy Different from Colonoscopy?

Virtual colonoscopy and colonoscopy are different in several ways:

- Virtual colonoscopy is an X-ray test, takes less time, and you don't need anesthesia

- With virtual colonoscopy, your doctor doesn't view the entire length of your colon

- Virtual colonoscopy may not find certain polyps as easily as a colonoscopy can

- Doctors can't remove polyps or treat certain other problems during a virtual colonoscopy

- Your health insurance coverage may be different for the two procedures

Why Do Doctors Use Colonoscopy?

A colonoscopy can help a doctor find the cause of symptoms, such as:

- Bleeding from your anus

- Changes in your bowel activity, such as diarrhea

- Pain in your abdomen

- Unexplained weight loss

Doctors also use colonoscopy as a screening tool for colon polyps and cancer. Screening is testing for diseases when you have no symptoms.

Screening may find diseases at an early stage, when a doctor has a better chance of curing the disease.

Screening for Colon and Rectal Cancer

Your doctor will recommend screening for colon and rectal cancer—also called colorectal cancer—starting at age 50 if you don't have health problems or risk factors that make you more likely to develop colon cancer.

You have risk factors for colorectal cancer if you

- are male
- are African American or
- someone in your family has had polyps or colorectal cancer
- have a personal history of inflammatory bowel disease (IBD), such as ulcerative colitis (UC) and Crohn's disease
- have Lynch syndrome, or another genetic disorder that increases the risk of colorectal cancer
- have other factors, such as that you weigh too much or smoke cigarettes

If you are more likely to develop colorectal cancer, your doctor may recommend screening at a younger age, and more often.

If you are older than age 75, talk with your doctor about whether you should be screened.

Government health insurance plans, such as Medicare, and private insurance plans sometimes change whether and how often they pay for cancer screening tests. Check with your insurance plan to find out how often your plan will cover a screening colonoscopy.

What Preparation Is Required for Undergoing Colonoscopy?

To prepare for a colonoscopy, you will need to talk with your doctor, change your diet for a few days, clean out your bowel, and arrange for a ride home after the procedure.

Talk with Your Doctor

You should talk with your doctor about any health problems you have and all prescribed and over-the-counter (OTC) medicines, vitamins, and supplements you take, including:

- Arthritis medicines

- Aspirin or medicines that contain aspirin

- Blood thinners

- Diabetes medicines

- Nonsteroidal anti-inflammatory drugs (NSAIDs) such as ibuprofen or naproxen

- Vitamins that contain iron or iron supplements

Change Your Diet and Clean out Your Bowel

A healthcare professional will give you written bowel prep instructions to follow at home before the procedure so that little or no stool remains in your intestine. A complete bowel prep lets you pass stool that is clear and liquid. Stool inside your intestine can prevent your doctor from clearly seeing the lining.

You may need to follow a clear liquid diet for 1–3 days before the procedure. You should avoid red and purple-colored drinks or gelatin. The instructions will include details about when to start and stop the clear liquid diet. In most cases, you may drink or eat the following:

- Fat-free bouillon or broth

- Gelatin in flavors such as lemon, lime, or orange

- Plain coffee or tea, without cream or milk

- Sports drinks in flavors such as lemon, lime, or orange

- Strained fruit juice, such as apple or white grape—avoid orange juice

- Water

Different bowel preps may contain different combinations of laxatives—pills that you swallow or powders that you dissolve in water or clear liquids. Some people will need to drink a large amount, often a gallon, of liquid laxative over a scheduled amount of time—most often the night before and the morning of the procedure. Your doctor may also prescribe an enema.

The bowel prep will cause diarrhea, so you should stay close to a bathroom. You may find this part of the bowel prep hard; however, finishing the prep is very important. Call a healthcare professional if you have side effects that keep you from finishing the prep.

Your doctor will tell you how long before the procedure you should have nothing by mouth.

Arrange for a Ride Home

For safety reasons, you can't drive for 24 hours after the procedure, as the sedatives or anesthesia need time to wear off. You will need to make plans for getting a ride home after the procedure.

How Do Doctors Perform a Colonoscopy?

A doctor performs a colonoscopy in a hospital or an outpatient center. A colonoscopy usually takes 30–60 minutes.

A healthcare professional will place an intravenous (IV) needle in a vein in your arm or hand to give you sedatives, anesthesia, or pain medicine, so you won't be aware or feel pain during the procedure. The healthcare staff will check your vital signs and keep you as comfortable as possible.

For the procedure, you'll lie on a table while the doctor inserts a colonoscope through your anus and into your rectum and colon. The scope inflates your large intestine with air for a better view. The camera sends a video image to a monitor, allowing the doctor to examine your large intestine.

The doctor may move you several times on the table to adjust the scope for better viewing. Once the scope reaches the opening to your small intestine, the doctor slowly removes the scope and examines the lining of your large intestine again.

During the procedure, the doctor may remove polyps and will send them to a lab for testing. You will not feel the polyp removal. Colon polyps are common in adults and are harmless in most cases. However, most colon cancer begins as a polyp, so removing polyps early helps to prevent cancer.

If your doctor finds abnormal tissue, he or she may perform a biopsy. You won't feel the biopsy.

What to Expect after a Colonoscopy

After a colonoscopy, you can expect the following:

- The anesthesia takes time to wear off completely. You'll stay at the hospital or outpatient center for 1–2 hours after the procedure.

- You may feel cramping in your abdomen or bloating during the first hour after the procedure.

- After the procedure, you—or a friend or family member— will receive instructions on how to care for yourself after the procedure. You should follow all instructions.

- You'll need your prearranged ride home, since you won't be able to drive after the procedure.

- You should expect a full recovery and return to your normal diet by the next day.

After the sedatives or anesthesia wear off, your doctor may share what was found during the procedure with you or, if you choose, with a friend or family member.

If the doctor removed polyps or performed a biopsy, you may have light bleeding from your anus. This bleeding is normal. A pathologist will examine the biopsy tissue, and results take a few days or longer to come back. A healthcare professional will call you or schedule an appointment to go over the results.

What Are the Risks of Colonoscopy?

The risks of colonoscopy include:

- Bleeding

- Perforation of the colon

- A reaction to the sedative, including breathing or heart problems

- Severe pain in your abdomen

- Death, although this risk is rare

A study of screening colonoscopies found roughly 4–8 serious complications for every 10,000 procedures.

Bleeding and perforation are the most common complications from colonoscopy. Most cases of bleeding occur in patients who have polyps removed. The doctor can treat bleeding that happens during the colonoscopy right away.

You may have delayed bleeding up to 2 weeks after the procedure. The doctor can diagnose and treat delayed bleeding with a repeat colonoscopy. The doctor may need to treat perforation with surgery.

Seek Care Right Away

If you have any of the following symptoms after a colonoscopy, seek medical care right away:

- Severe pain in your abdomen

- Fever

- Bloody bowel movements that do not get better

- Bleeding from the anus that does not stop

- Dizziness

- Weakness

Section 33.5

Cystoscopy and Ureteroscopy

This section includes text excerpted from "Cystoscopy and Ureteroscopy," National Institute of Diabetes and Digestive and Kidney Diseases (NIDDK), June 2015.

What Are Cystoscopy and Ureteroscopy?

Cystoscopy and ureteroscopy are common procedures performed by a urologist to look inside the urinary tract. A urologist is a doctor who specializes in urinary tract problems.

Cystoscopy. Cystoscopy uses a cystoscope to look inside the urethra and bladder. A cystoscope is a long, thin optical instrument with an eyepiece at one end, a rigid or flexible tube in the middle, and a tiny lens and light at the other end of the tube. By looking through the cystoscope, the urologist can see detailed images of the lining of the urethra and bladder. The urethra and bladder are part of the urinary tract.

Ureteroscopy. Ureteroscopy uses a ureteroscope to look inside the ureters and kidneys. Like a cystoscope, a ureteroscope has an eyepiece at one end, a rigid or flexible tube in the middle, and a tiny lens and light at the other end of the tube. However, a ureteroscope is longer and thinner than a cystoscope so the urologist can see detailed images of the lining of the ureters and kidneys. The ureters and kidneys are also part of the urinary tract.

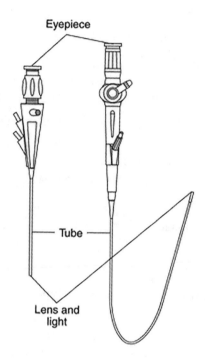

Figure 33.1. *Rigid Cystoscope and Flexible Ureteroscope*

Why Is a Cystoscopy or Ureteroscopy Performed?

A urologist performs a cystoscopy or ureteroscopy to find the cause of, and sometimes treat, urinary tract problems.

Cystoscopy. A urologist performs a cystoscopy to find the cause of urinary tract problems such as:

- Frequent urinary tract infections (UTIs)

- Hematuria—blood in the urine

- Urinary frequency—urination eight or more times a day

- Urinary urgency—the inability to delay urination

- Urinary retention—the inability to empty the bladder completely

- Urinary incontinence—the accidental loss of urine

- Pain or burning before, during, or after urination

- Trouble starting urination, completing urination, or both

- Abnormal cells, such as cancer cells, found in a urine sample

During a cystoscopy, a urologist can see:

- Stones—solid pieces of material in the bladder that may have formed in the kidneys or in the bladder when substances that are normally in the urine become highly concentrated

- Abnormal tissue, polyps, tumors, or cancer in the urethra or bladder

- Stricture, a narrowing of the urethra. Stricture can be a sign of an enlarged prostate in men or of scar tissue in the urethra.

During a cystoscopy, a urologist can treat problems such as bleeding in the bladder and blockage in the urethra. A urologist may also use a cystoscopy to:

- Remove a stone in the bladder or urethra

- Remove or treat abnormal tissue, polyps, and some types of tumors

- Take small pieces of urethral or bladder tissue for examination with a microscope—a procedure called a biopsy

- Inject material into the wall of the urethra to treat urinary leakage

- Inject medication into the bladder to treat urinary leakage

- Obtain urine samples from the ureters

- Perform retrograde pyelography—an X-ray procedure in which a urologist injects a special dye, called contrast medium, into a ureter to the kidney to create images of urinary flow. The test can show causes of obstruction, such as kidney stones and tumors.

- Remove a stent that was placed in the ureter after a ureteroscopy with biopsy or stone removal. A stent is a small, soft tube.

Ureteroscopy. In addition to the causes of urinary tract problems he or she can find with a cystoscope, a urologist performs a ureteroscopy to find the cause of urine blockage in a ureter or to evaluate other abnormalities inside the ureters or kidneys.

During a ureteroscopy, a urologist can see:

• A stone in a ureter or kidney

• Abnormal tissue, polyps, tumors, or cancer in a ureter or in the lining of a kidney

During a ureteroscopy, a urologist can treat problems such as urine blockage in a ureter. The urologist can also:

• Remove a from a ureter or kidney

• Remove or treat stone abnormal tissue, polyps, and some types of tumors

• Perform a biopsy of a ureter or kidney

After a ureteroscopy, the urologist may need to place a stent in a ureter to drain urine from the kidney to the bladder while swelling in the ureter goes away. The stent, which is completely inside the body, may cause some discomfort in the kidney or bladder area. The discomfort is generally mild. The stent may be left in the ureter for a few days to a week or more. The urologist may need to perform a cystoscopy to remove the stent in the ureter.

How Does a Patient Prepare for a Cystoscopy or Ureteroscopy?

In many cases, a patient does not need special preparations for a cystoscopy. A healthcare provider may ask the patient to drink plenty of liquids before the procedure, as well as urinate immediately before the procedure.

The patient may need to give a urine sample to test for a UTI. If the patient has a UTI, the urologist may treat the infection with antibiotics before performing a cystoscopy or ureteroscopy. A healthcare provider will provide instructions before the cystoscopy or ureteroscopy. These instructions may include:

• When to stop certain medications, such as blood thinners

• When to stop eating and drinking

- When to empty the bladder before the procedure

- Arranging for a ride home after the procedure

The urologist will ask about the patient's medical history, current prescription and over-the-counter (OTC) medications, and allergies to medications, including anesthetics. The urologist will talk about which anesthetic is best for the procedure and explain what the patient can expect after the procedure.

How Is a Cystoscopy or Ureteroscopy Performed?

A urologist performs a cystoscopy or ureteroscopy during an office visit or in an outpatient center or a hospital. For some patients, the urologist will apply an anesthetic gel around the urethral opening or inject a local anesthetic into the urethra. Some patients may require sedation or general anesthesia. The urologist often gives patients sedatives and general anesthesia for a:

- Ureteroscopy

- Cystoscopy with biopsy

- Cystoscopy to inject material into the wall of the urethra

- Cystoscopy to inject medication into the bladder

For sedation and general anesthesia, a nurse or technician places an intravenous (IV) needle in a vein in the arm or hand to give the medication. Sedation helps the patient relax and be comfortable. General anesthesia puts the patient into a deep sleep during the procedure. The medical staff will monitor the patient's vital signs and try to make him or her as comfortable as possible. During both procedures, a woman will lie on her back with the knees up and spread apart. During a cystoscopy, a man can lie on his back or be in a sitting position.

After the anesthetic has taken effect, the urologist gently inserts the tip of the cystoscope or ureteroscope into the urethra and slowly glides it through the urethra and into the bladder. A sterile liquid—water or salt water, called saline—flows through the cystoscope or ureteroscope to slowly fill the bladder and stretch it so the urologist has a better view of the bladder wall. As the bladder fills with liquid, the patient may feel some discomfort and the urge to urinate. The urologist may remove some of the liquid from the bladder during the procedure. As soon as the procedure is over, the urologist may remove the liquid from the bladder or the patient may empty the bladder.

For a cystoscopy, the urologist examines the lining of the urethra as he or she passes the cystoscope into the bladder. The urologist then examines the lining of the bladder. The urologist can insert small instruments through the to treat problems in the urethra and bladder or perform a biopsy.

For a ureteroscopy, the urologist passes the ureteroscope through the bladder and into a ureter. The urologist then examines the lining of the ureter. He or she may pass the ureteroscope all the way up into the kidney. The urologist can insert small instruments through the ureteroscope to treat problems in the ureter or kidney or perform a biopsy.

When a urologist performs a cystoscopy or a ureteroscopy to make a diagnosis, both procedures—including preparation—take 15–30 minutes. The time may be longer if the urologist removes a stone in the bladder or a ureter or if he or she performs a biopsy.

What Can a Patient Expect after a Cystoscopy or Ureteroscopy?

After a cystoscopy or ureteroscopy, a patient may:

- Have a mild burning feeling when urinating

- See small amounts of blood in the urine

- Have mild discomfort in the bladder area or kidney area when urinating

- Need to urinate more frequently or urgently

These problems should not last more than 24 hours. The patient should tell a healthcare provider right away if bleeding or pain is severe or if problems last more than a day.

The healthcare provider may recommend that the patient:

- Drink 16 ounces of water each hour for 2 hours after the procedure

- Take a warm bath to relieve the burning feeling

- Hold a warm, damp washcloth over the urethral opening to relieve discomfort

- Take an OTC pain reliever

The healthcare provider may prescribe an antibiotic to take for 1 or 2 days to prevent an infection. A patient should report any signs of infection—including severe pain, chills, or fever—right away to the healthcare provider.

Most patients go home the same day as the procedure. Recovery depends on the type of anesthesia. A patient who receives only a local anesthetic can go home immediately. A patient who receives general anesthesia may have to wait 1–4 hours before going home. A healthcare provider usually asks the patient to urinate before leaving. In some cases, the patient may need to stay overnight in the hospital. A healthcare provider will provide discharge instructions for rest, driving, and physical activities after the procedure.

What Are the Risks of Cystoscopy and Ureteroscopy?

The risks of cystoscopy and ureteroscopy include:

- UTIs
- Abnormal bleeding
- Abdominal pain
- A burning feeling or pain during urination
- Injury to the urethra, bladder, or ureters
- Urethral narrowing due to scar tissue formation
- The inability to urinate due to swelling of surrounding tissues
- Complications from anesthesia

Seek Immediate Medical Care

A patient who has any of the following symptoms after a cystoscopy or ureteroscopy should call or see a healthcare provider right away:

- The inability to urinate and the feeling of a full bladder
- Burning or painful urination that lasts more than 2 days
- Bright red urine or blood clots in the urine
- A fever, with or without chills
- Severe discomfort

Section 33.6

Endoscopic Ultrasound (EUS)

This section includes text excerpted from "Endoscopic Ultrasound," U.S. Department of Veterans Affairs (VA), May 12, 2015.

Emerging technologies has allowed for the development of a specialized endoscope that has ultrasound capabilities. This enables the physician to visualize the internal layers of the wall of the esophagus, stomach, first part of the small intestine, liver and pancreas. Being able to see an ultrasound image of the structures beyond the wall of the esophagus, stomach, and small intestine, allows the doctor to pass a small needle through the scope to take biopsy samples of pancreatic tumors, lymph nodes and other types of abnormalities. This technology can also be used in the staging of cancerous tumors of the esophagus, stomach, pancreas, and liver providing valuable information to the physicians for planning their patients care and treatment.

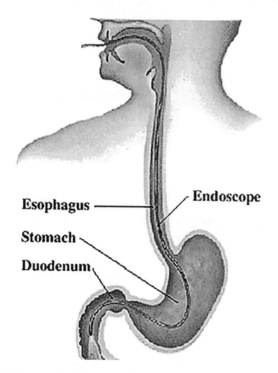

Figure 33.2. *Endoscopic Ultrasound*

Preparing for Endoscopic Ultrasound (EUS)

Follow these and any other instructions you are given before your endoscopic ultrasound (EUS). If you don't follow the doctor's instructions carefully, the test may need to be canceled or done over.

- Do not eat or drink anything after midnight the night before your exam.

- If your exam is in the afternoon, drink only clear liquids in the morning, and do not eat or drink anything for 6 hours before the exam.

- Bring your X-rays and any other test results you have.

- Because you will be sedated, arrange for an adult to drive you home after the exam.

- Tell your healthcare provider before the exam if you are taking any medications or have any medical problems.

The Procedure

EUS is performed in the following manner:

- You lie on the endoscopy table.

- Your throat may be numbed with a spray or gargle. You are given sedating (relaxing) medication through an intravenous (IV) line.

- You swallow the ultrasound scope. This is thinner than most pieces of food that you swallow. It will not affect your breathing. The medication helps keep you from gagging.

- Air is inserted to expand your GI tract. It can make you burp.

- The ultrasound scope carries images of your upper GI tract to a video screen. If you are awake, you may be able to look at the images.

- After the procedure is done, you rest for a time. An adult must drive you home.

Section 33.7

Upper Endoscopy

This section includes text excerpted from "Upper GI Endoscopy," National Institute of Diabetes and Digestive and Kidney Diseases (NIDDK), July 2017.

What Is Upper Gastrointestinal (GI) Endoscopy?

Upper gastrointestinal (GI) endoscopy is a procedure in which a doctor uses an endoscope—a flexible tube with a camera—to see the lining of your upper GI tract. A gastroenterologist, surgeon, or other trained healthcare professional performs the procedure, most often while you receive light sedation to help you relax.

Healthcare professionals may also call the procedure endoscopy, upper endoscopy, EGD or esophagogastroduodenoscopy.

Why Do Doctors Use Upper GI Endoscopy?

Doctors use upper GI endoscopy to help diagnose and treat symptoms and conditions that affect the esophagus, stomach, and upper intestine or duodenum.

Upper GI endoscopy can help find the cause of unexplained symptoms, such as:

- Persistent heartburn

- Bleeding

- Nausea and vomiting

- Pain

- Problems swallowing

- Unexplained weight loss

Upper GI endoscopy can be used to identify many different diseases:

- Gastroesophageal reflux disease

- Ulcers

- Cancer

- Inflammation, or swelling

- Precancerous abnormalities such as Barrett esophagus

371

- Celiac disease

- Strictures or narrowing of the esophagus

- Blockages

Upper GI endoscopy can check for damage after a person eats or drinks harmful chemicals.

During upper GI endoscopy, a doctor obtains biopsies by passing an instrument through the endoscope to obtain a small piece of tissue for testing. Biopsies are needed to diagnose conditions such as:

- Cancer

- Celiac disease

- Gastritis

Doctors also use upper GI endoscopy to:

- Treat conditions such as bleeding from ulcers, esophageal varices, or other conditions

- Dilate or open up strictures with a small balloon passed through the endoscope

- Remove objects, including food, that may be stuck in the upper GI tract

- Remove polyps or other growths

- Place feeding tubes or drainage tubes

Doctors are also starting to use upper GI endoscopy to perform weight loss procedures for some people with obesity.

How Does a Patient Prepare for an Upper GI Endoscopy?

Talk with Your Doctor

You should talk with your doctor about your medical history, including medical conditions and symptoms you have, allergies, and all prescribed and over-the-counter (OTC) medicines, vitamins, and supplements you take, including:

- Aspirin or medicines that contain aspirin

- Arthritis medicines

- Blood thinners

- Blood pressure medicines

- Diabetes medicines

- Nonsteroidal anti-inflammatory drugs (NSAIDS) such as ibuprofen and naproxen

You can take most medicines as usual, but you may need to adjust or stop some medicines for a short time before your upper GI endoscopy. Your doctor will tell you about any necessary changes to your medicines before the procedure.

Arrange for a Ride Home

For safety reasons, you can't drive for 24 hours after the procedure, as the sedatives used during the procedure need time to wear off. You will need to make plans for getting a ride home after the procedure.

Do Not Eat or Drink before the Procedure

To see your upper GI tract clearly, your doctor will most likely ask you not to eat or drink up to 8 hours before the procedure.

How Do Doctors Perform an Upper GI Endoscopy?

A doctor performs an upper GI endoscopy in a hospital or an outpatient center. Before the procedure, you will likely get a sedative or a medicine to help you stay relaxed and comfortable during the procedure. The sedative will be given to you through an intravenous (IV) needle in your arm. In some cases, the procedure can be done without getting a sedative. You may also be given a liquid medicine to gargle or a spray to numb your throat and help prevent you from gagging during the procedure. The healthcare staff will monitor your vital signs and keep you as comfortable as possible.

You'll be asked to lie on your side on an exam table. The doctor will carefully pass the endoscope down your esophagus and into your stomach and duodenum. A small camera mounted on the endoscope will send a video image to a monitor, allowing close examination of the lining of your upper GI tract. The endoscope pumps air into your stomach and duodenum, making them easier to see.

During the upper GI endoscopy, the doctor may:

- Take small samples of tissue, cells, or fluid in your upper GI tract for testing

- Stop any bleeding

- Perform other procedures, such as opening up strictures

The upper GI endoscopy most often takes between 15–30 minutes. The endoscope does not interfere with your breathing, and many people fall asleep during the procedure.

What You Should Expect after an Upper GI Endoscopy?

After an upper GI endoscopy, you can expect the following:

- To stay at the hospital or outpatient center for 1–2 hours after the procedure so the sedative can wear off

- To rest at home for the rest of the day

- Bloating or nausea for a short time after the procedure

- A sore throat for 1–2 days

- To go back to your normal diet once your swallowing returns to normal

After the procedure, you—or a friend or family member who is with you if you're still groggy—will receive instructions on how to care for yourself when you are home. You should follow all instructions.

Some results from an upper GI endoscopy are available right away. Your doctor will share these results with you or, if you choose, with your friend or family member. A pathologist will examine the samples of tissue, cells, or fluid that were taken to help make a diagnosis. Biopsy results take a few days or longer to come back. The pathologist will send a report to your healthcare professional to discuss with you.

What Are the Risks of an Upper GI Endoscopy?

Upper GI endoscopy is considered a safe procedure. The risks of complications from an upper GI endoscopy are low, but may include:

- Bleeding from the site where the doctor took the tissue samples or removed a polyp

- Perforation in the lining of your upper GI tract

- An abnormal reaction to the sedative, including breathing or heart problems

Bleeding caused by the procedure often is minor and stops without treatment. Serious complications such as perforation are uncommon. Your doctor may need to perform surgery to treat some complications. Your doctor can also treat an abnormal reaction to a sedative with medicines or IV fluids during or after the procedure.

Seek Care Right Away

If you have any of the following symptoms after an upper GI endoscopy, seek medical care right away:

- Chest pain
- Problems breathing
- Problems swallowing or throat pain that gets worse
- Vomiting—particularly if your vomit is bloody or looks like coffee grounds
- Pain in your abdomen that gets worse
- Bloody or black, tar-colored stool
- Fever

Section 33.8

Laryngoscopy

"Laryngoscopy," © 2018 Omnigraphics.
Reviewed July 2018.

What Is Laryngoscopy?

A laryngoscopy is a close-up examination of your larynx, which is located at the top of your windpipe, and is also known as the voice box. The vibration of your vocal cords, which are located in your larynx, produces sound and enables you to speak. An "ear, nose, and throat" (ENT) specialist will use an instrument called laryngoscope to view your throat. This process is called laryngoscopy.

Why Is a Laryngoscopy Done?

A laryngoscopy is performed if you have one of the following conditions:

- Voice problems, such as a hoarse or weak voice

- Throat or ear pain that does not go away

- A lump in the neck region

- Bad breath or a cough that does not go away

- Breathing or swallowing problems

A laryngoscopy can also be used to

- Remove a sample of tissue from the throat or vocal cords so that the tissue can be looked at under a microscope (this medical test is called a biopsy)

- Check the throat for redness, swelling, or blockage

- Remove something that is lodged in the throat

Risk Factors

Laryngoscopy is considered a safe procedure; however, risks associated with the procedure may include:

- Breathing and heart problems

- Spasm of the vocal cords

- Ulcers in the lining of the mouth or throat

- Injury to the tongue or lips

- Major bleeding

How Do I Prepare for a Laryngoscopy?

Your physician might want to take X-rays or other imaging tests before taking a laryngoscopy. In the case of a direct laryngoscopy, you will be advised not to eat or drink anything before you go to the medical center. You will also be asked to stop taking some or all of your medications for at least a week prior to the procedure or as directed by the physician.

The Procedure

Your physician will determine if you need an indirect or direct laryngoscopy.

Indirect laryngoscopy is a simple procedure; a small mirror is held at the back of your throat and the physician shines a light on the mirror to view the throat. A medicine is applied to numb your throat as you are awake and lying down during the procedure. This procedure is not recommended for infants, young children, or those who have been diagnosed with acute epiglottitis.

Direct laryngoscopy allows the physician to use a tube called a laryngoscope to examine your throat. General anesthesia given in the medical center will keep you in a state of sleep during the procedure. The physician may use a flexible or a stiff tube to remove any foreign object stuck in the throat.

Results

The doctor might collect a tissue specimen or remove a growth or a foreign object during the laryngoscopy procedure. A biopsy performed on the tissue specimen or growth may take three to five days to complete. Your doctor will explain your results with you and, if needed, discuss treatment options with you or refer you to another doctor.

Normal Result

If your throat, larynx, and vocal cords look normal, then your test result is normal.

Abnormal Result

The following conditions may indicate an abnormal result:

- Redness or swelling of the vocal chords (usually caused by acid reflux)

- Thinning of the muscles and tissues in the voice box

- Inflammation in the throat

- Nodules or polyps on the vocal chords

- Cancer of the throat or voice box

Follow-Up Care

Gargling with salt water can ease a sore throat. Over-the-counter (OTC) pain relievers or throat lozenges are effective as well.

References

1. "A Close-Up Look at Laryngoscopy," Healthline Media, April 20, 2016.

2. "Laryngoscopy," Canadian Cancer Society, July 11, 2017.

Section 33.9

Flexible Sigmoidoscopy

This section includes text excerpted from "Flexible Sigmoidoscopy," National Institute of Diabetes and Digestive and Kidney Diseases (NIDDK), July 2016.

What Is Flexible Sigmoidoscopy?

Flexible sigmoidoscopy is a procedure in which a trained medical professional uses a flexible, narrow tube with a light and tiny camera on one end, called a sigmoidoscope or scope, to look inside your rectum and lower colon, also called the sigmoid colon and descending colon. Flexible sigmoidoscopy can show irritated or swollen tissue, ulcers, polyps, and cancer.

Why Do Doctors Use Flexible Sigmoidoscopy?

A flexible sigmoidoscopy can help a doctor find the cause of unexplained symptoms, such as:

- Bleeding from your anus
- Changes in your bowel activity such as diarrhea
- Pain in your abdomen
- Unexplained weight loss

Doctors also use flexible sigmoidoscopy as a screening tool for colon polyps and colon and rectal cancer. Screening may find diseases at an early stage, when a doctor has a better chance of curing the disease.

Screening for Colon and Rectal Cancer

Your doctor will recommend screening for colon and rectal cancer at age 50 if you don't have health problems or other factors that make you more likely to develop colon cancer.

Factors that make you more likely to develop colorectal cancer include:

- Someone in your family has had polyps or cancer of the colon or rectum

- A personal history of inflammatory bowel disease (IBD), such as ulcerative colitis (UC) or Crohn's disease

- Other factors, such as if you weigh too much or smoke cigarettes

If you are more likely to develop colorectal cancer, your doctor may recommend screening at a younger age, and you may need to be tested more often.

If you are older than age 75, talk with your doctor about whether you should be screened.

Most doctors recommend colonoscopy to screen for colon cancer because colonoscopy shows the entire colon and can remove colon polyps. However, preparing for and performing a flexible sigmoidoscopy may take less time and you may not need anesthesia. Healthcare providers may combine flexible sigmoidoscopy with other tests.

If your doctor finds abnormal tissue or one or more polyps during a flexible sigmoidoscopy, you should have a colonoscopy to examine the rest of your colon.

Government health insurance plans, such as Medicare, and private health insurance plans sometimes change whether and how often they pay for cancer screening tests. Check with your insurance plan to find out how often your insurance will cover a screening flexible sigmoidoscopy.

How Should You Prepare for a Flexible Sigmoidoscopy?

To prepare for a flexible sigmoidoscopy, you will need to talk with your doctor, change your diet, and clean out your bowel.

Talk with Your Doctor

You should talk with your doctor about any medical conditions you have and all prescribed and over-the-counter (OTC) medicines, vitamins, and supplements you take, including:

- Arthritis medicines

- Aspirin or medicines that contain aspirin

- Blood thinners

- Diabetes medicines

- Nonsteroidal anti-inflammatory drugs (NSAIDs), such as ibuprofen or naproxen

- Vitamins that contain iron or iron supplements

Change Your Diet and Clean out Your Bowel

A healthcare professional will give you written bowel prep instructions to follow at home before the procedure. A healthcare professional orders a bowel prep so that little or no stool is present in your intestine. A complete bowel prep lets you pass stool that is clear and liquid. Stool inside your colon can prevent your doctor from clearly seeing the lining of your intestine.

You may need to follow a clear liquid diet the day before the procedure. The instructions will provide specific direction about when to start and stop the clear liquid diet. In most cases, you may drink or eat the following:

- Fat-free bouillon or broth

- Gelatin in flavors such as lemon, lime, or orange

- Plain coffee or tea, without cream or milk

- Sports drinks in flavors such as lemon, lime, or orange

- Strained fruit juice, such as apple or white grape—doctors recommend avoiding orange juice and red or purple liquids.

- Water

Your doctor will tell you how long before the procedure you should have nothing by mouth.

A healthcare professional will ask you to follow the directions for a bowel prep before the procedure. The bowel prep will cause diarrhea, so you should stay close to a bathroom.

Different bowel preps may contain different combinations of laxatives—pills that you swallow or powders that you dissolve in water and other clear liquids—and enemas. Some people will need to drink a large amount, often a gallon, of liquid laxative over a scheduled amount of time—most often the night before the procedure.

You may find this part of the bowel prep difficult; however, completing the prep is very important. Your doctor will not be able to see your sigmoid colon clearly if the prep is incomplete.

Call a healthcare professional if you have side effects that prevent you from finishing the prep.

How Do Doctors Perform a Flexible Sigmoidoscopy?

A trained medical professional performs a flexible sigmoidoscopy during an office visit or at a hospital or an outpatient center. You typically do not need sedatives or anesthesia, and the procedure takes about 20 minutes.

For the procedure, you'll be asked to lie on a table while the doctor inserts a sigmoidoscope into your anus and slowly guides it through your rectum and into your sigmoid colon. The scope pumps air into your large intestine to give the doctor a better view. The camera sends a video image of your intestinal lining to a monitor, allowing the doctor to examine the tissues lining your sigmoid colon and rectum. The doctor may ask you to move several times on the table to adjust the scope for better viewing. Once the scope has reached your transverse colon, the doctor slowly withdraws it and examines the lining of your sigmoid colon again.

During the procedure, your doctor may remove polyps and send them to a lab for testing. Colon polyps are common in adults and are harmless in most cases. However, most colon cancer begins as a polyp, so removing polyps early is an effective way to prevent cancer.

If your doctor finds abnormal tissue, he or she may perform a biopsy. You won't feel the biopsy.

If your doctor found polyps or other abnormal tissue during a flexible sigmoidoscopy, your doctor may suggest you return for a colonoscopy.

What You Can Expect after a Flexible Sigmoidoscopy

After a flexible sigmoidoscopy, you can expect the following:

- You may have cramping in your abdomen or bloating during the first hour after the procedure

- You can resume regular activities right away after the procedure.

- You can return to a normal diet

A healthcare professional will give you written instructions on how to take care of yourself after the procedure and will review them with you. You should follow all instructions.

If the doctor removed polyps or performed a biopsy, you may have light bleeding from your anus. This bleeding is normal. Some results from a flexible sigmoidoscopy are available right after the procedure, and your doctor will share these results with you. A pathologist will examine the biopsy tissue. Biopsy results take a few days or longer to come back.

What Are the Risks of a Flexible Sigmoidoscopy?

The risks of a flexible sigmoidoscopy include:

- Bleeding

- Perforation of the colon

- Severe pain in your abdomen

- Death, although this risk is rare

Bleeding and perforation are the most common complications from flexible sigmoidoscopy. Most cases of bleeding occur in patients who have polyps removed. The doctor can treat bleeding that occurs during the flexible sigmoidoscopy right away. However, you may have delayed bleeding up to 2 weeks after the procedure. The doctor diagnoses and treats delayed bleeding with a colonoscopy or repeat flexible sigmoidoscopy. The doctor may need to treat perforation with surgery.

Seek Care Right Away

If you have any of the following symptoms after a flexible sigmoidoscopy, seek care right away:

- Severe pain in your abdomen

- Fever

- Continued bloody bowel movements or continued bleeding from your anus

- Dizziness

- Weakness

Section 33.10

Endoscopic Retrograde Cholangiopancreatography (ERCP)

This section includes text excerpted from "Endoscopic Retrograde Cholangiopancreatography (ERCP)," National Institute of Diabetes and Digestive and Kidney Diseases (NIDDK), June 2016.

What Is Endoscopic Retrograde Cholangiopancreatography (ERCP)?

Endoscopic retrograde cholangiopancreatography (ERCP) is a procedure that combines upper gastrointestinal (GI) endoscopy and X-rays to treat problems of the bile and pancreatic ducts.

Why Do Doctors Use ERCP?

Doctors use ERCP to treat problems of the bile and pancreatic ducts. Doctors also use ERCP to diagnose problems of the bile and pancreatic ducts if they expect to treat problems during the procedure. For diagnosis alone, doctors may use noninvasive tests—tests that do not physically enter the body—instead of ERCP. Noninvasive tests such as magnetic resonance cholangiopancreatography (MRCP)—a type of magnetic resonance imaging (MRI)—are safer and can also diagnose many problems of the bile and pancreatic ducts.

Doctors perform ERCP when your bile or pancreatic ducts have become narrowed or blocked because of:

- Gallstones that form in your gallbladder and become stuck in your common bile duct

- Infection

- Acute pancreatitis

- Chronic pancreatitis

- Trauma or surgical complications in your bile or pancreatic ducts

- Pancreatic pseudocysts

- Tumors or cancers of the bile ducts

- Tumors or cancers of the pancreas

How to Prepare Yourself for ERCP

To prepare for ERCP, talk with your doctor, arrange for a ride home, and follow your doctor's instructions.

Talk with Your Doctor

You should talk with your doctor about any allergies and medical conditions you have and all prescribed and over-the-counter medicines, vitamins, and supplements you take, including:

- Arthritis medicines

- Aspirin or medicines that contain aspirin

- Blood thinners

- Blood pressure medicines

- Diabetes medicines

- Nonsteroidal anti-inflammatory drugs (NSAIDs) such as ibuprofen and naproxen

Your doctor may ask you to temporarily stop taking medicines that affect blood clotting or interact with sedatives. You typically receive sedatives during ERCP to help you relax and stay comfortable.

Tell your doctor if you are, or may be, pregnant. If you are pregnant and need ERCP to treat a problem, the doctor performing the procedure may make changes to protect the fetus from X-rays. Research has found that ERCP is generally safe during pregnancy.

Arrange for a Ride Home

For safety reasons, you can't drive for 24 hours after ERCP, as the sedatives or anesthesia used during the procedure needs time to wear off. You will need to make plans for getting a ride home after ERCP.

Don't Eat, Drink, Smoke, or Chew Gum

To see your upper GI tract clearly, your doctor will most likely ask you not to eat, drink, smoke, or chew gum during the 8 hours before ERCP.

How Do Doctors Perform ERCP?

Doctors who have specialized training in ERCP perform this procedure at a hospital or an outpatient center. An intravenous (IV) needle will be placed in your arm to provide a sedative. Sedatives help you stay relaxed and comfortable during the procedure. A healthcare professional will give you a liquid anesthetic to gargle or will spray anesthetic on the back of your throat. The anesthetic numbs your throat and helps prevent gagging during the procedure. The healthcare staff will monitor your vital signs and keep you as comfortable as possible. In some cases, you may receive general anesthesia.

You'll be asked to lie on an examination table. The doctor will carefully feed the endoscope down your esophagus, through your stomach, and into your duodenum. A small camera mounted on the endoscope will send a video image to a monitor. The endoscope pumps air into your stomach and duodenum, making them easier to see.

During ERCP, the doctor:

- Locates the opening where the bile and pancreatic ducts empty into the duodenum

- Slides a thin, flexible tube called a catheter through the endoscope and into the ducts

- Injects a special dye, also called contrast medium, into the ducts through the catheter to make the ducts more visible on X-rays

- Uses a type of X-ray imaging, called fluoroscopy, to examine the ducts and look for narrowed areas or blockages

The doctor may pass tiny tools through the endoscope to:

- Open blocked or narrowed ducts
- Break up or remove stones
- Perform a biopsy or remove tumors in the ducts
- Insert stents—tiny tubes that a doctor leaves in narrowed ducts to hold them open. A doctor may also insert temporary stents to stop bile leaks that can occur after gallbladder surgery.

The procedure most often takes between 1–2 hours.

What to Expect after ERCP?

After ERCP, you can expect the following:

- You will most often stay at the hospital or outpatient center for 1–2 hours after the procedure so the sedation or anesthesia can wear off. In some cases, you may need to stay overnight in the hospital after ERCP.

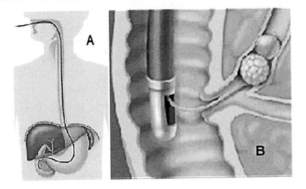

Figure 33.3. *Endoscopic Retrograde Cholangiopancreatography*
(Source: "Endoscopic Retrograde Cholangiopancreatography," U.S. Department of Veterans Affairs (VA).)

Figure A shows the endoscope moves from the mouth, through the upper digestive tract, to the common bile duct opening. Figure B shows a balloon at the tip of a catheter opens above the stone. The stone is pulled out of the duct and leaves your body through stool.

- You may have bloating or nausea for a short time after the procedure

- You may have a sore throat for 1–2 days

- You can go back to a normal diet once your swallowing has returned to normal

- You should rest at home for the remainder of the day

Following the procedure, you—or a friend or family member who is with you if you're still groggy—will receive instructions on how to care for yourself after the procedure. You should follow all instructions.

Some results from ERCP are available right away after the procedure. After the sedative has worn off, the doctor will share results with you or, if you choose, with your friend or family member.

If the doctor performed a biopsy, a pathologist will examine the biopsy tissue. Biopsy results take a few days or longer to come back.

What Are the Risks of ERCP?

The risks of ERCP include complications such as the following:

- Pancreatitis

- Infection of the bile ducts or gallbladder

- Excessive bleeding, called hemorrhage
- An abnormal reaction to the sedative, including respiratory or cardiac problems
- Perforation in the bile or pancreatic ducts, or in the duodenum near the opening where the bile and pancreatic ducts empty into it
- Tissue damage from X-ray exposure
- Death, although this complication is rare

Research has found that these complications occur in about 5–10 percent of ERCP procedures. People with complications often need treatment at a hospital.

Seek Care Right Away

If you have any of the following symptoms after ERCP, seek medical attention right away:

- Bloody or black, tar-colored stool
- Chest pain
- Fever
- Pain in your abdomen that gets worse
- Problems breathing
- Problems swallowing or throat pain that gets worse
- Vomiting—particularly if your vomit is bloody or looks like coffee grounds

Chapter 34

Electrocardiogram (EKG)

An electrocardiogram, also called an ECG or EKG, is a simple, painless test that detects and records your heart's electrical activity.

What Does an Electrocardiogram (EKG) Show?

Many heart problems change the heart's electrical activity in distinct ways. An EKG can help detect these heart problems.

EKG recordings can help doctors diagnose heart attacks that are in progress or have happened in the past. This is especially true if doctors can compare a current EKG recording to an older one.

An EKG also can show:

- Lack of blood flow to the heart muscle (coronary heart disease or CHD)

- A heartbeat that's too fast, too slow, or irregular (arrhythmia)

- A heart that doesn't pump forcefully enough (heart failure)

- Heart muscle that's too thick or parts of the heart that are too big (cardiomyopathy)

- Birth defects in the heart (congenital heart defects)

- Problems with the heart valves (heart valve disease)

- Inflammation of the sac that surrounds the heart (pericarditis)

This chapter includes text excerpted from "Electrocardiogram," National Heart, Lung, and Blood Institute (NHLBI), September 4, 2012. Reviewed July 2018.

An EKG can reveal whether the heartbeat starts in the correct place in the heart. The test also shows how long it takes for electrical signals to travel through the heart. Delays in signal travel time may suggest heart block or long QT syndrome (LQTS).

Who Needs an EKG?

Your doctor may recommend an EKG if you have signs or symptoms that suggest a heart problem. Examples of such signs and symptoms include:

- Chest pain
- Heart pounding, racing, or fluttering, or the sense that your heart is beating unevenly
- Breathing problems
- Tiredness and weakness
- Unusual heart sounds when your doctor listens to your heartbeat

You may need to have more than one EKG so your doctor can diagnose certain heart conditions.

An EKG also may be done as part of a routine health exam. The test can screen for early heart disease that has no symptoms. Your doctor is more likely to look for early heart disease if your mother, father, brother, or sister had heart disease—especially early in life.

You may have an EKG so your doctor can check how well heart medicine or a medical device, such as a pacemaker, is working. The test also may be used for routine screening before major surgery. Your doctor also may use EKG results to help plan your treatment for a heart condition.

What to Expect before an EKG

You don't need to take any special steps before having an EKG. However, tell your doctor or his or her staff about the medicines you're taking. Some medicines can affect EKG results.

What to Expect during an EKG?

An EKG is painless and harmless. A nurse or technician will attach soft, sticky patches called electrodes to the skin of your chest, arms, and legs. The patches are about the size of a quarter.

Often, 12 patches are attached to your body. This helps detect your heart's electrical activity from many areas at the same time. The nurse may have to shave areas of your skin to help the patches stick.

After the patches are placed on your skin, you'll lie still on a table while the patches detect your heart's electrical signals. A machine will record these signals on graph paper or display them on a screen.

The entire test will take about 10 minutes.

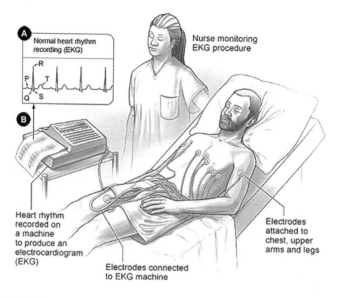

Figure 34.1. *Electrocardiogram*

The image shows the standard setup for an EKG. In figure A, a normal heart rhythm recording shows the electrical pattern of a regular heartbeat. In figure B, a patient lies in a bed with EKG electrodes attached to his chest, upper arms, and legs. A nurse monitors the painless procedure.

Special Types of Electrocardiogram

The standard EKG described above, called a resting 12-lead EKG, only records seconds of heart activity at a time. It will show a heart problem only if the problem occurs during the test.

Many heart problems are present all the time, and a resting 12-lead EKG will detect them. But some heart problems, like those related to an irregular heartbeat, can come and go. They may occur only for a few minutes a day or only while you exercise.

Doctors use special EKGs, such as stress tests and Holter and event monitors, to help diagnose these kinds of problems.

Stress Test

Some heart problems are easier to diagnose when your heart is working hard and beating fast. During stress testing, you exercise to make your heart work hard and beat fast while an EKG is done. If you can't exercise, you'll be given medicine to make your heart work hard and beat fast.

Holter and Event Monitors

Holter and event monitors are small, portable devices. They record your heart's electrical activity while you do your normal daily activities. A Holter monitor records your heart's electrical activity for a full 24- or 48-hour period.

An event monitor records your heart's electrical activity only at certain times while you're wearing it. For many event monitors, you push a button to start the monitor when you feel symptoms. Other event monitors start automatically when they sense abnormal heart rhythms.

What to Expect after an EKG

After an EKG, the nurse or technician will remove the electrodes (soft patches) from your skin. You may develop a rash or redness where the EKG patches were attached. This mild rash often goes away without treatment.

You usually can go back to your normal daily routine after an EKG.

What Are the Risks of an EKG?

An EKG has no serious risks. It's a harmless, painless test that detects the heart's electrical activity. EKGs don't give off electrical charges, such as shocks.

You may develop a mild rash where the electrodes (soft patches) were attached. This rash often goes away without treatment.

Chapter 35

Electroencephalogram (EEG)

What Is Electroencephalogram (EEG)?

An electroencephalogram (EEG), also known as a brain wave test, is used to evaluate the electrical activity of the brain. This activity appears as a series of squiggles/waves called traces. Each trace corresponds to different regions of the brain. The EEG can be analyzed to help make a diagnosis or to monitor brain activity. This procedure will not harm you.

What You Should Do before EEG

Before the EEG you are expected to do some preparation. Some of the things that you need to do are:

- Wash your hair with mild shampoo the night before or the day of the EEG. Do not use hair sprays, oils, or gels at least 24 hours before the test.

- If possible, eat a meal or light snack within four hours of your EEG

- Avoid food and drinks containing caffeine at least eight hours before the test

This chapter includes text excerpted from "Electroencephalogram (EEG)—NIH Clinical Center Patient Education Material," Clinical Center (CC), National Institutes of Health (NIH), November 2015.

- Continue taking your regular medications unless your doctor tells you otherwise

- Sometimes, the EEG gives better results when the patient has had less than the usual amount of sleep. Your doctor may ask you to stay awake for all or part of the night before your EEG.

Please arrive on time for your appointment at the EEG laboratory.

What to Expect during EEG

During EEG you can expect the following to happen:

- The EEG technician will measure and mark your scalp where small metal discs (electrodes) will be placed or fit you with a special cap containing the electrodes.

- The technician will rub your scalp with a mild, scratchy cleanser that may temporarily cause a little discomfort.

- The technician will then attach the electrodes to your body with a cream or gel. They may use an adhesive to attach the discs more securely to improve the quality of the recording.

- A special instrument connected to the electrodes amplifies the brain signals and records them on computer equipment. You will not feel anything during the recording.

- Your heart and eye movements will be monitored during the procedure.

- For better results and to ensure a good recording, you will lie on a bed or in a comfortable chair.

- From time to time, the technician may ask you to open and close your eyes. The technician will instruct you to perform a breathing exercise and will shine a special light in front of your eyes.

- The entire EEG procedure usually takes about 90 minutes.

What to Expect after EEG

After the EEG procedure is completed, you can expect the following:

- The technician will remove the gel with water. Shampoo your hair to clean out any other material.

- Some patients are sensitive to the gel or cream. You may experience some mild irritation from the rubbing of the scalp.

- If you did not receive sedation, you may return to your normal activities.

- If you received sedation, it will take a little while for the medication to wear off. Arrange to have someone drive you home. You should rest the remainder of the day.

- If you have questions about the procedure, please ask. Your nurse and doctor are ready to help you at all times.

Chapter 36

Holter and Event Monitors

Holter and event monitors are small, portable electrocardiogram devices that record your heart's electrical activity for long periods of time while you do your normal activities.

What Does a Holter or Event Monitor Show?

A Holter or event monitor may show what's causing symptoms of an arrhythmia. An arrhythmia is a problem with the rate or rhythm of the heartbeat.

A Holter or event monitor also can show whether a heart rhythm problem is harmless or requires treatment. The monitor might alert your doctor to medical conditions that can result in heart failure, stroke, or sudden cardiac arrest.

If the symptoms of a heart rhythm problem occur often, a Holter or event monitor has a good chance of recording them. You may not have symptoms while using a monitor. Even so, your doctor can learn more about your heart rhythm from the test results.

Sometimes Holter and event monitors can't help doctors diagnose heart rhythm problems. If this happens, talk with your doctor about other steps you can take.

One option might be to try a different type of monitor. Wireless Holter monitors and implantable loop recorders have longer recording

This chapter includes text excerpted from "Holter and Event Monitors," National Heart, Lung, and Blood Institute (NHLBI), December 12, 2016.

periods. This may allow your doctor to get the data he or she needs to make a diagnosis.

Who Needs a Holter or Event Monitor?

Your doctor may recommend a Holter or event monitor if he or she thinks you have an arrhythmia. An arrhythmia is a problem with the rate or rhythm of the heartbeat.

Holter and event monitors most often are used to detect arrhythmias in people who have:

- Issues with fainting or feeling dizzy. A monitor might be used if causes other than a heart rhythm problem has been ruled out.

- Palpitations that recur with no known cause. Palpitations are feelings that your heart is skipping a beat, fluttering, or beating too hard or fast. You may have these feelings in your chest, throat, or neck.

People who are being treated for heart rhythm problems also may need to use Holter or event monitors. The monitors can show how well their treatments are working.

Heart rhythm problems may occur only during certain activities, such sleeping or physical exertion. Holter and event monitors record your heart rhythm while you do your normal daily routine. This allows your doctor to see how your heart responds to various activities.

What to Expect before Using a Holter or Event Monitor

Your doctor will do a physical exam before giving you a Holter or event monitor. He or she may:

- Check your pulse to find out how fast your heart is beating (your heart rate) and whether your heart rhythm is steady or irregular

- Measure your blood pressure

- Check for swelling in your legs or feet. Swelling could be a sign of an enlarged heart or heart failure, which may cause an arrhythmia. An arrhythmia is a problem with the rate or rhythm of the heartbeat.

- Look for signs of other diseases that might cause heart rhythm problems, such as thyroid disease

You may have an EKG (electrocardiogram) test before your doctor sends you home with a Holter or event monitor.

An EKG is a simple test that records your heart's electrical activity for a few seconds. The test shows how fast your heart is beating and its rhythm (steady or irregular). An EKG also records the strength and timing of electrical signals as they pass through your heart.

A standard EKG won't detect heart rhythm problems that don't happen during the test. For this reason, your doctor may give you a Holter or event monitor. These monitors are portable. You can wear one while doing your normal daily activities. This increases the chance of recording symptoms that only occur once in a while.

Your doctor will explain how to wear and use the Holter or event monitor. Usually, you'll leave the office wearing it.

Each type of monitor is slightly different, but most have sensors (called electrodes) that attach to the skin on your chest using sticky patches. The sensors need good contact with your skin. Poor contact can cause poor results.

What to Expect while Using a Holter or Event Monitor

Your experience while using a Holter or event monitor depends on the type of monitor you have. However, most monitors have some factors in common.

Recording the Heart's Electrical Activity

All monitors record the heart's electrical activity. Thus, maintaining a clear signal between the sensors (electrodes) and the recording device is important.

In most cases, the sensors are attached to your chest using sticky patches. Wires connect the sensors to the monitor. You usually can clip the monitor to your belt or carry it in your pocket. (Postevent recorders and implantable loop recorders don't have chest sensors.)

A good stick between the patches and your skin helps provide a clear signal. Poor contact leads to a poor recording that's hard for your doctor to read.

Oil, too much sweat, and hair can keep the patches from sticking to your skin. You may need to shave the area where your doctor will attach the patches. If you have to replace the patches, you'll need to clean the area with a special prep pad that your doctor will provide.

You may need to use a small amount of special paste or gel to help the patches stick to your skin. Some patches come with paste or gel on them.

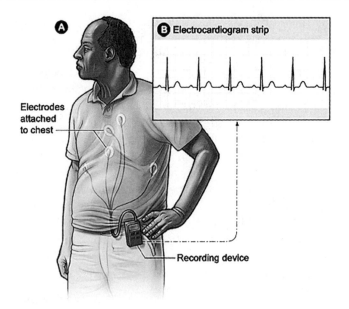

Figure 36.1. *Holter or Event Monitor*

Figure A shows how a Holter or event monitor attaches to a patient. In this example, the monitor is clipped to the patient's belt and electrodes are attached to his chest. Figure B shows an electrocardiogram strip, which maps the data from the Holter or event monitor.

Too much movement can pull the patches away from your skin or create "noise" on the EKG (electrocardiogram) strip. An EKG strip is a graph showing the pattern of the heartbeat. Noise looks like a lot of jagged lines; it makes it hard for your doctor to see the real rhythm of your heart.

When you have a symptom, stop what you're doing. This will ensure that the recording shows your heart's activity rather than your movement.

Your doctor will tell you whether you need to adjust your activity level during the testing period. If you exercise, choose a cool location to avoid sweating too much. This will help the patches stay sticky.

Other everyday items also can disrupt the signal between the sensors and the monitor. These items include magnets; metal detectors; microwave ovens; and electric blankets, toothbrushes, and razors. Avoid using these items. Also avoid areas with high voltage.

Cell phones and MP3 players (such as iPods) may interfere with the signal between the sensors and the monitor if they're too close to the monitor. When using any electronic device, try to keep it at least 6 inches away from the monitor.

Keeping a Diary

While using a Holter or event monitor, your doctor will advise you to keep a diary of your symptoms and activities. Write down what type of symptoms you're having, when they occur, and what you were doing at the time.

The most common symptoms of heart rhythm problems include:

• Fainting or feeling dizzy

• Palpitations. These are feelings that your heart is skipping a beat, fluttering, or beating too hard or fast. You may have these feelings in your chest, throat, or neck.

Make sure to note the time that symptoms occur, because your doctor will match the data with the information in your diary. This allows your doctor to see whether certain activities trigger changes in your heart rate and rhythm.

Also, include details in your diary about when you take any medicine or if you feel stress at certain times during the testing period.

What to Expect with Specific Monitors

Holter Monitors

Holter monitors are about the size of a large deck of cards. You'll wear one for 24–48 hours. You can't get your monitor wet, so you won't be able to bathe or shower. You can take a sponge bath if needed. When the testing period is done, you'll return the device to your doctor's office. The results will be stored on the device.

The recording period for a standard Holter monitor might be too short to capture a heart rhythm problem. If this is the case, your doctor may recommend a wireless Holter monitor.

Wireless Holter Monitors

Wireless Holter monitors can record for a longer time than standard Holter monitors. You can use a wireless Holter monitor for days or even weeks, until signs or symptoms of a heart rhythm problem occur.

Wireless monitors record for a preset amount of time. Then they automatically send data to your doctor's office or a company that checks the data.

These monitors use wireless cellular technology to send data. However, they still have wires that connect the device to the sensors stuck to your chest.

The batteries in the wireless monitor must be changed every 1–2 days. You'll need to detach the sensors to shower or bathe and then reattach them.

Event Monitors

Event monitors are slightly smaller than Holter monitors. They can be worn for weeks or until symptoms occur. Most event monitors are worn like Holter monitors—clipped to a belt or carried in a pocket.

When you have symptoms, you simply push a button on your monitor to start recording. Some event monitors start automatically if they detect abnormal heart rhythms.

Postevent Recorders

Postevent recorders can be worn like a wristwatch or carried in a pocket. The pocket version is about the size of a thick credit card. These recorders don't have wires that connect the device to chest sensors.

To start the recorder when you feel a symptom, you hold it to your chest. To start the wristwatch version, you touch a button on the side of the watch.

You send the stored data to your doctor's office using a telephone. Your doctor will explain how to use the monitor before you leave his or her office.

Autodetect Recorders

Autodetect recorders are about the size of the palm of your hand. Wires connect the device to sensors on your chest.

You don't need to start an autodetect recorder. This type of monitor automatically starts recording if it detects abnormal heart rhythms. It then sends the data to your doctor's office.

Implantable Loop Recorders

Implantable loop recorders are about the size of a pack of gum. This type of event monitor is inserted under the skin on your chest. Your doctor will discuss the procedure with you. No chest sensors are used with implantable loop recorders.

Your doctor can program the device to record when you start it during symptoms or automatically if it detects an abnormal heart rhythm. Devices may differ, so your doctor will tell you how to use your recorder. Sometimes a special card is held close to the device to start it.

What to Expect after Using a Holter or Event Monitor

After you're finished using a Holter or event monitor, you'll return it to your doctor's office or the place where you picked it up. If you were using an implantable loop recorder, your doctor will need to remove it from your chest. He or she will discuss the procedure with you.

Your doctor will tell you when to expect the results. Once your doctor has reviewed the recordings, he or she will discuss the results with you.

What Are the Risks of Using a Holter or Event Monitor?

The sticky patches used to attach the sensors (electrodes) to your chest have a small risk of skin irritation. You also may have an allergic reaction to the paste or gel that's sometimes used to attach the patches. The irritation will go away once the patches are removed.

If you're using an implantable loop recorder, you may get an infection or have pain where the device is placed under the skin. Your doctor can prescribe medicine to treat these problems.

Chapter 37

Stress Testing

What Is Stress Testing?

Stress testing provides information about how your heart works during physical stress. Some heart problems are easier to diagnose when your heart is working hard and beating fast.

During stress testing, you exercise (walk or run on a treadmill or pedal a stationary bike) to make your heart work hard and beat fast. Tests are done on your heart while you exercise.

You might have arthritis or another medical problem that prevents you from exercising during a stress test. If so, your doctor may give you medicine to make your heart work hard, as it would during exercise. This is called a pharmacological stress test.

Doctors usually use stress testing to help diagnose coronary heart disease (CHD). They also use stress testing to find out the severity of CHD.

CHD is a disease in which a waxy substance called plaque builds up in the coronary arteries. These arteries supply oxygen-rich blood to your heart.

Plaque narrows the arteries and reduces blood flow to your heart muscle. The buildup of plaque also makes it more likely that blood clots will form in your arteries. Blood clots can mostly or completely

This chapter includes text excerpted from "Stress Testing," National Heart, Lung, and Blood Institute (NHLBI), December 15, 2011. Reviewed July 2018.

block blood flow through an artery. This can lead to chest pain called angina or a heart attack.

You may not have any signs or symptoms of CHD when your heart is at rest. But when your heart has to work harder during exercise, it needs more blood and oxygen. Narrow arteries can't supply enough blood for your heart to work well. As a result, signs, and symptoms of CHD may occur only during exercise.

A stress test can detect the following problems, which may suggest that your heart isn't getting enough blood during exercise:

- Abnormal changes in your heart rate or blood pressure

- Symptoms such as shortness of breath or chest pain, especially if they occur at low levels of exercise

- Abnormal changes in your heart's rhythm or electrical activity

During a stress test, if you can't exercise for as long as what is considered normal for someone your age, it may be a sign that not enough blood is flowing to your heart. However, other factors besides CHD can prevent you from exercising long enough (for example, lung disease, anemia, or poor general fitness).

Doctors also may use stress testing to assess other problems, such as heart valve disease or heart failure.

Types of Stress Testing

The two main types of stress testing are a standard exercise stress test and an imaging stress test.

Standard Exercise Stress Test

A standard exercise stress test uses an EKG (electrocardiogram) to detect and record the heart's electrical activity.

An EKG shows how fast your heart is beating and the heart's rhythm (steady or irregular). It also records the strength and timing of electrical signals as they pass through your heart.

During a standard stress test, your blood pressure will be checked. You also may be asked to breathe into a special tube during the test. This allows your doctor to see how well you're breathing and measure the gases that you breathe out.

A standard stress test shows changes in your heart's electrical activity. It also can show whether your heart is getting enough blood during exercise.

Imaging Stress Test

As part of some stress tests, pictures are taken of your heart while you exercise and while you're at rest. These imaging stress tests can show how well blood is flowing in your heart and how well your heart pumps blood when it beats.

One type of imaging stress test involves echocardiography (echo). This test uses sound waves to create a moving picture of your heart. An exercise stress echo can show how well your heart's chambers and valves are working when your heart is under stress.

A stress echo also can show areas of poor blood flow to your heart, dead heart muscle tissue, and areas of the heart muscle wall that aren't contracting well. These areas may have been damaged during a heart attack, or they may not be getting enough blood.

Other imaging stress tests use radioactive dye to create pictures of blood flow to your heart. The dye is injected into your bloodstream before the pictures are taken. The pictures show how much of the dye has reached various parts of your heart during exercise and while you're at rest.

Tests that use radioactive dye include a thallium or sestamibi stress test and a positron emission tomography (PET) stress test. The amount of radiation in the dye is considered safe for you and those around you. However, if you're pregnant, you shouldn't have this test because of risks it might pose to your unborn child.

Imaging stress tests tend to detect CHD better than standard (non-imaging) stress tests. Imaging stress tests also can predict the risk of a future heart attack or premature death.

An imaging stress test might be done first (as opposed to a standard exercise stress test) if you:

- Can't exercise for enough time to get your heart working at its hardest (Medical problems, such as arthritis or leg arteries clogged by plaque, might prevent you from exercising long enough)

- Have abnormal heartbeats or other problems that prevent a standard exercise stress test from giving correct results

- Had a heart procedure in the past, such as coronary artery bypass grafting (CABG) or percutaneous coronary intervention (PCI), also known as coronary angioplasty, and stent placement

Other Names

- Exercise echocardiogram or exercise stress echo

- Exercise test

407

- Myocardial perfusion imaging (MPI)
- Nuclear stress test
- PET stress test
- Pharmacological stress test
- Sestamibi stress test
- Stress EKG or electrocardiography (ECG)
- Treadmill test

Who Needs Stress Testing?

You may need stress testing if you've had chest pains, shortness of breath, or other symptoms of limited blood flow to your heart.

Imaging stress tests, especially, can show whether you have coronary heart disease (CHD) or a heart valve problem. (Heart valves are like doors; they open and shut to let blood flow between the heart's chambers and into the heart's arteries. So, like CHD, faulty heart valves can limit the amount of blood reaching your heart.)

If you've been diagnosed with CHD or recently had a heart attack, a stress test can show whether you can handle an exercise program. If you've had a percutaneous coronary intervention, also known as coronary angioplasty, (with or without stent placement) or coronary artery bypass grafting, a stress test can show how well the treatment relieves your CHD symptoms.

You also may need a stress test if, during exercise, you feel faint, have a rapid heartbeat or a fluttering feeling in your chest, or have other symptoms of an arrhythmia (an irregular heartbeat).

If you don't have chest pain when you exercise but still get short of breath, your doctor may recommend a stress test. The test can help show whether a heart problem, rather than a lung problem or being out of shape, is causing your breathing problems.

For such testing, you breathe into a special tube. This allows a technician to measure the gases you breathe out. Breathing into the tube during stress testing also is done before a heart transplant to help assess whether you're a candidate for the surgery.

Stress testing shouldn't be used as a routine screening test for CHD. Usually, you have to have symptoms of CHD before a doctor will recommend stress testing.

However, your doctor may want to use a stress test to screen for CHD if you have diabetes. This disease increases your risk of CHD.

Currently, though, no evidence shows that having a stress test will improve your outcome if you have diabetes.

What to Expect before Stress Testing

Stress testing is done in a doctor's office or at a medical center or hospital. You should wear shoes and clothes in which you can exercise comfortably. Sometimes you're given a gown to wear during the test.

Your doctor might ask you to fast (not eat or drink anything but water) for a short time before the test. If you're diabetic, ask your doctor whether you need to adjust your medicines on the day of the test.

For some stress tests, you can't drink coffee or other caffeinated drinks for a day before the test. Certain over-the-counter (OTC) or prescription medicines also may interfere with some stress tests. Ask your doctor whether you need to avoid certain drinks or food or change how you take your medicine before the test.

If you use an inhaler for asthma or other breathing problems, bring it to the test. Make sure you let the doctor know that you use it.

What to Expect during Stress Testing

During all types of stress testing, a doctor, nurse, or technician will always be with you to closely check your health status.

Before you start the "stress" part of a stress test, the nurse will put sticky patches called electrodes on the skin of your chest, arms, and legs. To help an electrode stick to the skin, the nurse may have to shave a patch of hair where the electrode will be attached.

The electrodes will be connected to an EKG (electrocardiogram) machine. This machine records your heart's electrical activity. It shows how fast your heart is beating and the heart's rhythm (steady or irregular). An EKG also records the strength and timing of electrical signals as they pass through your heart.

The nurse will put a blood pressure cuff on your arm to check your blood pressure during the stress test. (The cuff will feel tight on your arm when it expands every few minutes.) Also, you might have to breathe into a special tube so the gases you breathe out can be measured.

Next, you'll exercise on a treadmill or stationary bike. If such exercise poses a problem for you, you might turn a crank with your arms instead. During the test, the exercise level will get harder. You can stop whenever you feel the exercise is too much for you.

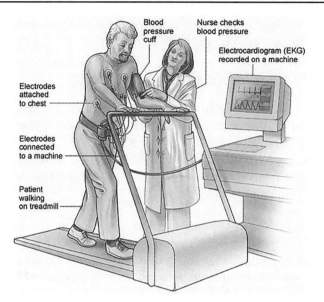

Figure 37.1. *Stress Testing*

The figure shows a patient having a stress test. Electrodes are attached to the patient's chest and connected to an EKG (electrocardiogram) machine. The EKG records the heart's electrical activity. A blood pressure cuff is used to record the patient's blood pressure while he walks on a treadmill.

If you can't exercise, medicine might be injected into a vein in your arm or hand. The medicine will increase blood flow through your coronary arteries and make your heart beat fast, as it would during exercise. You can then have the stress test.

The medicine may make you flushed and anxious, but the effects go away as soon as the test is over. The medicine also may give you a headache.

While you're exercising or getting medicine to make your heart work harder, the nurse will ask you how you're feeling. You should tell him or her if you feel chest pain, short of breath, or dizzy.

The exercise or medicine infusion will continue until you reach a target heart rate, or until you:

- Feel moderate to severe chest pain

- Get too out of breath to continue

- Develop abnormally high or low blood pressure or an arrhythmia (an irregular heartbeat)

- Become dizzy

The nurse will continue to check your heart functions and blood pressure after the test until they return to normal levels.

The "stress" part of a stress test (when your heart is working hard) usually lasts about 15 minutes or less.

However, there's prep time before the test and monitoring time afterward. Both extend the total test time to about an hour for a standard stress test, and up to 3 hours or more for some imaging stress tests.

Exercise Stress Echocardiogram Test

For an exercise stress echocardiogram (echo) test, the nurse will take pictures of your heart using echocardiography before you exercise and as soon as you finish.

A sonographer (a person who specializes in using ultrasound techniques) will apply gel to your chest. Then, he or she will briefly put a transducer (a wand-like device) against your chest and move it around.

The transducer sends and receives high-pitched sounds that you probably won't hear. The echoes from the sound waves are converted into moving pictures of your heart on a screen.

You might be asked to lie on your side on an exam table for this test. Some stress echo tests also use dye to improve imaging. The dye is injected into your bloodstream while the test occurs.

Sestamibi or Other Imaging Stress Tests Involving Radioactive Dye

For a sestamibi stress test or other imaging stress test that uses radioactive dye, the nurse will inject a small amount of dye into your bloodstream. This is done through a needle placed in a vein in your arm or hand.

You'll get the dye about a half-hour before you start exercising or take medicine to make your heart work hard. The amount of radiation in the dye is considered safe for you and those around you. However, if you're pregnant, you shouldn't have this test because of risks it might pose to your unborn child.

Pictures will be taken of your heart at least two times: when it's at rest and when it's working its hardest. You'll lie down on a table, and a special camera or scanner that can detect the dye in your bloodstream will take pictures of your heart.

Some pictures may not be taken until you lie quietly for a few hours after the stress test. Some patients may even be asked to return in a day or so for more pictures.

411

What to Expect after Stress Testing

After stress testing, you'll be able to return to your normal activities. If you had a test that involved radioactive dye, your doctor may ask you to drink plenty of fluids to flush it out of your body. You shouldn't have certain other imaging tests until the dye is no longer in your body. Your doctor can advise you further.

What Does Stress Testing Show?

Stress testing shows how your heart works during physical stress (exercise) and how healthy your heart is.

A standard exercise stress test uses an EKG (electrocardiogram) to monitor changes in your heart's electrical activity. Imaging stress tests take pictures of blood flow throughout your heart. They also show your heart valves and the movement of your heart muscle.

Doctors use both types of stress tests to look for signs that your heart isn't getting enough blood flow during exercise. Abnormal test results may be due to coronary heart disease (CHD) or other factors, such as poor physical fitness.

If you have a standard exercise stress test and the results are normal, you may not need further testing or treatment. But if your test results are abnormal, or if you're physically unable to exercise, your doctor may want you to have an imaging stress test or other tests.

Even if your standard exercise stress test results are normal, your doctor may want you to have an imaging stress test if you continue having symptoms (such as shortness of breath or chest pain).

Imaging stress tests are more accurate than standard exercise stress tests, but they're much more expensive.

Imaging stress tests show how well blood is flowing in the heart muscle and reveal parts of the heart that aren't contracting strongly. They also can show the parts of the heart that aren't getting enough blood, as well as dead tissue in the heart, where no blood flows. (A heart attack can cause heart tissue to die.)

If your imaging stress test suggests significant CHD, your doctor may want you to have more testing and treatment.

What Are the Risks of Stress Testing?

Stress tests pose little risk of serious harm. The chance of these tests causing a heart attack or death is about 1 in 5,000. More common, but less serious side effects linked to stress testing include:

- An arrhythmia (irregular heartbeat). Often, an arrhythmia will go away quickly once you're at rest. But if it persists, you may need monitoring or treatment in a hospital.

- Low blood pressure, which can cause you to feel dizzy or faint. This problem may go away once your heart stops working hard; it usually doesn't require treatment.

- Jitteriness or discomfort while getting medicine to make your heart work hard and beat fast (you may be given medicine if you can't exercise). These side effects usually go away shortly after you stop getting the medicine. Sometimes the symptoms may last a few hours.

Also, some of the medicines used for pharmacological stress tests can cause wheezing, shortness of breath, and other asthma-like symptoms. Sometimes these symptoms are severe and require treatment.

Chapter 38

Transesophageal Echocardiography

What Is Transesophageal Echocardiography (TEE)?

Transesophageal echocardiography, or TEE, is a test that uses sound waves to create high-quality moving pictures of the heart and its blood vessels.

TEE is a type of echocardiography (echo). Echo shows the size and shape of the heart and how well the heart chambers and valves are working.

Echo can pinpoint areas of heart muscle that aren't contracting well because of poor blood flow or injury from a previous heart attack.

Echo also can detect possible blood clots inside the heart, fluid build up in the pericardium (the sac around the heart), and problems with the aorta. The aorta is the main artery that carries oxygen-rich blood from your heart to your body.

During echo, a device called a transducer is used to send sound waves (called ultrasound) to the heart. As the ultrasound waves bounce off the structures of the heart, a computer in the echo machine converts them into pictures on a screen.

This chapter includes text excerpted from "Transesophageal Echocardiography," National Heart, Lung, and Blood Institute (NHLBI), February 20, 2010. Reviewed July 2018.

TEE involves a flexible tube (probe) with a transducer at its tip. Your doctor will guide the probe down your throat and into your esophagus (the passage leading from your mouth to your stomach). This approach allows your doctor to get more detailed pictures of your heart because the esophagus is directly behind the heart.

TEE can help doctors diagnose heart and blood vessel diseases and conditions in adults and children. Doctors also may use TEE to guide cardiac catheterization, help prepare for surgery, or assess a patient's status during or after surgery.

Doctors may use TEE in addition to transthoracic echo (TTE), the most common type of echo. If TTE pictures don't give doctors enough information, they may recommend TEE to get more detailed pictures.

TEE has a low risk of complications in both adults and children. Even newborns can have TEE.

Types of TEE

Standard transesophageal echocardiography (TEE) pictures are two-dimensional (2D). It's also possible to get three-dimensional (3D) pictures from TEE. These pictures provide even more details about the structure and function of the heart and its blood vessels.

Doctors can use 3D TEE to help diagnose heart problems, such as congenital heart disease and heart valve disease. Doctors also may use this technology to assist with heart surgery.

Who Needs TEE

Doctors may recommend transesophageal echocardiography (TEE) to help diagnose a heart or blood vessel disease or condition. TEE can be used for adults and children.

Doctors also may use TEE to guide cardiac catheterization, help prepare for surgery, or assess a patient's status during or after surgery.

TEE helps doctors detect problems with the structure and function of the heart and its blood vessels.

In general, transthoracic echo (TTE) is the first echo test used to diagnose heart and blood vessel problems. However, you might have TEE if your doctor needs more information or more detailed pictures than TTE can provide.

For TTE, the transducer (the device that sends the sound waves) is placed on the chest, outside of the body. This means the sound waves may not always have a clear path to the heart and blood vessels. For example, obesity, scarring from previous heart surgery, or certain lung problems (such as a collapsed lung) may block the sound waves.

For TEE, the transducer is at the tip of a flexible tube (probe). Your doctor will guide the probe down your throat and into your esophagus (the passage leading from your mouth to your stomach).

This approach allows your doctor to get more detailed pictures of your heart because the esophagus is directly behind the heart.

Doctors may use TEE to help diagnose:

- Coronary heart disease (CHD)

- Congenital heart disease

- Heart attack

- Aortic aneurysm

- Endocarditis

- Cardiomyopathy

- Heart valve disease

- Injury to the heart or aorta (the main artery that carries oxygen-rich blood from your heart to your body)

TEE also can show blood clots that may have caused a stroke or that may affect treatment for atrial fibrillation (AF), a type of arrhythmia.

TEE and Cardiac Catheterization

Cardiac catheterization is a medical procedure used to diagnose and/or treat certain heart conditions. During this procedure, a long, thin, flexible tube called a catheter is put into a blood vessel in your arm, groin (upper thigh), or neck and threaded to your heart.

Doctors may use TEE to help guide the catheter while they're doing the procedure.

Through the catheter, doctors can do tests and treatments on your heart. For example, cardiac catheterization might be used to repair holes in the heart, heart valve disease, and abnormal heart rhythms.

TEE and Surgery

Doctors may use TEE to prepare for a patient's surgery and identify possible risks. For example, they may use TEE to look for possible sources of blood clots in the heart or aorta. Blood clots can cause a stroke during surgery.

TEE might be used in the operating room after a patient receives medicine to make him or her sleep during the surgery. The test can show the heart's structure and function and help guide the surgery.

TEE also helps doctors assess a patient's status during surgery. For example, TEE can help check for blood flow and blood pressure problems.

At the end of surgery, TEE might be used again to check how well the surgery worked. For example, TEE can show whether heart valves are working well. TEE also can show how well the heart is pumping.

People having surgery that isn't related to the heart also may have TEE to check their heart function if they have known heart disease or a critical illness.

What to Expect before TEE

Transesophageal echocardiography (TEE) most often is done in a hospital. You usually will need to fast (not eat or drink) for several hours prior to the test. Your doctor will let you know exactly how long you should fast.

You should let your doctor know whether you're taking any blood-thinning medicines, have trouble swallowing, or are allergic to any medicines. If you have dentures or oral prostheses, you'll need to remove them before the test.

You may be given medicine to help you relax during TEE. If so, you'll have to arrange for a ride home after the test because the medicine can make you sleepy.

Talk with your doctor about whether you need to take any special steps before having TEE. Your doctor can tell you whether you need to change how you take your regular medicines on the day of the test or whether you need to make other changes.

What to Expect during TEE

During transesophageal echocardiography (TEE), your doctor or your child's doctor will use a probe with a transducer at its tip. The transducer sends sound waves (ultrasound) to the heart. Probes come in many sizes; smaller probes are used for children and newborns.

The back of your mouth will be numbed with gel or spray before the probe is put down your throat. You may feel some discomfort as the probe is guided into your esophagus (the passage leading from your mouth to your stomach).

Adults having TEE may get medicine to help them relax during the test. The medicine will be injected into a vein.

Children always receive medicine to help them relax or sleep if they're having TEE. This helps them remain still so the doctor can safely insert the probe and take good pictures of the heart and blood vessels.

Your doctor will insert the probe into your mouth or nose. He or she will then gently guide it down your throat into your esophagus. Your esophagus lies directly behind your heart. During this process, your doctor will take care to protect your teeth and mouth from injury.

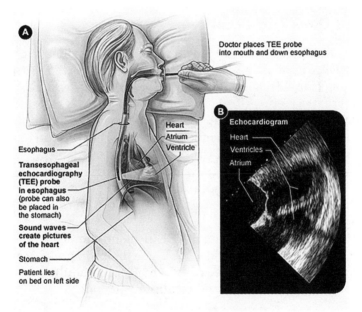

Figure 38.1. *Transesophageal Echocardiography*

Figure A shows a transesophageal echocardiography probe in the esophagus, which is located behind the heart. Sound waves from the probe create high-quality pictures of the heart. Figure B shows an echocardiogram of the heart's lower and upper chambers (ventricles and atrium, respectively).

Your blood pressure, blood oxygen level, and other vital signs will be checked during the test. You may be given oxygen through a tube in your nose.

TEE takes less than an hour. However, if you received medicine to help you relax, you might be watched for a few hours after the test for side effects from the medicine.

What to Expect after TEE

After having transesophageal echocardiography (TEE), your or your child's blood pressure, blood oxygen level, and other vital signs will continue to be closely watched. You can likely go home a few hours after having the test.

After the TEE, you may have a sore throat for a few hours. You shouldn't eat or drink for 30–60 minutes after having TEE. Most people can return to their normal activities within about 24 hours of the test.

Talk with your doctor or your child's doctor to learn more about what to expect after having TEE.

What Does TEE Show?

Transesophageal echocardiography (TEE) provides high-quality moving pictures of your heart and blood vessels. These pictures help doctors detect and treat heart and blood vessel diseases and conditions.

TEE creates pictures from inside the esophagus (the passage leading from the mouth to the stomach) or, sometimes, from inside the stomach. Because the esophagus lies directly behind the heart, TEE provides close-up pictures of the heart.

TEE also offers different views and may provide more detailed pictures than transthoracic echocardiography (TTE), the most common type of echo. (For TTE, the transducer is placed on the chest, outside of the body.)

Your doctor may recommend TEE if he or she needs more information than TTE can provide. TEE can help diagnose and assess heart and blood vessel diseases and conditions in adults and children. Examples of these diseases and conditions include:

- Coronary heart disease (CHD)

- Congenital heart disease

- Heart attack

- Aortic aneurysm

- Endocarditis

- Cardiomyopathy

- Heart valve disease

- Injury to the heart or aorta (the main artery that carries oxygen-rich blood from your heart to your body)

TEE also can show blood clots that may have caused a stroke or that may affect treatment for atrial fibrillation, a type of arrhythmia.

Doctors also may use TEE during cardiac catheterization. TEE can help doctors guide the catheter (thin, flexible tube) through the blood vessels. TEE also can help doctors prepare for surgery or assess a patient's status during or after surgery.

What Are the Risks of TEE?

Transesophageal echocardiography (TEE) has a very low risk of serious complications in both adults and children. To reduce your risk, your healthcare team will carefully check your heart rate and other vital signs during and after the test.

Some risks are associated with the medicine that might be used to help you relax during TEE. You may have a bad reaction to the medicine, problems breathing, or nausea (feeling sick to your stomach). Usually, these problems go away without treatment.

Your throat also might be sore for a few hours after the test. Although rare, the probe used during TEE can damage the esophagus (the passage leading from your mouth to your stomach).

Part Five

Screening and Assessments for Specific Conditions and Diseases

Chapter 39

Allergy Testing

Chapter Contents

Section 39.1

Allergy Blood Test

This section includes text excerpted from "Allergy Blood Test," MedlinePlus, National Institutes of Health (NIH), September 6, 2017.

What Is an Allergy Blood Test?

Allergies are a common and chronic condition that involves the body's immune system. Normally, your immune system works to fight off viruses, bacteria, and other infectious agents. When you have an allergy, your immune system treats a harmless substance, like dust or pollen, as a threat. To fight this perceived threat, your immune system makes antibodies called immunoglobulin E (IgE).

Substances that cause an allergic reaction are called allergens. Besides dust and pollen, other common allergens include animal dander, foods, including nuts and shellfish, and certain medicines, such as penicillin. Allergy symptoms can range from sneezing and a stuffy nose to a life-threatening complication called anaphylactic shock. Allergy blood tests measure the amount of IgE antibodies in the blood. A small amount of IgE antibodies is normal. A larger amount of IgE may mean you have an allergy.

Other names: IgE allergy test, Quantitative IgE, Immunoglobulin E, Total IgE, Specific IgE

What Is It Used For?

Allergy blood tests are used to find out if you have an allergy. One type of test called a total IgE test measures the overall number of IgE antibodies in your blood. Another type of allergy blood test called a specific IgE test measures the level of IgE antibodies in response to individual allergens.

Why Do I Need an Allergy Blood Test?

Your healthcare provider may order allergy testing if you have symptoms of an allergy. These include:

- Stuffy or runny nose
- Sneezing

426

- Itchy, watery eyes
- Hives (a rash with raised red patches)
- Diarrhea
- Vomiting
- Shortness of breath
- Coughing
- Wheezing

What Happens during an Allergy Blood Test?

A healthcare professional will take a blood sample from a vein in your arm, using a small needle. After the needle is inserted, a small amount of blood will be collected into a test tube or vial. You may feel a little sting when the needle goes in or out. This usually takes less than five minutes.

Will I Need to Do Anything to Prepare for the Test?

You don't need any special preparations for an allergy blood test.

Are There Any Risks to the Test?

There is very little risk to having an allergy blood test. You may have slight pain or bruising at the spot where the needle was put in, but most symptoms go away quickly.

What Do the Results Mean?

If your total IgE levels are higher than normal, it likely means you have some kind of allergy. But it does not reveal what you are allergic to. A specific IgE test will help identify your particular allergy. If your results indicate an allergy, your healthcare provider may refer you to an allergy specialist or recommend a treatment plan.

Your treatment plan will depend on the type and severity of your allergy. People at risk for anaphylactic shock, a severe allergic reaction that can cause death, need to take extra care to avoid the allergy-causing substance. They may need to carry an emergency epinephrine treatment with them at all times.

Be sure to talk to your healthcare provider if you have questions about your test results and/or your allergy treatment plan.

Is There Anything Else I Need to Know about an Allergy Blood Test?

An IgE skin test is another way to detect allergies, by measuring IgE levels and looking for a reaction directly on the skin. Your healthcare provider may order an IgE skin test instead of, or in addition to, an IgE allergy blood test.

Section 39.2

Patch Tests for Allergies

This section includes text excerpted from "Allergenics —
Allergen Patch Tests," Child Welfare Information Gateway,
U.S. Food and Drug Administration (FDA), March 7, 2017.

What Is Allergen Patch Tests?

Allergen patch tests are diagnostic tests applied to the surface of the skin. Patch tests are used by healthcare providers to determine the specific cause of contact dermatitis, and are manufactured from natural substances or chemicals (such as nickel, rubber, and fragrance mixes) that are known to cause contact dermatitis.

Indications and Usage

T.R.U.E. TEST® is an epicutaneous patch test indicated for use as an aid in the diagnosis of allergic contact dermatitis (ACD) in persons 6 years of age and older whose history suggests sensitivity to one or more of the 35 allergens and allergen mixes included on the T.R.U.E. TEST panels.

Dosage and Administration

Dose

T.R.U.E. TEST contains three adhesive panels consisting of 35 allergen and allergen mix patches and a 15 negative control.

Administration

T.R.U.E. TEST should only be applied to healthy skin. Test sites should be free of scars, acne, dermatitis, or other conditions that may interfere with test result interpretation. Avoid application of T.R.U.E. TEST panels to tanned or sun exposed skin because this may increase the risk of false negatives. Avoid patch testing for three (3) weeks after ultraviolet (UV) treatments, heavy sun, or tanning bed exposure. Avoid using alcohol or other irritating substances on the skin prior to testing. Avoid excessive sweating during the testing period to maintain sufficient adhesion to the skin. Avoid excessive physical activity to maintain sufficient adhesion and to prevent actual loss of patch test material. Avoid getting the panels and surrounding area wet. If excessive body hair exists at the test site, remove with an electric shaver (do not use razors). Very oily skin may be cleaned with mild soap and water prior to testing.

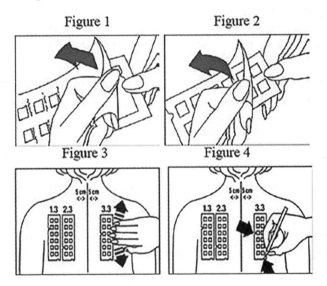

Figure 39.1. *T.R.U.E. Test Procedure*

Test panels should be applied as follows:

1. Peel open the package and remove the test panel (Figure 1).

2. Remove the protective plastic covering from the test surface of the panel (Figure 2). Be careful not to touch the test allergens or allergen mixes.

3. Position test Panel 1.3 on the patient's back as shown in Figure 3. Allergen number 1 should be in the upper left corner. Avoid applying the panel on the margin of the scapula or directly over the midline of the spine. Ensure that each patch of the allergen panel is in contact with the skin by smoothing the panel outward from the center to the edge (as illustrated for Panel 3.3 in Figure 3).

4. With a medical marking pen, indicate on the skin the location of the two notches on the panel (as illustrated for Panel 3.3 in Figure 4).

5. Repeat the process with test Panel 2.3. Position the test Panel 2.3 beside Panel 1.3, on the left side of the patient's back so that the number 13 allergen is in the upper left corner. Apply test Panel 2.3 five (5) cm from the midline of the spine (Figure 3).

6. Repeat the process with Panel 3.3 positioning the panel on the right side of the patient's back so that the number 25 allergen is in the upper left corner. Apply test Panel 3.3 five (5) cm from the midline of 54 the spine (Figure 3).

7. If needed, hypoallergenic surgical tape, appropriate for patch testing, may be used for increased adhesion around the outside edges of the panels.

Timing of Test Readings

Patients are scheduled to return approximately 48 hours after patch test application to have the panels removed. Prior to removal of the panels, use a medical marking pen to remark the notches found on the panels. The patch test reaction on the patient's skin may be evaluated at 48 hours, but an additional reading(s) at 72 and/or 96 hours is necessary. Late positive reactions may occur 7–21 days after application of the panels.

Interpretation Instructions

An identification template is provided for each of the three (3) panels for quick identification of any allergen that causes a reaction. To assure correct positioning, marks on the skin made with the medical marking pen should correlate with the notches on the template. The interpretation method, similar to the one recommended by the

International Contact Dermatitis Research Group (ICDRG), is as follows:

- ? Doubtful reaction: faint macular erythema only
- + Weak positive reaction: nonvesicular with erythema, infiltration, possibly papules
- ++ Strong positive reaction: vesicular, erythema, infiltration, papules
- +++ Extreme positive reaction: bullous or ulcerative reaction
- – Negative reaction
- IR Irritant reaction: Pustules as well as patchy follicular or homogeneous erythema without infiltrations are usually signs of irritation and do not indicate allergy.

Itching is a subjective symptom that is expected to accompany a positive reaction.

False Negatives

False negative results may be due to insufficient patch contact with the skin and/or premature evaluation of the test. Repeat testing may be indicated. The effect of repetitive testing with T.R.U.E. TEST is unknown.

False Positives

A false positive result may occur when an irritant reaction cannot be differentiated from an allergic reaction. A positive test reaction should meet the criteria for an allergic reaction. If an irritant reaction cannot be distinguished from a true positive reaction or if a doubtful reaction is present, a retest may be considered. The effect of repetitive testing with T.R.U.E. TEST is unknown.

Chapter 40

Autism Spectrum Disorder (ASD) Testing

Medical Tests and Evaluations Used to Diagnose Autism Spectrum Disorder (ASD)

The first signs of an autism spectrum disorder (ASD) often appear before a child reaches the age of two. These signs usually take the form of developmental delays in early language skills and social interactions. If a baby does not point or use other intentional gestures by 12 months, for instance, or use two-word spontaneous phrases by 24 months, he or she should be evaluated for an ASD. Identifying these signs as soon as possible is key to early diagnosis and treatment, which can improve skill and language development and help the child reach his or her full potential.

Under recommendations issued by the American Academy of Pediatrics, pediatricians and other healthcare providers are trained to screen children for ASDs during regular well-child visits. If they notice signs of developmental delays or symptoms of an ASD, they will usually refer the child to a specialist—such as a developmental pediatrician, child psychologist, pediatric neurologist, psychiatrist, or speech pathologist—for a complete evaluation.

"Medical Tests and Evaluations Used to Diagnose ASD," © 2016 Omnigraphics. Reviewed July 2018.

Since autism is a spectrum disorder with varying degrees of severity, it can be difficult to diagnose. No single medical test can determine whether a child has an ASD. Instead, specialists typically conduct a series of assessments to figure out whether the developmental delays they have identified in a child are caused by an ASD or another condition that may present similar symptoms, such as a personality disorder, hearing problems, lead poisoning, or fragile X syndrome.

Medical Tests to Diagnose ASD

Specialists use various types of behavioral evaluations and physical assessments to gather the information needed to make a diagnosis of ASD. Some of the common types of behavioral evaluations include:

- Application of the American Association of Childhood and Adolescent Psychiatry (AACAP) guidelines for assessing whether a child's behavior indicates an ASD

- Compilation of a complete medical and developmental history through interviews or questionnaires with parents or other caregivers

- Observations of the child's behavior, social interactions, and communication skills in different situations over time

- Administration of structured tests covering developmental level, intelligence, communication, behavior, and social interaction to determine whether the child's developmental delays affect his or her thinking, problem-solving, and decision-making abilities

Specialists may also perform physical examinations and laboratory tests to help determine whether a child's symptoms indicate ASD or may be related to a physical problem. Some of these assessments include:

- A complete physical examination—including height, weight, and head measurements—to see whether the child's growth is following a normal pattern

- An ear examination and hearing tests to see whether speech and language delays or issues with social skills and behavior may be caused by a hearing problem

- Blood tests for lead poisoning, which can cause developmental delays

- Chromosomal analysis to determine whether signs of intellectual disability may be related to a genetic disorder, such as fragile X syndrome

- Brain scans, such as an electroencephalograph (EEG) or magnetic resonance imaging (MRI), to see whether differences in brain structure may be causing regression in the child's development or behavior

All of these medical tests and evaluations are intended to rule out other conditions and pinpoint ASD as the cause of the child's developmental delays. Once the diagnosis has been made, ASD specialists can design a program of treatments and interventions to help address any deficits and enable the child to reach his or her full potential.

Reference

"Autism: Exams and Tests," WebMD, November 14, 2014.

Chapter 41

Bladder and Kidney Function Tests

Chapter Contents

Section 41.1

Albumin Blood Test

This section includes text excerpted from "Albumin Blood Test," MedlinePlus, National Institutes of Health (NIH), December 19, 2017.

What Is an Albumin Blood Test?

An albumin blood test measures the amount of albumin in your blood. Albumin is a protein made by your liver. Albumin helps keep fluid in your bloodstream so it doesn't leak into other tissues. It also carries various substances throughout your body, including hormones, vitamins, and enzymes. Low albumin levels can indicate a problem with your liver or kidneys.

What Is It Used For?

An albumin blood test is a type of liver function test. Liver function tests are blood tests that measure different enzymes and proteins in the liver, including albumin. An albumin test may also be part of a comprehensive metabolic panel, a test that measures several substances in your blood. These substances include electrolytes, glucose, and proteins such as albumin.

Why Do You Need an Albumin Blood Test?

Your healthcare provider may have ordered liver function tests or a comprehensive metabolic panel, which include tests for albumin, as part your regular checkup. You may also need this test if you have symptoms of liver or kidney disease.

Symptoms of liver disease include:

- jaundice, a condition that causes your skin and eyes to turn yellow

- fatigue

- weight loss

- loss of appetite

- dark-colored urine

- pale-colored stool

Symptoms of kidney disease include:

- swelling around the abdomen, thighs, or face
- more frequent urination, especially at night
- foamy, bloody, or coffee-colored urine
- nausea
- itchy skin

What Happens during an Albumin Blood Test?

A healthcare professional will take a blood sample from a vein in your arm, using a small needle. After the needle is inserted, a small amount of blood will be collected into a test tube or vial. You may feel a little sting when the needle goes in or out. This usually takes less than five minutes.

Will You Need to Do Anything to Prepare for the Test?

You don't need any special preparations to test for albumin in blood. If your healthcare provider has ordered other blood tests, you may need to fast (not eat or drink) for several hours before the test. Your healthcare provider will let you know if there are any special instructions to follow.

Are There Any Risks to the Test?

There is very little risk to having a blood test. You may have slight pain or bruising at the spot where the needle was put in, but most symptoms go away quickly.

What Do the Results Mean?

If your albumin levels are lower than normal, it may indicate one of the following conditions:

- liver disease, including cirrhosis
- kidney disease
- malnutrition
- infection

- inflammatory bowel disease (IBD)

- thyroid disease

Higher than normal levels of albumin may indicate dehydration or severe diarrhea.

If your albumin levels are not in the normal range, it doesn't necessarily mean you have a medical condition needing treatment. Certain drugs, including steroids, insulin, and hormones, can raise albumin levels. Other drugs, including birth control pills, can lower your albumin levels.

Section 41.2

Blood Urea Nitrogen (BUN) Test

This section includes text excerpted from "BUN (Blood Urea Nitrogen)," MedlinePlus, National Institutes of Health (NIH), December 19, 2017.

What Is a Blood Urea Nitrogen (BUN) Test?

A BUN, or blood urea nitrogen test, can provide important information about your kidney function. The main job of your kidneys is to remove waste and extra fluid from your body. If you have kidney disease, this waste material can build up in your blood and may lead to serious health problems, including high blood pressure, anemia, and heart disease.

The test measures the amount of urea nitrogen in your blood. Urea nitrogen is one of the waste products removed from your blood by your kidneys. Higher than normal BUN levels may be a sign that your kidneys aren't working efficiently.

People with early kidney disease may not have any symptoms. A BUN test can help uncover kidney problems at an early stage when treatment can be more effective.

What Is BUN Test Used For?

A BUN test is often part of a series of tests called a comprehensive metabolic panel, and can be used to help diagnose or monitor a kidney disease or disorder.

Why Do You Need a BUN Test?

Your healthcare provider may order a BUN test as part of a routine checkup or if you have or are at risk for a kidney problem. Although early kidney disease usually does not have any signs or symptoms, certain factors can put you at a higher risk. These include:

- family history of kidney problems

- diabetes

- high blood pressure

- heart disease

In addition, your BUN levels may be checked if you are experiencing symptoms of later stage kidney disease, such as:

- needing to go the bathroom (urinate) frequently or infrequently

- itching

- recurring fatigue

- swelling in your arms, legs, or feet

- muscle cramps

- trouble sleeping

What Happens during a BUN Test?

A healthcare professional will take a blood sample from a vein in your arm, using a small needle. After the needle is inserted, a small amount of blood will be collected into a test tube or vial. You may feel a little sting when the needle goes in or out. This usually takes less than five minutes.

Will You Need to Do Anything to Prepare for the BUN Test?

You don't need any special preparations for a BUN test. If your healthcare provider has also ordered other blood tests, you may need to fast (not eat or drink) for several hours before the test. Your healthcare provider will let you know if there are any special instructions to follow.

Are There Any Risks to the BUN Test?

There is very little risk to having a blood test. You may have slight pain or bruising at the spot where the needle was put in, but most symptoms go away quickly.

What Do the BUN Test Results Mean?

Normal BUN levels can vary, but generally a high level of blood urea nitrogen is a sign that your kidneys are not working correctly. However, abnormal results don't always indicate that you have a medical condition needing treatment. Higher than normal BUN levels can also be caused by dehydration, burns, certain medications, a high protein diet, or other factors. To learn what your results mean, talk to your healthcare provider.

Is There Anything Else You Need to Know about the BUN Test?

A BUN test is only one type of measurement of kidney function. If your healthcare provider suspects you have kidney disease, additional tests may be recommended. These may include a measurement of creatinine, which is another waste product filtered by your kidneys, and a test called a GFR (Glomerular Filtration Rate), which estimates how well your kidneys are filtering blood.

Section 41.3

Calcium Blood Test

This section includes text excerpted from "Calcium Blood Test,"
MedlinePlus, National Institutes of Health (NIH), October 11, 2017.

What Is a Calcium Blood Test?

A calcium blood test measures the amount of calcium in your blood. Calcium is one of the most important minerals in your body. You need calcium for healthy bones and teeth. Calcium is also essential for proper functioning of your nerves, muscles, and heart. About 99 percent of your body's calcium is stored in your bones. The remaining 1 percent circulates in the blood. If there is too much or too little calcium in the blood, it may be a sign of bone disease, thyroid disease, kidney disease, or other medical conditions.

What Is Calcium Blood Test Used For?

There are two types of calcium blood tests:

1. **Total calcium,** which measures the calcium attached to specific proteins in your blood.

2. **Ionized calcium,** which measures the calcium that is unattached or "free" from these proteins.

Total calcium is often part of a routine screening test called a basic metabolic panel. A basic metabolic panel is a test that measures different minerals and other substances in the blood, including calcium.

Why Do You Need a Calcium Blood Test?

Your healthcare provider may have ordered a basic metabolic panel, which includes a calcium blood test, as part of your regular checkup, or if you have symptoms of abnormal calcium levels.

Symptoms of high calcium levels include:

- nausea and vomiting
- more frequent urination
- increased thirst
- constipation
- abdominal pain
- loss of appetite

Symptoms of low calcium levels include:

- tingling in the lips, tongue, fingers, and feet
- muscle cramps
- muscle spasms
- irregular heartbeat

Many people with high or low calcium levels do not have any symptoms. Your healthcare provider may order a calcium test if you have a preexisting condition that may affect your calcium levels. These include:

- kidney disease

- thyroid disease

- malnutrition

- certain types of cancer

What Happens during a Calcium Blood Test?

A healthcare professional will take a blood sample from a vein in your arm, using a small needle. After the needle is inserted, a small amount of blood will be collected into a test tube or vial. You may feel a little sting when the needle goes in or out. This usually takes less than five minutes.

Will You Need to Do Anything to Prepare for the Calcium Blood Test?

You don't need any special preparations for a calcium blood test or a basic metabolic panel. If your healthcare provider has ordered more tests on your blood sample, you may need to fast (not eat or drink) for several hours before the test. Your healthcare provider will let you know if there are any special instructions to follow.

Are There Any Risks to the Calcium Blood Test?

There is very little risk to having a blood test. You may have slight pain or bruising at the spot where the needle was put in, but most symptoms go away quickly.

What Do the Calcium Blood Test Results Mean?

If your results show higher than normal calcium levels, it may indicate:

- hyperparathyroidism, a condition in which your parathyroid glands produce too much parathyroid hormone

- Paget disease of the bone, a condition that causes your bones to become too big, weak, and prone to fractures

- overuse of antacids that contain calcium

- excessive intake of calcium from vitamin d supplements or milk

- certain types of cancer

If your results show lower than normal calcium levels, it may indicate:

- hypoparathyroidism, a condition in which your parathyroid glands produce too little parathyroid hormone

- vitamin D deficiency

- magnesium deficiency

- inflammation of the pancreas (pancreatitis)

- kidney disease

If your calcium test results are not in the normal range, it doesn't necessarily mean that you have a medical condition needing treatment. Other factors, such as diet and certain medicines, can affect your calcium levels. If you have questions about your results, talk to your healthcare provider.

Is There Anything Else You Need to Know about a Calcium Blood Test?

A calcium blood test does not tell you how much calcium is in your bones. Bone health can be measured with a type of X-ray called a bone density scan, or dexa scan. A dexa scan measures the mineral content, including calcium, and other aspects of your bones.

Section 41.4

Calcium in Urine Test

This section includes text excerpted from "Calcium in Urine Test," MedlinePlus, National Institutes of Health (NIH), October 3, 2017.

What Is a Calcium in Urine Test?

A calcium in urine test measures the amount of calcium in your urine. Calcium is one of the most important minerals in your body. You need calcium for healthy bones and teeth. Calcium is also essential for proper functioning of your nerves, muscles, and heart. Almost all of your body's calcium is stored in your bones. A small amount circulates in the blood, and the remainder is filtered by the kidneys and passed into your urine. If urine calcium levels are too high or too low, it may mean you have a medical condition, such as kidney disease or kidney stones. Kidney stones are hard, pebble-like substances that can form in one or both kidneys when calcium or other minerals build up in the urine. Most kidney stones are formed from calcium.

Too much or too little calcium in the blood can also indicate a kidney disorder, as well as certain bone diseases, and other medical problems. So if you have symptoms of one of these disorders, your healthcare provider may order a calcium blood test, along with a calcium in urine test. In addition, a calcium blood test is often included as part of a regular check-up.

What Is Calcium in Urine Test Used For?

A calcium in urine test may be used to diagnose or monitor kidney function or kidney stones. It may also be used to diagnose disorders of the parathyroid, a gland near the thyroid that helps regulate the amount of calcium in your body.

Why Do You Need a Calcium in Urine Test?

You may need a calcium in urine test if you have symptoms of a kidney stone. These symptoms include:

• severe back pain

• abdominal pain

• nausea and vomiting

- blood in the urine

- frequent urination

You may also need a calcium in urine test if you have symptoms of a parathyroid disorder.

Symptoms of too much parathyroid hormone include:

- nausea and vomiting

- loss of appetite

- abdominal pain

- fatigue

- frequent urination

- bone and joint pain

Symptoms of too little parathyroid hormone include:

- abdominal pain

- muscle cramps

- tingling fingers

- dry skin

- brittle nails

What Happens during a Calcium in Urine Test?

You'll need to collect all your urine during a 24-hour period. This is called a 24-hour urine sample test. Your healthcare provider or a laboratory professional will give you a container to collect your urine in and instructions on how to collect and store your samples. A 24-hour urine sample test generally includes the following steps:

- Empty your bladder in the morning and flush that urine down. Do not collect this urine. Record the time.

- For the next 24 hours, save all your urine in the container provided.

- Store your urine container in a refrigerator or a cooler with ice.

- Return the sample container to your health provider's office or the laboratory as instructed.

Will You Need to Do Anything to Prepare for the Calcium in Urine Test?

You don't need any special preparations for a calcium in urine test. Be sure to carefully follow all the instructions for providing a 24-hour urine sample.

Are There Any Risks to the Calcium in Urine Test?

There is no known risk to having a calcium in urine test.

What Do the Calcium in Urine Test Results Mean?

If your results show higher than normal calcium levels in your urine, it may indicate:

- risk for or the presence of a kidney stone

- hyperparathyroidism, a condition in which your parathyroid gland produces too much parathyroid hormone

- sarcoidosis, a disease that causes inflammation in the lungs, lymph nodes, or other organs

- too much calcium in your diet from vitamin D supplements or milk

If your results show lower than normal calcium levels in your urine, it may indicate:

- hypoparathyroidism, a condition in which your parathyroid gland produces too little parathyroid hormone

- vitamin D deficiency

- a kidney disorder

Is There Anything Else You Need to Know about a Calcium in Urine Test?

A calcium in urine test does not tell you how much calcium is in your bones. Bone health can be measured with a type of X-ray called a bone density scan, or dexa scan. A dexa scan measures the mineral content, including calcium, and other aspects of your bones.

Section 41.5

Chloride Blood Test

This section includes text excerpted from "Chloride
Blood Test," MedlinePlus, National Institutes of
Health (NIH), October 11, 2017.

What Is a Chloride Blood Test?

A chloride blood test measures the amount of chloride in your
blood. Chloride is a type of electrolyte. Electrolytes are electrically
charged minerals that help control the amount of fluids and the
balance of acids and bases in your body. Chloride is often measured
along with other electrolytes to diagnose or monitor conditions
such as kidney disease, heart failure, liver disease, and high blood
pressure.

What Is Chloride Blood Test Used For?

A chloride test is not normally given as an individual test. You
usually get a chloride test as part of a routine blood screening or to
help diagnose a condition related to an imbalance of acids or fluids in
your body.

Why Do You Need a Chloride Blood Test?

Your healthcare provider may have ordered a chloride blood test
as part of an electrolyte panel, which is a routine blood test. An electrolyte panel is a test that measures chloride and other electrolytes,
such as potassium, sodium, and bicarbonate. You may also need a
chloride blood test if you have symptoms of an acid or fluid imbalance,
including:

- vomiting over a long period of time

- diarrhea

- fatigue

- weakness

- dehydration

- trouble breathing

What Happens during a Chloride Blood Test?

A healthcare professional will take a blood sample from a vein in your arm, using a small needle. After the needle is inserted, a small amount of blood will be collected into a test tube or vial. You may feel a little sting when the needle goes in or out. This usually takes less than five minutes.

Will You Need to Do Anything to Prepare for the Chloride Blood Test?

You don't need any special preparations for a chloride blood test or an electrolyte panel. If your healthcare provider has ordered other blood tests, you may need to fast (not eat or drink) for several hours before the test. Your healthcare provider will let you know if there are any special instructions to follow.

Are There Any Risks to the Chloride Blood Test?

There is very little risk to having a blood test. You may have slight pain or bruising at the spot where the needle was put in, but most symptoms go away quickly.

What Do the Chloride Blood Test Results Mean?

There are many reasons why your chloride levels may not be in the normal range. High levels of chloride may indicate:

- dehydration

- kidney disease

- acidosis, a condition in which you have too much acid in your blood. It can cause nausea, vomiting, and fatigue.

- alkalosis, a condition in which you have too much base in your blood. It can cause irritability, muscle twitching, and tingling in the fingers and toes.

Low levels of chloride may indicate:

- heart failure

- lung diseases

- Addison disease, a condition in which your body's adrenal glands don't produce enough of certain types of hormones. It can cause

450

a variety of symptoms, including weakness, dizziness, weight loss, and dehydration.

If your chloride levels are not the normal range, it doesn't necessarily mean you have a medical problem needing treatment. Many factors can affect your chloride levels. If you have taken in too much fluid or have lost fluid because of vomiting or diarrhea, it can affect your chloride levels. Also, certain medicines such as antacids can cause abnormal results. To learn what your results mean, talk to your healthcare provider.

Is There Anything Else You Need to Know about a Chloride Blood Test?

Urine also contains some chloride. Your healthcare provider may recommend a urine chloride test in addition to the blood test to get more information about your chloride levels.

Section 41.6

Urodynamic Testing

This section includes text excerpted from "Urodynamic Testing," National Institute of Diabetes and Digestive and Kidney Diseases (NIDDK), February 2014. Reviewed July 2018.

What Is Urodynamic Testing?

Urodynamic testing is any procedure that looks at how well the bladder, sphincters, and urethra are storing and releasing urine. Most urodynamic tests focus on the bladder's ability to hold urine and empty steadily and completely. Urodynamic tests can also show whether the bladder is having involuntary contractions that cause urine leakage. A healthcare provider may recommend urodynamic tests if symptoms suggest problems with the lower urinary tract. Lower urinary tract symptoms (LUTS) include:

- urine leakage

- frequent urination

- painful urination

- sudden, strong urges to urinate

- problems emptying the bladder completely

- recurrent urinary tract infections

Urodynamic tests range from simple observation to precise measurements using sophisticated instruments. For simple observation, a healthcare provider may record:

- the length of time it takes a person to produce a urinary stream

- the volume of urine produced

- ability or inability to stop the urine flow in midstream

For precise measurements, imaging equipment takes pictures of the bladder filling and emptying, pressure monitors record the pressures inside the bladder, and sensors record muscle and nerve activity. The healthcare provider will decide the type of urodynamic test based on the person's health information, physical exam, and LUTS. The urodynamic test results help diagnose the cause and nature of a lower urinary tract problem.

Most urodynamic tests do not involve special preparations, though some tests may require a person to make a change in fluid intake or to stop taking certain medications. Depending on the test, a person may be instructed to arrive for testing with a full bladder.

What Does Urodynamic Tests Include?

Urodynamic tests include:

- Uroflowmetry

- Postvoid residual measurement

- Cystometric test

- Leak point pressure measurement

- Pressure flow study

- Electromyography

- Video urodynamic tests

Uroflowmetry

Uroflowmetry is the measurement of urine speed and volume. Special equipment automatically measures the amount of urine and the flow rate—how fast the urine comes out. Uroflowmetry equipment includes a device for catching and measuring urine and a computer to record the data. During a uroflowmetry test, the person urinates privately into a special toilet or funnel that has a container for collecting the urine and a scale. The equipment creates a graph that shows changes in flow rate from second to second so the healthcare provider can see when the flow rate is the highest and how many seconds it takes to get there. Results of this test will be abnormal if the bladder muscles are weak or urine flow is blocked. Another approach to measuring flow rate is to record the time it takes to urinate into a special container that accurately measures the volume of urine. Uroflowmetry measurements are performed in a healthcare provider's office; no anesthesia is needed.

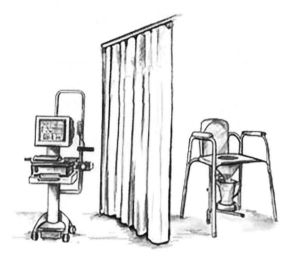

Figure 41.1. *Uroflowmetry Equipment*

Postvoid Residual Measurement

This urodynamic test measures the amount of urine left in the bladder after urination. The remaining urine is called the postvoid residual. Postvoid residual can be measured with ultrasound equipment that uses harmless sound waves to create a picture of the bladder. Bladder ultrasounds are performed in a healthcare provider's office, radiology center, or hospital by a specially trained technician and interpreted by a doctor, usually a radiologist. Anesthesia is not needed. Postvoid residual can also be measured using a catheter—a thin flexible tube. A healthcare provider inserts the catheter through the urethra up into the bladder to remove and measure the amount of remaining urine. A postvoid residual of 100 milliliters or more is a sign that the bladder is not emptying completely. Catheter measurements are performed in a healthcare provider's office, clinic, or hospital with local anesthesia.

Cystometric Test

A cystometric test measures how much urine the bladder can hold, how much pressure builds up inside the bladder as it stores urine, and how full it is when the urge to urinate begins. A catheter is used to empty the bladder completely. Then a special, smaller catheter is placed in the bladder. This catheter has a pressure-measuring device called a manometer. Another catheter may be placed in the rectum to record pressure there.

Once the bladder is emptied completely, the bladder is filled slowly with warm water. During this time, the person is asked to describe how the bladder feels and indicate when the need to urinate arises. When

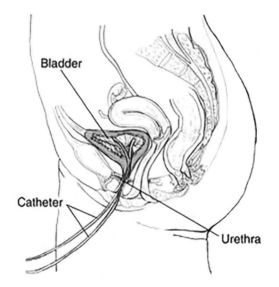

Figure 41.2. *Cystometric Test*

the urge to urinate occurs, the volume of water and the bladder pressure are recorded. The person may be asked to cough or strain during this procedure to see if the bladder pressure changes. A cystometric test can also identify involuntary bladder contractions. Cystometric tests are performed in a healthcare provider's office, clinic, or hospital with local anesthesia.

Leak Point Pressure (LPP) Measurement

This urodynamic test measures pressure at the point of leakage during a cystometric test. While the bladder is being filled for the cystometric test, it may suddenly contract and squeeze some water out without warning. The manometer measures the pressure inside the bladder when this leakage occurs. This reading may provide information about the kind of bladder problem that exists. The person may be asked to apply abdominal pressure to the bladder by coughing, shifting position, or trying to exhale while holding the nose and mouth. These actions help the healthcare provider evaluate the sphincters.

Pressure Flow Study

A pressure flow study measures the bladder pressure required to urinate and the flow rate a given pressure generates. After the cystometric test, the person empties the bladder, during which time a manometer is used to measure bladder pressure and flow rate. This pressure flow study helps identify bladder outlet blockage that men may experience with prostate enlargement. Bladder outlet blockage is less common in women but can occur with a cystocele or, rarely, after a surgical procedure for urinary incontinence. Pressure flow studies are performed in a healthcare provider's office, clinic, or hospital with local anesthesia.

Electromyography (EMG)

Electromyography (EMG) uses special sensors to measure the electrical activity of the muscles and nerves in and around the bladder and the sphincters. If the healthcare provider thinks the urinary problem is related to nerve or muscle damage, the person may be given an electromyography. The sensors are placed on the skin near the urethra and rectum or on a urethral or rectal catheter. Muscle and nerve activity is recorded on a machine. The patterns of the nerve impulses show whether the messages sent to the bladder and sphincters are coordinated correctly. Electromyography is performed by a specially trained technician in a healthcare provider's office, outpatient clinic, or hospital. Anesthesia is not needed if sensors are placed on the skin. Local anesthesia is needed if sensors are placed on a urethral or rectal catheter.

Video Urodynamic Tests

Video urodynamic tests take pictures and videos of the bladder during filling and emptying. The imaging equipment may use X-rays or ultrasound. If X-ray equipment is used, the bladder will be filled with a special fluid, called contrast medium, that shows up on X-rays. X-rays are performed by an X-ray technician in a healthcare provider's office, outpatient facility, or hospital; anesthesia is not needed. If ultrasound equipment is used, the bladder is filled with warm water and harmless sound waves are used to create a picture of the bladder. The pictures and videos show the size and shape of the bladder and help the healthcare provider understand the problem. Bladder ultrasounds are performed in a healthcare provider's office, radiology center, or hospital by a specially trained technician and interpreted by a doctor, usually a radiologist. Although anesthesia is not needed for the ultrasound, local anesthesia is needed to insert the catheter to fill the bladder.

What Happens after Urodynamic Tests?

After having urodynamic tests, a person may feel mild discomfort for a few hours when urinating. Drinking an 8-ounce glass of water every half-hour for 2 hours may help to reduce the discomfort. The healthcare provider may recommend taking a warm bath or holding a warm, damp washcloth over the urethral opening to relieve the discomfort.

An antibiotic may be prescribed for 1 or 2 days to prevent infection, but not always. People with signs of infection—including pain, chills, or fever—should call their healthcare provider immediately.

How Soon will Urodynamic Tests Results Be Available?

Results for simple tests such as cystometry and uroflowmetry are often available immediately after the test. Results of other tests such as electromyography and video urodynamic tests may take a few days to come back. A healthcare provider will talk with the patient about the results and possible treatments.

Section 41.7

Tracking Chronic Kidney Disease

This section includes text excerpted from "Chronic
Kidney Disease Tests and Diagnosis," National
Institute of Diabetes and Digestive and Kidney
Diseases (NIDDK), October 2016.

How Can You Tell If You Have Kidney Disease?

Early kidney disease usually doesn't have any symptoms. Testing is
the only way to know how well your kidneys are working. Get checked
for kidney disease if you have:

- diabetes

- high blood pressure

- heart disease

- a family history of kidney failure

If you have diabetes, get checked every year. If you have high blood
pressure, heart disease, or a family history of kidney failure, talk
with your healthcare provider about how often you should get tested.
The sooner you know you have kidney disease, the sooner you can get
treatment to help protect your kidneys.

What Tests Do Doctors Use to Diagnose and Monitor Kidney Disease?

To check for kidney disease, healthcare providers use

- a blood test that checks how well your kidneys are filtering your
  blood, called GFR. GFR stands for glomerular filtration rate

- a urine test to check for albumin. Albumin is a protein that can
  pass into the urine when the kidneys are damaged

If you have kidney disease, your healthcare provider will use the
same two tests to help monitor your kidney disease and make sure
your treatment plan is working.

Blood Test for Glomerular Filtration Rate (GFR)

Your healthcare provider will use a blood test to check your kidney function. The results of the test mean the following:

- A glomerular filtration rate (GFR) of 60 or more is in the normal range. Ask your healthcare provider when your GFR should be checked again.

- A GFR of less than 60 may mean you have kidney disease. Talk with your healthcare provider about how to keep your kidney health at this level.

- A GFR of 15 or less is called kidney failure. Most people below this level need dialysis or a kidney transplant. Talk with your healthcare provider about your treatment options.

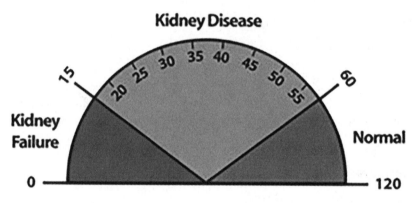

Figure 41.3. *Glomerular Filtration Rate (GFR)*

GFR results show whether your kidneys are filtering at a normal level.

You can't raise your GFR, but you can try to keep it from going lower.

Creatinine. Creatinine is a waste product from the normal breakdown of muscles in your body. Your kidneys remove creatinine from your blood. Providers use the amount of creatinine in your blood to estimate your GFR. As kidney disease gets worse, the level of creatinine goes up.

Urine Test for Albumin

If you are at risk for kidney disease, your provider may check your urine for albumin.

Albumin is a protein found in your blood. A healthy kidney doesn't let albumin pass into the urine. A damaged kidney lets some albumin pass into the urine. The less albumin in your urine, the better. Having albumin in the urine is called albuminuria.

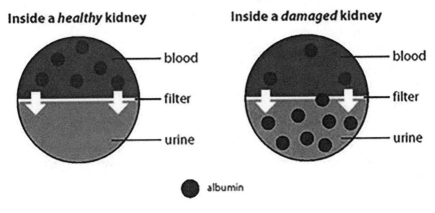

Figure 41.4. *Albumin Level*

A healthy kidney doesn't let albumin pass into the urine. A damaged kidney lets some albumin pass into the urine.

A healthcare provider can check for albumin in your urine in two ways:

1. **Dipstick test for albumin.** A provider uses a urine sample to look for albumin in your urine. You collect the urine sample in a container in a healthcare provider's office or lab. For the test, a provider places a strip of chemically treated paper, called a dipstick, into the urine. The dipstick changes color if albumin is present in the urine.

2. **Urine albumin-to-creatinine ratio (UACR).** This test measures and compares the amount of albumin with the amount of creatinine in your urine sample. Providers use your UACR to estimate how much albumin would pass into your urine over 24 hours. A urine albumin result of:

   - 30 mg/g or less is normal

   - more than 30 mg/g may be a sign of kidney disease

If you have albumin in your urine, your provider may want you to repeat the urine test one or two more times to confirm the results. Talk with your provider about what your specific numbers mean for you.

If you have kidney disease, measuring the albumin in your urine helps your provider know which treatment is best for you. A urine albumin level that stays the same or goes down may mean that treatments are working.

How Do You Know If Your Kidney Disease Is Getting Worse?

You can keep track of your test results over time. You can tell that your treatments are working if your:

- GFR stays the same

- urine albumin stays the same or goes down

Your healthcare provider will work with you to manage your kidney disease.

Chapter 42

Cancer Screening Tests

Chapter Contents

Section 42.1

Cancer Screening Overview

This section includes text excerpted from "Cancer Screening Overview (PDQ®)—Patient Version," National Cancer Institute (NCI), April 25, 2017.

Cancer screening is looking for cancer before a person has any symptoms. Screening tests can help find cancer at an early-stage, before symptoms appear. When abnormal tissue or cancer is found early, it may be easier to treat or cure. By the time symptoms appear, the cancer may have grown and spread. This can make the cancer harder to treat or cure.

It is important to remember that when your doctor suggests a screening test, it does not always mean he or she thinks you have cancer. Screening tests are done when you have no cancer symptoms.

Types of Screening Tests

Screening tests include the following:

- **Physical exam and history.** An exam of the body to check general signs of health, including checking for signs of disease, such as lumps or anything else that seems unusual. A history of the patient's health habits and past illnesses and treatments will also be taken.

- **Laboratory tests.** Medical procedures that test samples of tissue, blood, urine, or other substances in the body

- **Imaging procedures.** Procedures that make pictures of areas inside the body

- **Genetic tests.** Tests that look for certain gene mutations (changes) that are linked to some types of cancer

Risks of Screening Tests

Not all screening tests are helpful and most have risks. It is important to know the risks of the test and whether it has been proven to decrease the chance of dying from cancer.

Some screening tests can cause serious problems. Some screening procedures can cause bleeding or other problems. For example, colon cancer screening with sigmoidoscopy, or colonoscopy can cause tears in the lining of the colon.

False-positive test results are possible. Screening test results may appear to be abnormal even though there is no cancer. A false-positive test result (one that shows there is cancer when there really isn't) can cause anxiety and is usually followed by more tests and procedures, which also have risks.

False-negative test results are possible. Screening test results may appear to be normal even though there is cancer. A person who receives a false-negative test result (one that shows there is no cancer when there really is) may delay seeking medical care even if there are symptoms.

Finding the cancer may not improve the person's health or help the person live longer. Some cancers never cause symptoms or become life-threatening, but if found by a screening test, the cancer may be treated. There is no way to know if treating the cancer would help the person live longer than if no treatment were given. In both teenagers and adults, there is an increased risk of suicide in the first year after being diagnosed with cancer. Also, treatments for cancer have side effects.

For some cancers, finding and treating the cancer early does not improve the chance of a cure or help the person live longer.

Informed and Shared Decision-Making

It is important that you understand the benefits and harms of screening tests and make an informed choice about which screening tests are right for you.

Before having any screening test, it is important that you discuss the test with your doctor or other healthcare provider. Every screening test has both benefits and harms. Your healthcare provider should talk to you about the benefits and harms of a screening test and include you in the decision about whether the screening test is right for you. This is called informed and shared decision-making.

1. Your healthcare provider will talk to you about the possible benefits, harms, and unknowns of a screening test. This may include information about the benefits of finding a cancer early or the harms related to false test results, overdiagnosis, and overtreatment. Your healthcare provider may also give you information in a leaflet, booklet, video, website, or other material.

2. After you understand the benefits and harms of a screening test, you can decide whether or not you want to have the screening test based on what is best for you. Sometimes the harms and benefits are closely matched and the decision about whether to have a screening test is hard to make.

3. Your healthcare provider will write your decision down in your medical record and order the screening test, if that was your decision.

Goals of Screening Tests

Screening tests have many goals. A screening test that works the way it should and is helpful does the following:

- finds cancer before symptoms appear

- screens for a cancer that is easier to treat and cure when found early

- has few false-negative test results and false-positive test results

- decreases the chance of dying from cancer

Screening tests are not meant to diagnose cancer. Screening tests usually do not diagnose cancer. If a screening test result is abnormal, more tests may be done to check for cancer. For example, a screening mammogram may find a lump in the breast. A lump may be cancer or something else. More tests need to be done to find out if the lump is cancer. These are called diagnostic tests. Diagnostic tests may include a biopsy, in which cells or tissues are removed so a pathologist can check them under a microscope for signs of cancer.

Who Needs to Be Screened?

Anything that increases the chance of cancer is called a cancer risk factor. Having a risk factor does not mean that you will get cancer; not having risk factors doesn't mean that you will not get cancer.

Some screening tests are used only for people who have known risk factors for certain types of cancer. People known to have a higher risk of cancer than others include those who:

- have had cancer in the past; or

- have a family history of cancer.; or

- have certain gene mutations (changes) that have been linked to cancer.

People who have a high risk of cancer may need to be screened more often or at an earlier age than other people.

Cancer screening research includes finding out who has an increased risk of cancer. Scientists are trying to better understand who is likely to get certain types of cancer. They study the things we do and the things around us to see if they cause cancer. This information helps doctors figure out who should be screened for cancer, which screening tests should be used, and how often the tests should be done.

Since 1973, the Surveillance, Epidemiology, and End Results (SEER) Program of the National Cancer Institute (NCI) has been collecting information on people with cancer from different parts of the United States. Information from SEER, research studies, and other sources is used to study who is at risk.

How Cancer Risk Is Measured

Cancer risk is measured in different ways. The findings from surveys and studies about cancer risk are studied and the results are explained in different ways. Some of the ways risk is explained include absolute risk, relative risk, and odds ratios.

Absolute Risk

This is the risk a person has of developing a disease, in a given population (for example, the entire U.S. population) over a certain period of time. Researchers estimate the absolute risk by studying a large number of people that are part of a certain population (for example, women in a given age group). Researchers count the number of people in the group who get a certain disease over a certain period of time. For example, a group of 100,000 women between the ages of 20–29 are observed for one year, and 4 of them get breast cancer during that time. This means that the one-year absolute risk of breast cancer for a woman in this age group is 4 in 100,000 or 4 chances in 100,000.

Relative Risk

This is often used in research studies to find out whether a trait or a factor can be linked to the risk of a disease. Researchers compare two groups of people who are a lot alike. However, the people in one of the groups must have the trait or factor being studied (they have been "exposed"). The people in the other group do not have it (they have not been exposed). To figure out relative risk, the percentage of people in the exposed group who have the disease is divided by the percentage of people in the unexposed group who have the disease.

Relative risks can be:

- **Larger than 1:** The trait or factor is linked to an increase in risk

- **Equal to 1:** The trait or factor is not linked to risk

- **Less than 1:** The trait or factor is linked to a decrease in risk

Relative risks are also called risk ratios.

Odds Ratio

In some types of studies, researchers don't have enough information to figure out relative risks. They use something called an odds ratio instead. An odds ratio can be an estimate of relative risk.

One type of study that uses an odds ratio instead of relative risk is called a case-control study. In a case-control study, two groups of people are compared. However, the individuals in each group are chosen based on whether or not they have a certain disease. Researchers look at the odds that the people in each group were exposed to something (a trait or factor) that might have caused the disease. Odds describes the number of times the trait or factor was present or happened, divided by the number of times it wasn't present or didn't happen. To get an odds ratio, the odds for one group are divided by the odds for the other group.

Odds ratios can be:

- **Larger than 1:** The trait or factor is linked to an increase in risk

- **Equal to 1:** The trait or factor is not linked to risk

- **Less than 1:** The trait or factor is linked to a decrease in risk

Looking at traits and exposures in people with and without cancer can help find possible risk factors. Knowing who is at an increased risk for certain types of cancer can help doctors decide when and how often they should be screened.

Does Screening Help People Live Longer?

Finding some cancers at an early stage (before symptoms appear) may help decrease the chance of dying from those

cancers. For many cancers, the chance of recovery depends on the stage (the amount or spread of cancer in the body) of the cancer when it was diagnosed. Cancers that are diagnosed at earlier stages are often easier to treat or cure.

Studies of cancer screening compare the death rate of people screened for a certain cancer with the death rate from that cancer in people who were not screened. Some screening tests have been shown to be helpful both in finding cancers early and in decreasing the chance of dying from those cancers. These include mammograms for breast cancer and sigmoidoscopy and fecal occult blood testing for colorectal cancer. Other tests are used because they have been shown to find a certain type of cancer in some people before symptoms appear, but they have not been proven to decrease the risk of dying from that cancer. If a cancer is fast-growing and spreads quickly, finding it early may not help the person survive the cancer.

Screening studies are done to see whether deaths from cancer decrease when people are screened. When collecting information on how long cancer patients live, some studies define survival as living five years after the diagnosis. This is often used to measure how well cancer treatments work. However, to see if screening tests are useful, studies usually look at whether deaths from the cancer decrease in people who were screened. Over time, signs that a cancer screening test is working include:

- an increase in the number of early-stage cancers found
- a decrease in the number of late-stage cancers found
- a decrease in the number of deaths from the cancer

The number of deaths from cancer is lower today than it was in the past. It is not always clear if this is because screening tests found the cancers earlier or because cancer treatments have gotten better, or both. The SEER program of the NCI collects and reports information on survival times of people with cancer in the United States. This information is studied to see if finding cancer early affects how long these people live.

Certain factors may cause survival times to look like they are getting better when they are not. These factors include lead-time bias and overdiagnosis.

- **Lead-time bias.** Survival time for cancer patients is usually measured from the day the cancer is diagnosed until the day they die. Patients are often diagnosed after they have signs and symptoms of cancer. If a screening test leads to a diagnosis before a patient has any symptoms, the patient's survival time is increased because the date of diagnosis is earlier. This increase in survival time makes it seem as though screened patients are living longer when that may not be happening. This is called lead-time bias. It could be that the only reason the survival time appears to be longer is that the date of diagnosis is earlier for the screened patients. But the screened patients may die at the same time they would have without the screening test.

- **Overdiagnosis.** Sometimes, screening tests find cancers that don't matter because they would have gone away on their own or never caused any symptoms. These cancers would never have been found if not for the screening test. Finding these cancers is called overdiagnosis. Overdiagnosis can make it seem like more people are surviving cancer longer, but in reality, these are people who would not have died from cancer anyway.

How Screening Tests Become Standard Tests

Results from research studies help doctors decide when a screening test works well enough to be used as a standard test. Evidence about how safe, accurate, and useful cancer screening tests are comes from clinical trials (research studies with people) and other kinds of research studies. When enough evidence has been collected to show that a screening test is safe, accurate, and useful, it becomes a standard test. Examples of cancer screening tests that were once under study but are now standard tests include:

- Colonoscopy for colorectal cancer
- Mammograms for breast cancer
- Papanicolaou (Pap) tests (Pap smears) for cervical cancer

Different types of research studies are done to study cancer screening. Cancer screening trials study better ways of finding cancer in people before they have symptoms. Screening trials also study screening tests that may find cancer earlier or are more accurate than existing tests, or that may be easier, safer, or cheaper to use. Screening trials are designed to find the possible benefits and possible harms of cancer screening tests. Different clinical trial designs are used to study cancer screening tests.

The strongest evidence about screening comes from research done in clinical trials. However, clinical trials cannot always be used to study questions about screening. Findings from other types of studies can give useful information about how safe, useful, and accurate cancer screening tests are.

Types of Studies That Are Used to Get Information about Cancer Screening Tests

Randomized Controlled Trials

Randomized controlled trials give the highest level of evidence about how safe, accurate, and useful cancer screening tests are. In these trials, volunteers are assigned randomly (by chance) to one of two or more groups. The people in one group (the control group) may be given a standard screening test (if one exists) or no screening test. The people in the other group(s) are given the new screening test(s). Test results for the groups are then compared to see if the new screening test works better than the standard test, and to see if there are any harmful side effects.

Using chance to assign people to groups means that the groups will probably be very much alike and that the trial results won't be affected by human choices or something else.

Nonrandomized Controlled Trials

In nonrandomized clinical trials, volunteers are not assigned randomly (by chance) to different groups. They choose which group they want to be in or the study leaders assign them. Evidence from this type of research is not as strong as evidence from randomized controlled trials.

Cohort Studies

A cohort study follows a large number of people over time. The people are divided into groups, called cohorts, based on whether or not they have had a certain treatment or been exposed to certain things. In cohort studies, the information is collected and studied after certain outcomes (such as cancer or death) have occurred. For example, a cohort study might follow a group of women who have regular Pap tests, and divide them into those who test positive for the human papillomavirus (HPV) and those who test negative for HPV. The cohort

469

study would show how the cervical cancer rates are different for the two groups over time.

Case-Control Studies

Case-control studies are like cohort studies but are done in a shorter time. They do not include many years of follow-up. Instead of looking forward in time, they look backward. In case-control studies, information is collected from cases (people who already have a certain disease) and compared with information collected from controls (people who do not have the disease). For example, a group of patients with melanoma and a group without melanoma might be asked about how they check their skin for abnormal growths and how often they check it. Based on the different answers from the two groups, the study may show that checking your skin is a useful screening test to decrease the number of melanoma cases and deaths from melanoma.

Evidence from case-control studies is not as strong as evidence from clinical trials or cohort studies.

Ecologic Studies

Ecologic studies report information collected on entire groups of people, such as people in one city or county. Information is reported about the whole group, not about any single person in the group. These studies may give some evidence about whether a screening test is useful.

Expert Opinions

Expert opinions can be based on the experiences of doctors or reports of expert committees or panels. Expert opinions do not give strong evidence about the usefulness of screening tests.

Section 42.2

Bladder and Other Urothelial Cancers Screening

This section includes text excerpted from "Bladder and
Other Urothelial Cancers Screening (PDQ®)—Patient Version,"
National Cancer Institute (NCI), March 9, 2018.

Bladder and other urothelial cancers are diseases in which malignant (cancer) cells form in the urothelium. The bladder is a hollow organ in the lower part of the abdomen. It is shaped like a small balloon and has a muscle wall that allows it to get larger or smaller to store urine made by the kidneys. There are two kidneys, one on each side of the backbone, above the waist. Tiny tubules in the kidneys filter and clean the blood. They take out waste products and make urine. The urine passes from each kidney through a long tube called a ureter into the bladder. The bladder holds the urine until it passes through the urethra and leaves the body.

The urothelium is a layer of tissue that lines the urethra, bladder, ureters, prostate, and renal pelvis. Cancer that begins in the urothelium of the bladder is much more common than cancer that begins in the urothelium of the urethra, ureters, prostate, or renal pelvis.

There are 3 types of cancer that begin in the urothelial cells of the bladder. These cancers are named for the type of cells that become malignant (cancerous):

1. **Transitional cell carcinoma.** Cancer that begins in cells in the innermost layer of the bladder urothelium. These cells are able to stretch when the bladder is full and shrink when it is emptied. Most bladder cancers begin in the transitional cells.

2. **Squamous cell carcinoma.** Cancer that forms in squamous cells, which are thin, flat cells that may form in the bladder urothelium after long-term infection or irritation.

3. **Adenocarcinoma.** Cancer that begins in glandular cells. Glandular cells in the bladder urothelium make substances such as mucus.

Screening for Bladder and Other Urothelial Cancers

Tests are used to screen for different types of cancer. Some screening tests are used because they have been shown to be helpful both in finding cancers early and in decreasing the chance of dying from these cancers. Other tests are used because they have been shown to find cancer in some people; however, it has not been proven in clinical trials that use of these tests will decrease the risk of dying from cancer.

Scientists study screening tests to find those with the fewest risks and most benefits. Cancer screening trials also are meant to show whether early detection (finding cancer before it causes symptoms) decreases a person's chance of dying from the disease. For some types of cancer, finding and treating the disease at an early-stage may result in a better chance of recovery.

There is no standard or routine screening test for bladder cancer. Screening for bladder cancer is under study and there are screening clinical trials taking place in many parts of the country. Two types of tests used to screen for bladder cancer in patients who have had bladder cancer in the past:

1. **Cystoscopy.** Cystoscopy is a procedure to look inside the bladder and urethra to check for abnormal areas. A cystoscope (a thin, lighted tube) is inserted through the urethra into the bladder. Tissue samples may be taken for biopsy.

2. **Urine cytology.** Urine cytology is a laboratory test in which a sample of urine is checked under a microscope for abnormal cells.

Hematuria tests may also be used to screen for bladder cancer. Hematuria (red blood cells in the urine) may be caused by cancer or by other conditions. A hematuria test is used to check for blood in a sample of urine by viewing it under a microscope or using a special test strip. The test may be repeated over time.

Risks of Screening for Bladder and Other Urothelial Cancers

Screening tests have risks. Decisions about screening tests can be difficult. Not all screening tests are helpful and most have risks. Before having any screening test, you may want to discuss the test with your doctor. It is important to know the risks of the test and whether it has been proven to reduce the risk of dying from cancer.

False-positive test results can occur. Screening test results may appear to be abnormal even though no cancer is present. A false-positive test result (one that shows there is cancer when there really isn't) can cause anxiety and is usually followed by more tests (such as cystoscopy or other invasive procedures), which also have risks. False-positive results often occur with hematuria testing; blood in the urine is usually caused by conditions other than cancer.

False-negative test results can occur. Screening test results may appear to be normal even though bladder cancer is present. A person who receives a false-negative test result (one that shows there is no cancer when there really is) may delay seeking medical care even if there are symptoms.

Your doctor can advise you about your risk for bladder cancer and your need for screening tests.

Section 42.3

Breast Cancer Screening

This section includes text excerpted from "Breast Cancer Screening (PDQ®)—Patient Version," National Cancer Institute (NCI), August 11, 2017.

Breast cancer is a disease in which malignant (cancer) cells form in the tissues of the breast. It is the second leading cause of death from cancer in American women. Women in the United States get breast cancer more than any other type of cancer except for skin cancer. Breast cancer is second only to lung cancer as a cause of cancer death in women.

Breast cancer occurs more often in white women than in black women. However, black women are more likely than white women to die from the disease. Breast cancer occurs in men also, but the number of cases is small.

Types of Screening

Some of the tests that are used by healthcare providers to screen for breast cancer are described below.

Mammogram

Mammography is the most common screening test for breast cancer. A mammogram is an X-ray of the breast. This test may find tumors that are too small to feel. A mammogram may also find ductal carcinoma in situ (DCIS). In DCIS, there are abnormal cells in the lining of a breast duct, which may become invasive cancer in some women.

Mammograms are less likely to find breast tumors in women younger than 50 years than in older women. This may be because younger women have denser breast tissue that appears white on a mammogram. Because tumors also appear white on a mammogram, they can be harder to find when there is dense breast tissue.

The following may affect whether a mammogram is able to detect (find) breast cancer:

- the size of the tumor

- how dense the breast tissue is

- the skill of the radiologist

Women aged 40–74 years who have screening mammograms have a lower chance of dying from breast cancer than women who do not have screening mammograms.

Clinical Breast Exam (CBE)

A clinical breast exam (CBE) is an exam of the breast by a doctor or other health professional. The doctor will carefully feel the breasts and under the arms for lumps or anything else that seems unusual. It is not known if having clinical breast exams decreases the chance of dying from breast cancer.

Breast self-exams may be done by women or men to check their breasts for lumps or other changes. It is important to know how your breasts usually look and feel. If you feel any lumps or notice any other changes, talk to your doctor. Doing breast self-exams has not been shown to decrease the chance of dying from breast cancer.

Magnetic Resonance Imaging (MRI)

Magnetic resonance imaging (MRI) is a procedure that uses a magnet, radio waves, and a computer to make a series of detailed pictures of areas inside the body. This procedure is also called nuclear magnetic resonance imaging (NMRI). MRI does not use any X-rays.

MRI is used as a screening test for women who have one or more of the following:

- certain gene changes, such as in the *BRCA1* or *BRCA2* genes

- a family history (first degree relative, such as a mother, daughter or sister) with breast cancer

- certain genetic syndromes, such as Li-Fraumeni (LF) or Cowden syndrome (CS)

MRIs find breast cancer more often than mammograms do, but it is common for MRI results to appear abnormal even when there isn't any cancer.

Screening Tests That Are Being Studied in Clinical Trials

Thermography

Thermography is a procedure in which a special camera that senses heat is used to record the temperature of the skin that covers the breasts. A computer makes a map of the breast showing the changes in temperature. Tumors can cause temperature changes that may show up on the thermogram.

There have been no clinical trials of thermography to find out how well it detects breast cancer or if having the procedure decreases the risk of dying from breast cancer.

Tissue Sampling

Breast tissue sampling is taking cells from breast tissue to check under a microscope. Abnormal cells in breast fluid have been linked to an increased risk of breast cancer in some studies. Scientists are studying whether breast tissue sampling can be used to find breast cancer at an early-stage or predict the risk of developing breast cancer. Three ways of taking tissue samples are being studied:

1. **Fine-needle aspiration (FNA).** A thin needle is inserted into the breast tissue around the areola (darkened area around the nipple) to take out a sample of cells and fluid.

2. **Nipple aspiration.** The use of gentle suction to collect fluid through the nipple. This is done with a device similar to the breast pumps used by women who are breastfeeding.

3. **Ductal lavage.** A hair-size catheter (tube) is inserted into the nipple and a small amount of salt water is released into the duct. The water picks up breast cells and is removed.

Risks of Breast Cancer Screening

Screening tests have risks. Decisions about screening tests can be difficult. Not all screening tests are helpful and most have risks. Before having any screening test, you may want to discuss the test with your doctor. It is important to know the risks of the test and whether it has been proven to reduce the risk of dying from cancer.

The risks of breast cancer screening tests include the following:

False-positive test results can occur. Screening test results may appear to be abnormal even though no cancer is present. A false-positive test result (one that shows there is cancer when there really isn't) is usually followed by more tests (such as biopsy), which also have risks.

When a breast biopsy result is abnormal, getting a second opinion from a different pathologist may improve the accuracy of a breast cancer diagnosis. Most abnormal test results turn out not to be cancer. False-positive results are more common in the following:

- younger women

- women who have had previous breast biopsies

- women with a family history of breast cancer

- women who take hormones, such as estrogen and progestin

False-positive results are more likely the first time a screening mammogram is done than with later screenings. Being able to compare a current mammogram with a past mammogram lowers the risk of a false-positive result.

The skill of the radiologist also can affect the chance of a false-positive result.

False-negative test results can occur. Screening test results may appear to be normal even though breast cancer is present. A woman who receives a false-negative test result (one that shows there is no cancer when there really is) may delay seeking medical care even if she has symptoms.

One in 5 cancers may be missed by mammography. False-negative results occur more often in younger women than in older women because the breast tissue of younger women is more dense. The chance of a false-negative result is also affected by the following:

- the size of the tumor
- the rate of tumor growth
- the level of hormones, such as estrogen, and progesterone, in the woman's body
- the skill of the radiologist

Finding breast cancer may not improve health or help a woman live longer. Screening may not help you if you have fast-growing breast cancer or if it has already spread to other places in your body. Also, some breast cancers found on a screening mammogram may never cause symptoms or become life-threatening. Finding these cancers is called overdiagnosis. When such cancers are found, treatment would not help you live longer and may instead cause serious side effects.

There may be pain or discomfort during a mammogram. During a mammogram, the breast is placed between 2 plates that are pressed together. Pressing the breast helps to get a better X-ray of the breast. Some women have pain or discomfort during a mammogram. Some women have more pain than others. The amount of pain depends on the following:

- the phase of the woman's menstrual cycle
- the woman's anxiety level
- how much pain the woman expected
- mammograms expose the breast to radiation

Being exposed to radiation is a risk factor for breast cancer. The risk of breast cancer from radiation exposure is higher in women who received radiation before age 30 and at high doses. For women older than 40 years, the benefits of an annual screening mammogram may be greater than the risks from radiation exposure.

Anxiety from additional testing may result from false positive results. Studies have shown that false-positive results from screening mammograms are usually followed by more testing that can lead to anxiety. In one study, women who had a false-positive screening mammogram followed by more testing reported feeling anxiety 3 months later, even though cancer was not diagnosed. Another study found that women who had a false-positive screening mammogram had anxiety right after screening, but it went away within a few months. A third study found that some women had anxiety several years after having a false-positive screening mammogram. However, several studies show that women who feel anxiety after false-positive test results are more likely to schedule regular breast screening exams in the future.

The risks and benefits of screening for breast cancer may be different in different age groups. The benefits of breast cancer screening may vary among age groups:

- In women who are expected to live 5 years or fewer, finding and treating early-stage breast cancer may reduce their quality of life without helping them live longer

- As with other women, in women older than 65 years, the results of a screening test may lead to more diagnostic tests and anxiety while waiting for the test results. Also, the breast cancers found are usually not life-threatening.

- It has not been shown that women with an average risk of developing breast cancer benefit from starting screening mammography before age 40

Women who have had radiation treatment to the chest, especially at a young age, are advised to have routine breast cancer screening. Yearly MRI screening may begin 8 years after treatment or by age 25 years, whichever is later. The benefits and risks of mammograms and MRIs for these women have not been studied.

There is no information on the benefits or risks of breast cancer screening in men. No matter how old you are, if you have risk factors for breast cancer you should ask for medical advice about when to begin having breast cancer screening tests and how often to have them.

Talk to your doctor about your risk of breast cancer and your need for screening tests.

Talk to your doctor or other healthcare provider about your risk of breast cancer, whether a screening test is right for you, and the benefits and harms of the screening test. You should take part in the decision about whether you want to have a screening test, based on what is best for you.

Section 42.4

Cervical Cancer Screening

This section includes text excerpted from "Cervical Cancer Screening (PDQ®)—Patient Version," National Cancer Institute (NCI), April 14, 2016.

Cervical cancer is a disease in which malignant (cancer) cells form in the cervix. Screening for cervical cancer using the Papanicolaou (Pap) test has decreased the number of new cases of cervical cancer and the number of deaths due to cervical cancer since 1950.

Cervical dysplasia occurs more often in women who are in their 20s–30s. Death from cervical cancer is rare in women younger than 30 years and in women of any age who have regular screenings with the Pap test. The Pap test is used to detect cancer and changes that may lead to cancer. The chance of death from cervical cancer increases with age. Deaths from cervical cancer occur more often in black women than in white women.

Types of Cervical Cancer Screening

Studies show that screening for cervical cancer helps decrease the number of deaths from the disease. Regular screening of women between the ages of 21–65 years with the Pap test decreases their chance of dying from cervical cancer.

Papanicolaou Test (Pap Test)

A Papanicolaou test (Pap test) is commonly used to screen for cervical cancer. A Pap test is a procedure to collect cells from the surface of the cervix and vagina. A piece of cotton, a brush, or a small wooden stick is used to gently scrape cells from the cervix and vagina. The cells are viewed under a microscope to find out if they are abnormal. This procedure is also called a Pap smear. A new method of collecting and viewing cells has been developed, in which the cells are placed into a liquid before being placed on a slide. It is not known if the new method will work better than the standard method to reduce the number of deaths from cervical cancer.

Human Papillomavirus (HPV) Test

After certain positive Pap test results, an human papillomavirus (HPV) test may be done. An HPV test is a laboratory test that is used to check the deoxyribonucleic acid (DNA) or ribonucleic acid (RNA) for certain types of HPV infection. Cells are collected from the cervix and DNA or RNA from the cells is checked to find out if there is an infection caused by a type of HPV that is linked to cervical cancer. This test may be done using the sample of cells removed during a Pap test. This test may also be done if the results of a Pap test show certain abnormal cervical cells. When both the HPV test and Pap test are done using cells from the sample removed during a Pap test, it is called a Pap/HPV cotest.

An HPV test may be done with or without a Pap test to screen for cervical cancer. Screening women aged 30 and older with both the Pap test and the HPV test every 5 years finds more cervical changes that can lead to cancer than screening with the Pap test alone. Screening with both the Pap test and the HPV test lowers the number of cases of cervical cancer.

An HPV DNA test may be used without a Pap test for cervical cancer screening in women aged 25 years and older.

Risks of Cervical Cancer Screening

Screening tests have risks. Decisions about screening tests can be difficult. Not all screening tests are helpful and most have risks. Before having any screening test, you may want to discuss the test with your doctor. It is important to know the risks of the test and whether it has been proven to reduce the risk of dying from cancer.

The risks of cervical cancer screening include the following:

Unnecessary follow-up tests may be done. In women younger than 21 years, screening with the Pap test may show changes in the cells of the cervix that are not cancer. This may lead to unnecessary follow-up tests and possibly treatment. Women in this age group have a very low risk of cervical cancer and it is likely that any abnormal cells will go away on their own.

False-negative test results can occur. Screening test results may appear to be normal even though cervical cancer is present. A woman who receives a false-negative test result (one that shows there is no cancer when there really is) may delay seeking medical care even if she has symptoms.

False-positive test results can occur. Screening test results may appear to be abnormal even though no cancer is present. Also, some abnormal cells in the cervix never become cancer. When a Pap test shows a false-positive result (one that shows there is cancer when there really isn't), it can cause anxiety and is usually followed by more tests and procedures (such as colposcopy, cryotherapy, or loop electrosurgical excision procedure (LEEP)), which also have risks. The long-term effects of these procedures on fertility and pregnancy are not known.

The HPV test finds many infections that will not lead to cervical dysplasia or cervical cancer, especially in women younger than 30 years.

When both the Pap test and the HPV test are done, false-positive test results are more common.

Your doctor can advise you about your risk for cervical cancer and your need for screening tests. Studies show that the number of cases of cervical cancer and deaths from cervical cancer are greatly reduced by screening with Pap tests. Many doctors recommend a Pap test be done every year. Studies have shown that after a woman has a Pap test and the results show no sign of abnormal cells, the Pap test can be repeated every 2–3 years.

The Pap test is not a helpful screening test for cervical cancer in the following groups of women:

- women who are younger than 21 years

- women who have had a total hysterectomy (surgery to remove the uterus and cervix) for a condition that is not cancer

- women who are aged 65 years or older and have a Pap test result that shows no abnormal cells. These women are very unlikely to have abnormal Pap test results in the future.

The decision about how often to have a Pap test is best made by you and your doctor.

Section 42.5

Colorectal Cancer Screening

This section includes text excerpted from "Colorectal
Cancer Screening (PDQ®)—Patient Version," National
Cancer Institute (NCI), February 23, 2018.

Colorectal cancer is a disease in which malignant (cancer) cells form in the tissues of the colon or the rectum. Colorectal cancer is the second leading cause of death from cancer in the United States. The number of colorectal cancer cases and the number of deaths from colorectal cancer are decreasing a little bit each year in adults aged 55 years and older. But in adults younger than 55 years, there has been a small increase in the number of new cases and deaths from colorectal cancer in recent years. Colorectal cancer is found more often in men than in women.

Screening for Colorectal Cancer

For some types of cancer, finding and treating the disease at an early-stage may result in a better chance of recovery. Studies show that some screening tests for colorectal cancer help find cancer at an early-stage and may decrease the number of deaths from the disease.

Tests Used to Screen Colorectal Cancer

Fecal Occult Blood Test (FOBT)

A fecal occult blood test (FOBT) is a test to check stool (solid waste) for blood that can only be seen with a microscope. A small sample of stool is placed on a special card or in a special container and returned to the doctor or laboratory for testing. Blood in the stool may be a sign of polyps, cancer, or other conditions.

There are two types of FOBTs:

1. **Guaiac FOBT.** The sample of stool on the special card is tested with a chemical. If there is blood in the stool, the special card changes color.

2. **Immunochemical FOBT.** A liquid is added to the stool sample. This mixture is injected into a machine that contains antibodies that can detect blood in the stool. If there is blood in

the stool, a line appears in a window in the machine. This test is also called fecal immunochemical test or FIT.

Sigmoidoscopy

Sigmoidoscopy is a procedure to look inside the rectum and sigmoid (lower) colon for polyps, abnormal areas, or cancer. A sigmoidoscope is inserted through the rectum into the sigmoid colon. A sigmoidoscope is a thin, tube-like instrument with a light and a lens for viewing. It may also have a tool to remove polyps or tissue samples, which are checked under a microscope for signs of cancer.

Colonoscopy

Colonoscopy is a procedure to look inside the rectum and colon for polyps, abnormal areas, or cancer. A colonoscope is inserted through the rectum into the colon. A colonoscope is a thin, tube-like instrument with a light and a lens for viewing. It may also have a tool to remove polyps or tissue samples, which are checked under a microscope for signs of cancer.

Virtual Colonoscopy (VC)

Virtual colonoscopy (VC) is a procedure that uses a series of X-rays called computed tomography (CT) to make a series of pictures of the colon. A computer puts the pictures together to create detailed images that may show polyps and anything else that seems unusual on the inside surface of the colon. This test is also called computed tomography colonography (CTC).

Clinical trials are comparing virtual colonoscopy with other colorectal cancer screening tests. Some clinical trials are testing whether drinking a contrast material that coats the stool, instead of using laxatives to empty the colon, shows polyps clearly.

Deoxyribonucleic Acid (DNA) Stool Test

This test checks deoxyribonucleic acid (DNA) in stool cells for genetic changes that may be a sign of colorectal cancer.

Risks of Colorectal Cancer Screening

Screening tests have risks. Decisions about screening tests can be difficult. Not all screening tests are helpful and most have risks.

Different screening tests have different risks or harms. Screening tests may cause anxiety when you are thinking about or getting ready for the test or when there is a positive test result. Before having any screening test, you may want to discuss the test with your doctor. It is important to know the risks of the test and whether it has been proven to reduce the risk of dying from cancer.

Talk to your doctor about your risk for colorectal cancer and the need for screening tests.

False-negative test results can occur. Screening test results may appear to be normal even though colorectal cancer is present. A person who receives a false-negative test result (one that shows there is no cancer when there really is) may delay seeking medical care even if there are symptoms.

False-positive test results can occur. Screening test results may appear to be abnormal even though no cancer is present. A false-positive test result (one that shows there is cancer when there really isn't) can cause anxiety and is usually followed by more tests (such as biopsy), which also have risks.

The following colorectal cancer screening tests have risks:

- **Colonoscopy.** Serious problems caused by colonoscopy are rare, but can include tears in the lining of the colon and bleeding. These problems can be serious and need to be treated in a hospital. Tearing of the lining of the colon and bleeding occur more often when a biopsy or polypectomy is done. Sedation is used to decrease the discomfort from the procedure. Sedation may cause heart and lung problems, such as irregular heartbeat, heart attack, or trouble breathing.

- **Sigmoidoscopy.** There are fewer complications with a sigmoidoscopy than with a colonoscopy. Although tears in the lining of the colon and bleeding can occur, they are less common than with a colonoscopy. There is usually no sedation with sigmoidoscopy, lowering the risk of complications.

- **Virtual colonoscopy (VC).** Virtual colonoscopy has fewer possible physical harms than either colonoscopy or sigmoidoscopy. The harms of being exposed to radiation from X-rays used in virtual colonoscopy are not known. Virtual colonoscopy often finds problems with organs other than the colon, including the kidneys, chest, liver, ovaries, spleen, and pancreas. Some of these findings lead to more testing, such as colonoscopy, that may not improve the patient's health.

- **Fecal occult blood test (FOBT) or DNA stool test.** The results of an FOBT or DNA stool test may appear to be abnormal even though no cancer is found. A positive test result may lead to more testing, including colonoscopy.

Section 42.6

Esophageal Cancer Screening

This section includes text excerpted from "Esophageal Cancer Screening (PDQ®)—Patient Version," National Cancer Institute (NCI), March 9, 2018.

Esophageal cancer is a disease in which malignant (cancer) cells form in the tissues of the esophagus. Esophageal cancer starts in the inside lining of the esophagus and spreads outward through the other layers as it grows. The two most common types of esophageal cancer are named for the type of cells that become malignant (cancerous):

- **Squamous cell carcinoma.** Cancer that begins in squamous cells, the thin, flat cells lining the esophagus. This cancer is most often found in the upper and middle part of the esophagus but can occur anywhere along the esophagus. This is also called epidermoid carcinoma.

- **Adenocarcinoma.** Cancer that begins in glandular cells. Glandular cells in the lining of the esophagus produce and release fluids such as mucus. Adenocarcinomas usually form in the lower part of the esophagus, near the stomach.

Screening Tests for Esophageal Cancer

Some screening tests are used because they have been shown to be helpful both in finding cancers early and in decreasing the chance of dying from these cancers. Other tests are used because they have been shown to find cancer in some people; however, it has not been proven in clinical trials that use of these tests will decrease the risk of dying from cancer.

Scientists study screening tests to find those with the fewest risks and most benefits. Cancer screening trials also are meant to show whether early detection (finding cancer before it causes symptoms) decreases a person's chance of dying from the disease. For some types of cancer, the chance of recovery is better if the disease is found and treated at an early-stage.

There is no standard or routine screening test for esophageal cancer. Screening for esophageal cancer is under study with screening clinical trials taking place in many parts of the country.

Tests That May Detect (Find) Esophageal Cancer

Esophagoscopy

A procedure to look inside the esophagus to check for abnormal areas. An esophagoscope is inserted through the mouth or nose and down the throat into the esophagus. An esophagoscope is a thin, tube-like instrument with a light and a lens for viewing. It may also have a tool to remove tissue samples, which are checked under a microscope for signs of cancer.

Biopsy

The removal of cells or tissues so they can be viewed under a microscope by a pathologist to check for signs of cancer. Taking biopsy samples from several different areas in the lining of the lower part of the esophagus may detect early Barrett esophagus. This procedure may be used for patients who have risk factors for Barrett esophagus.

Brush Cytology

A procedure in which cells are brushed from the lining of the esophagus and viewed under a microscope to see if they are abnormal. This may be done during an esophagoscopy.

Balloon Cytology

A procedure in which cells are collected from the lining of the esophagus using a deflated balloon that is swallowed by the patient. The balloon is then inflated and pulled out of the esophagus. Esophageal cells on the balloon are viewed under a microscope to see if they are abnormal.

Chromoendoscopy

A procedure in which a dye is sprayed onto the lining of the esophagus during esophagoscopy. Increased staining of certain areas of the lining may be a sign of early Barrett esophagus.

Fluorescence Spectroscopy

A procedure that uses a special light to view tissue in the lining of the esophagus. The light probe is passed through an endoscope and shines on the lining of the esophagus. The light given off by the cells lining the esophagus is then measured. Malignant tissue gives off less light than normal tissue.

Risks of Esophageal Cancer Screening

Screening tests have risks. Decisions about screening tests can be difficult. Not all screening tests are helpful and most have risks. Before having any screening test, you may want to discuss the test with your doctor. It is important to know the risks of the test and whether it has been proven to reduce the risk of dying from cancer.

The risks of esophageal cancer screening tests include the following:

- finding esophageal cancer may not improve health or help a person live longer

- screening may not improve your health or help you live longer if you have advanced esophageal cancer or if it has already spread to other places in your body

Some cancers never cause symptoms or become life-threatening, but if found by a screening test, the cancer may be treated. It is not known if treatment of these cancers will help you live longer than if no treatment were given, and treatments for cancer may have serious side effects.

False-negative test results can occur. Screening test results may appear to be normal even though esophageal cancer is present. A person who receives a false-negative test result (one that shows there is no cancer when there really is) may delay seeking medical care even if there are symptoms.

False-positive test results can occur. Screening test results may appear to be abnormal even though no cancer is present. A false-positive test result (one that shows there is cancer when there really isn't) can cause anxiety and is usually followed by more tests (such as biopsy), which also have risks.

Side effects may be caused by the test itself. There are rare but serious side effects that may occur with esophagoscopy and biopsy. These include the following:

- a small hole (puncture) in the esophagus
- problems with breathing
- heart attack
- passage of food, water, stomach acid, or vomit into the airway
- severe bleeding that may need to be treated in a hospital

Section 42.7

Lung Cancer Screening

This section includes text excerpted from "Lung Cancer Screening (PDQ®)—Patient Version," National Cancer Institute (NCI), June 16, 2017.

Lung cancer is a disease in which malignant (cancer) cells form in the tissues of the lung.

There are two types of lung cancer: small cell lung cancer and non-small cell lung cancer.

Lung cancer is the leading cause of cancer death in the United States.

Lung cancer is the third most common type of nonskin cancer in the United States. Lung cancer is the leading cause of cancer death in men and in women.

Screening for Lung Cancer

The following screening tests have been studied to see if they decrease the risk of dying from lung cancer:

- **Low-dose spiral computed tomography (CT) scan (Low-dose computed tomography (LDCT) scan).** A procedure that uses low-dose radiation to make a series of very detailed pictures of areas inside the body. It uses an X-ray machine that scans the body in a spiral path. The pictures are made by a computer linked to the X-ray machine. This procedure is also called a low-dose helical CT scan.

- **Chest X-ray.** An X-ray of the organs and bones inside the chest. An X-ray is a type of energy beam that can go through the body and onto film, making a picture of areas inside the body.

- **Sputum cytology.** Sputum cytology is a procedure in which a sample of sputum (mucus that is coughed up from the lungs) is viewed under a microscope to check for cancer cells.

Screening with low-dose spiral CT scans has been shown to decrease the risk of dying from lung cancer in heavy smokers. The National Lung Screening Trial (NLST) studied people aged 55–74 years who had smoked at least 1 pack of cigarettes per day for 30 years or more. Heavy smokers who had quit smoking within the past 15 years were also studied. The trial used chest X-rays or low-dose spiral CT scans (LDCT) scans to check for signs of lung cancer. LDCT scans were better than chest X-rays at finding early-stage lung cancer. Screening with LDCT also decreased the risk of dying from lung cancer in current and former heavy smokers.

Current smokers whose LDCT scan result shows possible signs of cancer may be more likely to quit smoking.

Screening with chest X-rays and/or sputum cytology does not decrease the risk of dying from lung cancer. Chest X-ray and sputum cytology are two screening tests that have been used to check for signs of lung cancer. Screening with chest X-ray, sputum cytology, or both of these tests does not decrease the risk of dying from lung cancer.

Risks of Lung Cancer Screening

Screening tests have risks. Decisions about screening tests can be difficult. Not all screening tests are helpful and most have risks. Before having any screening test, you may want to discuss the test with your doctor. It is important to know the risks of the test and whether it has been proven to reduce the risk of dying from cancer.

The risks of lung cancer screening tests include the following:

Finding lung cancer may not improve health or help you live longer. Screening may not improve your health or help you live longer if you have lung cancer that has already spread to other places in your body.

When a screening test result leads to the diagnosis and treatment of a disease that may never have caused symptoms or become life-threatening, it is called overdiagnosis. It is not known if treatment of these cancers would help you live longer than if no treatment were given, and treatments for cancer may have serious side effects. Harms of treatment may happen more often in people who have medical problems caused by heavy or long-term smoking.

False-negative test results can occur. Screening test results may appear to be normal even though lung cancer is present. A person who receives a false-negative test result (one that shows there is no cancer when there really is) may delay seeking medical care even if there are symptoms.

False-positive test results can occur. Screening test results may appear to be abnormal even though no cancer is present. A false-positive test result (one that shows there is cancer when there really isn't) can cause anxiety and is usually followed by more tests (such as biopsy), which also have risks. A biopsy to diagnose lung cancer can cause part of the lung to collapse. Sometimes surgery is needed to reinflate the lung. Harms of diagnostic tests may happen more often in patients who have medical problems caused by heavy or long-term smoking.

Chest X-rays and low-dose spiral CT scans expose the chest to radiation. Radiation exposure from chest X-rays and low-dose spiral CT scans may increase the risk of cancer. Younger people and people at low risk for lung cancer are more likely to develop lung cancer caused by radiation exposure.

Talk to your doctor about your risk for lung cancer and your need for screening tests. Talk to your doctor or other healthcare provider about your risk for lung cancer, whether a screening test is right for you, and about the benefits and harms of the screening test. You should take part in the decision about whether a screening test is right for you.

Section 42.8

Oral Cavity, Pharyngeal, and Laryngeal Cancer Screening

This section includes text excerpted from "Oral Cavity, Pharyngeal, and Laryngeal Cancer Screening (PDQ®)—Patient Version," National Cancer Institute (NCI), April 12, 2018.

Oral cavity, pharyngeal, and laryngeal cancer are diseases in which malignant (cancer) cells form in the mouth and throat. Oral cavity, pharyngeal, and laryngeal cancers usually form in the squamous cells (thin, flat cells that line the oral cavity, pharynx, and larynx).

Oral cavity cancer forms in any of these tissues of the oral cavity:

- the lips

- the front two-thirds of the tongue

- the gingiva (gums)

- the buccal mucosa (the lining of the inside of the cheeks)

- the floor (bottom) of the mouth under the tongue

- the hard palate (the front of the roof of the mouth)

- the retromolar trigone (the small area behind the wisdom teeth)

Pharyngeal cancer forms in any of these tissues of the pharynx (throat):

- the nasopharynx (the upper part of the throat behind the nose)

- the oropharynx, which includes the following tissues:

  - the middle part of the throat behind the mouth

  - the back one-third of the tongue

  - the soft palate (the back of the roof of the mouth), including the uvula

  - the side and back walls of the throat

  - the tonsils

- the hypopharynx (the bottom part of the throat)

Laryngeal cancer forms in any of these tissues of the larynx (voice box):

- the supraglottis (the area above the vocal cords, including the epiglottis)

- the vocal cords (two small bands of muscle within the larynx that vibrate to produce the voice)

- the glottis (the middle part of the larynx, including the vocal cords)

- the subglottis (the lowest part of the larynx, from just below the vocal cords to the top of the trachea)

Screening of Oral Cavity, Pharyngeal, and Laryngeal Cancer

There is no standard or routine screening test for oral cavity, pharyngeal, and laryngeal cancer. No studies have shown that screening for oral cavity, pharyngeal, or laryngeal cancer would decrease the risk of dying from this disease.

A dentist or medical doctor may check the oral cavity during a routine check-up. The exam will include looking for lesions, including areas of leukoplakia (an abnormal white patch of cells) and erythroplakia (an abnormal red patch of cells). Leukoplakia and erythroplakia lesions on the mucous membranes may become cancerous.

If lesions are seen in the mouth, the following procedures may be used to find abnormal tissue that might become oral cavity cancer:

- **Toluidine blue stain.** A procedure in which lesions in the mouth are coated with a blue dye. Areas that stain darker are more likely to be cancer or become cancer.

- **Fluorescence staining.** A procedure in which lesions in the mouth are viewed using a special light. After the patient uses a fluorescent mouth rinse, normal tissue looks different from abnormal tissue when seen under the light.

- **Exfoliative cytology.** A procedure to collect cells from the oral cavity. A piece of cotton, a brush, or a small wooden stick is used to gently scrape cells from the lips, tongue, or mouth. The cells are viewed under a microscope to find out if they are abnormal.

- **Brush biopsy.** The removal of cells using a brush that is designed to collect cells from all layers of a lesion. The cells are viewed under a microscope to find out if they are abnormal.

More than half of oral cancers have already spread to lymph nodes or other areas by the time they are found.

Epstein-Barr virus (EBV) has been linked to nasopharyngeal cancer. Screening for nasopharyngeal cancer using the EBV antibody test or EBV deoxyribonucleic acid (DNA) test has been studied. These are laboratory tests used to check the blood for EBV antibodies or EBV DNA. If EBV antibodies or DNA are found in the blood more tests may be done to check for nasopharyngeal cancer. No studies have shown that screening would decrease the risk of dying from this disease.

Risks of Oral Cavity, Pharyngeal, and Laryngeal Cancer Screening

Screening tests have risks. Decisions about screening tests can be difficult. Not all screening tests are helpful and most have risks. Before having any screening test, you may want to discuss the test with your doctor. It is important to know the risks of the test and whether it has been proven to reduce the risk of dying from cancer.

The risks of oral cavity, pharyngeal, and laryngeal cancer screening include the following:

Finding oral cavity, pharyngeal, or laryngeal cancer may not improve health or help a person live longer. Some cancers never cause symptoms or become life-threatening, but if found by a screening test, the cancer may be treated. Finding these cancers is called overdiagnosis. It is not known if treatment of these cancers would help you live longer than if no treatment were given, and treatments for cancer, such as surgery and radiation therapy, may have serious side effects.

False-negative test results can occur. Screening test results may appear to be normal even though oral cavity, pharyngeal, or laryngeal cancer is present. A person who receives a false-negative test result (one that shows there is no cancer when there really is) may delay seeking medical care even if there are symptoms.

False-positive test results can occur. Screening test results may appear to be abnormal even though no cancer is present. A false-positive test result (one that shows there is cancer when there really isn't) can cause anxiety and is usually followed by more tests and procedures (such as biopsy), which also have risks.

493

Misdiagnosis can occur. A biopsy is needed to diagnose oral cavity, pharyngeal, and laryngeal cancer. Cells or tissues are removed from the oral cavity, pharynx, or larynx and viewed under a microscope by a pathologist to check for signs of cancer. When the cells are cancer and the pathologist reports them as not being cancer, the cancer is misdiagnosed. Cancer is also misdiagnosed when the cells are not cancer and the pathologist reports there is cancer. When cancer is misdiagnosed, treatment that is needed may not be given or treatment may be given that is not needed.

Section 42.9

Prostate Cancer Screening

This section includes text excerpted from "Prostate Cancer Screening (PDQ®)—Patient Version," National Cancer Institute (NCI), February 22, 2018.

Prostate cancer is a disease in which malignant (cancer) cells form in the tissues of the prostate. As men age, the prostate may get bigger. A bigger prostate may block the flow of urine from the bladder and cause problems with sexual function. This condition is called benign prostatic hyperplasia (BPH), and although it is not cancer, surgery may be needed to correct it. The symptoms of benign prostatic hyperplasia or of other problems in the prostate may be similar to symptoms of prostate cancer.

Prostate cancer is the most common nonskin cancer among men in the United States. It is found mainly in older men. Although the number of men with prostate cancer is large, most men diagnosed with this disease do not die from it. Prostate cancer causes more deaths in men than any other cancer except lung cancer. Prostate cancer occurs more often in African-American men than in white men. African-American men with prostate cancer are more likely to die from the disease than white men with prostate cancer.

Screening for Prostate Cancer

There is no standard or routine screening test for prostate cancer. Screening tests for prostate cancer are under study, and there are screening clinical trials taking place in many parts of the country.

Tests to Detect (Find) Prostate Cancer

Digital Rectal Exam (DRE)

Digital rectal exam (DRE) is an exam of the rectum. The doctor or nurse inserts a lubricated, gloved finger into the lower part of the rectum to feel the prostate for lumps or anything else that seems unusual.

Prostate-Specific Antigen (PSA) Test

A prostate-specific antigen (PSA) test is a test that measures the level of PSA in the blood. PSA is a substance made mostly by the prostate that may be found in an increased amount in the blood of men who have prostate cancer. The level of PSA may also be high in men who have an infection or inflammation of the prostate or benign prostatic hyperplasia (BPH; an enlarged, but noncancerous, prostate).

A PSA test or a DRE may be able to detect prostate cancer at an early-stage, but it is not clear whether early detection and treatment decrease the risk of dying from prostate cancer.

Studies are being done to find ways to make PSA testing more accurate for early cancer detection.

A prostate cancer gene 3 (PCA3) ribonucleic acid (RNA) test may be used for certain patients. If a man had a high PSA level and a biopsy of the prostate did not show cancer and the PSA level remains high after the biopsy, a prostate cancer gene 3 (PCA3) RNA test may be done. This test measures the amount of PCA3 RNA in the urine after a DRE. If the PCA3 RNA level is higher than normal, another biopsy may help diagnose prostate cancer.

Risks of Prostate Screening

The risks of prostate screening include the following:
Finding prostate cancer may not improve health or help a man live longer. Screening may not improve your health or help you live longer if you have cancer that has already spread to the area outside of the prostate or to other places in your body.

Some cancers never cause symptoms or become life-threatening, but if found by a screening test, the cancer may be treated. Finding these cancers is called overdiagnosis. It is not known if treatment of these cancers would help you live longer than if no treatment were given.

Treatments for prostate cancer, such as radical prostatectomy and radiation therapy, may have long-term side effects in many men. The most common side effects are erectile dysfunction and urinary incontinence.

Some studies of patients with newly diagnosed prostate cancer showed these patients had a higher risk of death from cardiovascular (heart and blood vessel) disease or suicide. The risk was greatest in the first weeks or months after diagnosis.

Follow-up tests, such as a biopsy, may be done to diagnose cancer. If a PSA test is higher than normal, a biopsy of the prostate may be done. Complications from a biopsy of the prostate may include fever, pain, blood in the urine or semen, and urinary tract infection. Even if a biopsy shows that a patient does not have prostate cancer, he may worry more about developing prostate cancer in the future.

False-negative test results can occur. Screening test results may appear to be normal even though prostate cancer is present. A man who receives a false-negative test result (one that shows there is no cancer when there really is) may delay seeking medical care even if he has symptoms.

False-positive test results can occur. Screening test results may appear to be abnormal even though no cancer is present. A false-positive test result (one that shows there is cancer when there really isn't) can cause anxiety and is usually followed by more tests, (such as biopsy) which also have risks.

Your doctor can advise you about your risk for prostate cancer and your need for screening tests.

Section 42.10

Skin Cancer Screening

This section includes text excerpted from "Skin Cancer Screening (PDQ®)—Patient Version," National Cancer Institute (NCI), February 23, 2018.

Skin cancer is a disease in which malignant (cancer) cells form in the tissues of the skin.

Skin cancer begins in the epidermis, which is made up of three kinds of cells:

1. **Squamous cells.** Thin, flat cells that form the top layer of the epidermis. cancer that forms in squamous cells is called squamous cell carcinoma of the skin.

2. **Basal cells.** Round cells under the squamous cells. cancer that forms in basal cells is called basal cell carcinoma.

3. **Melanocytes.** Found in the lower part of the epidermis, these cells make melanin, the pigment that gives skin its natural color. when skin is exposed to the sun, melanocytes make more pigment and cause the skin to tan, or darken. cancer that forms in melanocytes is called melanoma.

Nonmelanoma skin cancer is the most common cancer in the United States.

Screening for Skin Cancer

Having a skin exam to screen for skin cancer has not been shown to decrease your chance of dying from skin cancer. During a skin exam a doctor or nurse checks the skin for moles, birthmarks, or other pigmented areas that look abnormal in color, size, shape, or texture. Skin exams to screen for skin cancer have not been shown to decrease the number of deaths from the disease.

Regular skin checks by a doctor are important for people who have already had skin cancer. If you are checking your skin and find a worrisome change, you should report it to your doctor.

If an area on the skin looks abnormal, a biopsy is usually done. The doctor will remove as much of the suspicious tissue as possible with a local excision. A pathologist then looks at the tissue under a microscope to check for cancer cells. Because it is sometimes difficult to tell if a skin growth is benign (not cancer) or malignant (cancer), you may want to have the biopsy sample checked by a second pathologist.

Most melanomas in the skin can be seen by the naked eye. Usually, melanoma grows for a long time under the top layer of skin (the epidermis) but does not grow into the deeper layer of skin (the dermis). This allows time for skin cancer to be found early. Melanoma is easier to cure if it is found before it spreads.

Risks of Screening Tests

Decisions about screening tests can be difficult. Not all screening tests are helpful and most have risks. Before having any screening test, you may want to discuss the test with your doctor. It is important to know the risks of the test and whether it has been proven to reduce the risk of dying from cancer.

The risks of skin cancer screening tests include the following:

Finding skin cancer does not always improve health or help you live longer. Screening may not improve your health or help you live longer if you have advanced skin cancer. Some cancers never cause symptoms or become life-threatening, but if found by a screening test, the cancer may be treated. Treatments for cancer may have serious side effects.

False-negative test results can occur. Screening test results may appear to be normal even though cancer is present. A person who receives a false-negative test result (one that shows there is no cancer when there really is) may delay getting medical care even if there are symptoms.

False-positive test results can occur. Screening test results may appear to be abnormal even though no cancer is present. A false-positive test result (one that shows there is cancer when there really isn't) can cause anxiety and is usually followed by more tests (such as a biopsy), which also have risks.

A biopsy may cause scarring. When a skin biopsy is done, the doctor will try to leave the smallest scar possible, but there is a risk of scarring and infection.

Talk to your doctor about your risk for skin cancer and your need for screening tests.

Section 42.11

Testicular Cancer Screening

"Testicular Self-Examination," © 2017 Omnigraphics.
Reviewed July 2018.

Although testicular cancer has a relatively low rate of occurrence, accounting for just one percent of malignancies in all men, it is the most common neoplasm, or abnormal growth, in adolescent males and young men under 35 years of age. Testicular cancer is easily diagnosable and can be successfully treated, with a high survival rate of more than ten years in nearly 90 percent of patients. As with most types of cancer, the prognosis is particularly good with early detection. While significant advances have been made in developing treatments for testicular cancer in the last few decades, the benefits of early detection through self-examination have not received much attention, often resulting in delays before medical attention is sought.

In the absence of a standard or routine screening for testicular cancer, the condition is most often detected either by a doctor during a routine physical examination, or by an individual during the course of a self-exam. The outlook for testicular cancer depends on whether or not the disease has metastasized to lymph nodes, tissues, and organs, and this underscores the importance of early detection by TSE. Early detection involves the diagnosis of testicular cancer through Stages 1 and 2. Stage 1 refers to a "localized" tumor restricted to the primary site, the testes. Stage 2 is the term for a "regional" tumor, one that has spread to other areas. An early diagnosis resulting from a self-exam can greatly enhance treatment outcomes and also reduce the side effects commonly associated with chemotherapy, radiation, and surgery.

How to Perform a Self-Exam

It is important to perform a self-examination every month. This allows you to familiarize yourself with the size, shape, and consistency of your testes and sensitize you to any abnormality in the future. This also helps you to distinguish the epididymis—a highly coiled duct behind the testis for the temporary storage of sperm—from an abnormal lump or growth. Further, it is quite normal for most men to have testicular asymmetry. Differently sized testes with one hanging lower than the other is a normal anatomical feature and should not be construed as a sign of abnormality.

The ideal time to perform a self-exam is right after a warm shower when the scrotum is relaxed and can be easily drawn back to examine the testicles.

TSE is a simple procedure that takes no more than a couple of minutes:

- Hold the penis away from the scrotum to enable close examination of the testes.

- Hold the testicles between your thumb and fingers and roll gently.

- Feel each testicle for any painless lump, usually grain or pea-sized, in the front or sides, taking care not to confuse a lump with supporting tissues and blood vessels.

- If you detect any thickening, discomfort, or pain in the testicles or groin, contact your healthcare professional immediately.

Studies show that men often delay seeking medical attention because early symptoms are typically mild, and many men tend to believe that a lump is benign or harmless and may go away on its own. Concerns about loss of sexuality, or sterility, may also get in the way of seeking professional help when an abnormality is detected.

While the majority of scrotal and testicular irregularities may not be associated with malignancy, it is important for all men—especially those who carry a high risk for testicular tumors—to perform regular self-exams. A family history of testicular cancer and previous history of malignant tumors in one or both of the testes are regarded as high-risk factors, as are conditions such as *cryptorchidism*, a common birth defect associated with undescended testes.

References

1. "How to Perform a Testicular Self-Examination," The Nemours Foundation, 2012.

2. "Testicular Examination and Testicular Self-Examination (TSE)," Healthwise, Incorporated, June 4, 2014.

3. "SEER Stat Fact Sheets: Testis Cancer," National Institutes of Health (NIH), April 2016.

Section 42.12

Tumor Markers

This section includes text excerpted from "Tumor Markers,"
National Cancer Institute (NCI), November 4, 2015.

Tumor markers are substances that are produced by cancer or by other cells of the body in response to cancer or certain benign (noncancerous) conditions. Most tumor markers are made by normal cells as well as by cancer cells; however, they are produced at much higher levels in cancerous conditions. These substances can be found in the blood, urine, stool, tumor tissue, or other tissues or bodily fluids of some patients with cancer. Most tumor markers are proteins. However, patterns of gene expression and changes to deoxyribonucleic acid (DNA) have also begun to be used as tumor markers.

Many different tumor markers have been characterized and are in clinical use. Some are associated with only one type of cancer, whereas others are associated with two or more cancer types. No "universal" tumor marker that can detect any type of cancer has been found.

There are some limitations to the use of tumor markers. Sometimes, noncancerous conditions can cause the levels of certain tumor markers to increase. In addition, not everyone with a particular type of cancer will have a higher level of a tumor marker associated with that cancer. Moreover, tumor markers have not been identified for every type of cancer.

How Are Tumor Markers Used in Cancer Care?

Tumor markers are used to help detect, diagnose, and manage some types of cancer. Although an elevated level of a tumor marker may suggest the presence of cancer, this alone is not enough to diagnose cancer. Therefore, measurements of tumor markers are usually combined with other tests, such as biopsies, to diagnose cancer.

Tumor marker levels may be measured before treatment to help doctors plan the appropriate therapy. In some types of cancer, the level of a tumor marker reflects the stage (extent) of the disease and/or the patient's prognosis (likely outcome or course of disease).

Tumor markers may also be measured periodically during cancer therapy. A decrease in the level of a tumor marker or a return to the marker's normal level may indicate that the cancer is responding to treatment, whereas no change or an increase may indicate that the cancer is not responding.

Tumor markers may also be measured after treatment has ended to check for recurrence (the return of cancer).

How Are Tumor Markers Measured?

A doctor takes a sample of tumor tissue or bodily fluid and sends it to a laboratory, where various methods are used to measure the level of the tumor marker.

If the tumor marker is being used to determine whether treatment is working or whether there is a recurrence, the marker's level will be measured in multiple samples taken over time. Usually these "serial measurements," which show whether the level of a marker is increasing, staying the same, or decreasing, are more meaningful than a single measurement.

What Tumor Markers Are Being Used, and for Which Cancer Types?

A number of tumor markers are currently being used for a wide range of cancer types. Although most of these can be tested in laboratories that meet standards set by the Clinical Laboratory Improvement Amendments (CLIA), some cannot be and may, therefore, be considered experimental. Tumor markers that are in common use are listed below.

ALK *Gene Rearrangements and Overexpression*

- Cancer types: Nonsmall cell lung cancer and anaplastic large cell lymphoma (ALCL)
- Tissue analyzed: Tumor
- How used: To help determine treatment and prognosis

Alpha-Fetoprotein (AFP)

- Cancer types: Liver cancer and germ cell tumors
- Tissue analyzed: Blood
- How used: To help diagnose liver cancer and follow response to treatment; to assess stage, prognosis, and response to treatment of germ cell tumors

Beta-2-Microglobulin (B2M)

- Cancer types: Multiple myeloma, chronic lymphocytic leukemia (CLL), and some lymphomas

- Tissue analyzed: Blood, urine, or cerebrospinal fluid (CSF)

- How used: To determine prognosis and follow response to treatment

Beta-Human Chorionic Gonadotropin (Beta-hCG)

- Cancer types: Choriocarcinoma and germ cell tumors

- Tissue analyzed: Urine or blood

- How used: To assess stage, prognosis, and response to treatment

BRCA1 *and* **BRCA2** *Gene Mutations*

- Cancer type: Ovarian cancer

- Tissue analyzed: Blood

- How used: To determine whether treatment with a particular type of targeted therapy is appropriate

BCR-ABL Fusion Gene (Philadelphia Chromosome)

- Cancer type: Chronic myeloid leukemia (CML), acute lymphoblastic leukemia (ALL), and acute myelogenous leukemia (AML)

- Tissue analyzed: Blood and/or bone marrow

- How used: To confirm diagnosis, predict response to targeted therapy, and monitor disease status

BRAF V600 Mutations

- Cancer types: Cutaneous melanoma and colorectal cancer

- Tissue analyzed: Tumor

- How used: To select patients who are most likely to benefit from treatment with certain targeted therapies

C-kit / CD117

- Cancer types: Gastrointestinal stromal tumor (GIST) and mucosal melanoma
- Tissue analyzed: Tumor
- How used: To help in diagnosing and determining treatment

CA15-3 / CA27.29

- Cancer type: Breast cancer
- Tissue analyzed: Blood
- How used: To assess whether treatment is working or disease has recurred

CA19-9

- Cancer types: Pancreatic cancer, gallbladder cancer, bile duct cancer, and gastric cancer
- Tissue analyzed: Blood
- How used: To assess whether treatment is working

CA-125

- Cancer type: Ovarian cancer
- Tissue analyzed: Blood
- How used: To help in diagnosis, assessment of response to treatment, and evaluation of recurrence

Calcitonin

- Cancer type: Medullary thyroid cancer (MTC)
- Tissue analyzed: Blood
- How used: To aid in diagnosis, check whether treatment is working, and assess recurrence

Carcinoembryonic Antigen (CEA)

- Cancer types: Colorectal cancer and some other cancers
- Tissue analyzed: Blood

- How used: To keep track of how well cancer treatments are working or check if cancer has come back

CD20

- Cancer type: Non-Hodgkin lymphoma (NHL)
- Tissue analyzed: Blood
- How used: To determine whether treatment with a targeted therapy is appropriate

Chromogranin A (CgA)

- Cancer type: Neuroendocrine tumors
- Tissue analyzed: Blood
- How used: To help in diagnosis, assessment of treatment response, and evaluation of recurrence

Chromosomes 3, 7, 17, and 9p21

- Cancer type: Bladder cancer
- Tissue analyzed: Urine
- How used: To help in monitoring for tumor recurrence

Circulating Tumor Cells of Epithelial Origin (CELLSEARCH®)

- Cancer types: Metastatic breast, prostate, and colorectal cancers
- Tissue analyzed: Blood
- How used: To inform clinical decision making, and to assess prognosis

Cytokeratin Fragment 21–1

- Cancer type: Lung cancer
- Tissue analyzed: Blood
- How used: To help in monitoring for recurrence

EGFR *Gene Mutation Analysis*

- Cancer type: Nonsmall cell lung cancer
- Tissue analyzed: Tumor
- How used: To help determine treatment and prognosis

Estrogen Receptor (ER)/Progesterone Receptor (PR)

- Cancer type: Breast cancer
- Tissue analyzed: Tumor
- How used: To determine whether treatment with hormone therapy and some targeted therapies is appropriate

Fibrin/Fibrinogen

- Cancer type: Bladder cancer
- Tissue analyzed: Urine
- How used: To monitor progression and response to treatment

HE4

- Cancer type: Ovarian cancer
- Tissue analyzed: Blood
- How used: To plan cancer treatment, assess disease progression, and monitor for recurrence

HER2/Neu Gene Amplification or Protein Overexpression

- Cancer types: Breast cancer, gastric cancer, and gastroesophageal junction adenocarcinoma
- Tissue analyzed: Tumor
- How used: To determine whether treatment with certain targeted therapies is appropriate

Immunoglobulins

- Cancer types: Multiple myeloma and Waldenström macroglobulinemia (WM)
- Tissue analyzed: Blood and urine

- How used: To help diagnose disease, assess response to treatment, and look for recurrence

KRAS *Gene Mutation Analysis*

- Cancer types: Colorectal cancer and nonsmall cell lung cancer

- Tissue analyzed: Tumor

- How used: To determine whether treatment with a particular type of targeted therapy is appropriate

Lactate Dehydrogenase

- Cancer types: Germ cell tumors, lymphoma, leukemia, melanoma, and neuroblastoma

- Tissue analyzed: Blood

- How used: To assess stage, prognosis, and response to treatment

Neuron-Specific Enolase (NSE)

- Cancer types: Small cell lung cancer and neuroblastoma

- Tissue analyzed: Blood

- How used: To help in diagnosis and to assess response to treatment

Nuclear Matrix Protein 22

- Cancer type: Bladder cancer

- Tissue analyzed: Urine

- How used: To monitor response to treatment

Programmed Death Ligand 1 (PD-L1)

- Cancer type: Nonsmall cell lung cancer

- Tissue analyzed: Tumor

- How used: To determine whether treatment with a particular type of targeted therapy is appropriate

Prostate-Specific Antigen (PSA)

- Cancer type: Prostate cancer
- Tissue analyzed: Blood
- How used: To help in diagnosis, assess response to treatment, and look for recurrence

Thyroglobulin

- Cancer type: Thyroid cancer
- Tissue analyzed: Blood
- How used: To evaluate response to treatment and look for recurrence

Urokinase Plasminogen Activator (uPA) and Plasminogen Activator Inhibitor (PAI-1)

- Cancer type: Breast cancer
- Tissue analyzed: Tumor
- How used: To determine aggressiveness of cancer and guide treatment

5-Protein Signature (OVA1®)

- Cancer type: Ovarian cancer
- Tissue analyzed: Blood
- How used: To preoperatively assess pelvic mass for suspected ovarian cancer

21-Gene Signature (Oncotype DX®)

- Cancer type: Breast cancer
- Tissue analyzed: Tumor
- How used: To evaluate risk of recurrence

70-Gene Signature (Mammaprint®)

- Cancer type: Breast cancer
- Tissue analyzed: Tumor
- How used: To evaluate risk of recurrence

Can Tumor Markers Be Used in Cancer Screening?

Because tumor markers can be used to assess the response of a tumor to treatment and for prognosis, researchers have hoped that they might also be useful in screening tests that aim to detect cancer early, before there are any symptoms. For a screening test to be useful, it should have very high sensitivity (ability to correctly identify people who have the disease) and specificity (ability to correctly identify people who do not have the disease). If a test is highly sensitive, it will identify most people with the disease—that is, it will result in very few false-negative results. If a test is highly specific, only a small number of people will test positive for the disease who do not have it—in other words, it will result in very few false-positive results.

Although tumor markers are extremely useful in determining whether a tumor is responding to treatment or assessing whether it has recurred, no tumor marker identified to date is sufficiently sensitive or specific to be used on its own to screen for cancer.

For example, the prostate-specific antigen (PSA) test, which measures the level of PSA in the blood, is often used to screen men for prostate cancer. However, an increased PSA level can be caused by benign prostate conditions as well as by prostate cancer, and most men with an elevated PSA level do not have prostate cancer. Initial results from two large randomized controlled trials, the National Cancer Institute (NCI)-sponsored Prostate, Lung, Colorectal, and Ovarian Cancer Screening Trial (PLCO), and the European Randomized Study of Screening for Prostate Cancer (ERSPC), showed that PSA testing at best leads to only a small reduction in the number of prostate cancer deaths. Moreover, it is not clear whether the benefits of PSA screening outweigh the harms of follow-up diagnostic tests and treatments for cancers that in many cases would never have threatened a man's life.

Similarly, results from the PLCO trial showed that CA-125, a tumor marker that is sometimes elevated in the blood of women with ovarian cancer but can also be elevated in women with benign conditions, is not sufficiently sensitive or specific to be used together with transvaginal ultrasound to screen for ovarian cancer in women at average risk of the disease. An analysis of 28 potential markers for ovarian cancer in blood from women who later went on to develop ovarian cancer found that none of these markers performed even as well as CA-125 at detecting the disease in women at average risk.

509

Chapter 43

Celiac Disease Tests

Celiac disease is a digestive disorder that damages the small intestine. The disease is triggered by eating foods containing gluten. Gluten is a protein found naturally in wheat, barley, and rye, and is common in foods such as bread, pasta, cookies, and cakes. Many prepackaged foods, lip balms and lipsticks, hair and skin products, toothpastes, vitamin and nutrient supplements, and, rarely, medicines, contain gluten.

Celiac disease can be very serious. The disease can cause long-lasting digestive problems and keep your body from getting all the nutrients it needs. Celiac disease can also affect the body outside the intestine.

How Do Doctors Diagnose Celiac Disease?

Celiac disease can be hard to diagnose because some of the symptoms are like symptoms of other diseases, such as irritable bowel syndrome (IBS) and lactose intolerance. Your doctor may diagnose celiac disease with a medical and family history, physical exam, and tests. Tests may include blood tests, genetic tests, and biopsy.

Medical and Family History

Your doctor will ask you for information about your family's health—specifically, if anyone in your family has a history of celiac disease.

This chapter includes text excerpted from "Diagnosis of Celiac Disease," National Institute of Diabetes and Digestive and Kidney Diseases (NIDDK), June 2016.

Physical Exam

During a physical exam, a doctor most often:

- checks your body for a rash or malnutrition, a condition that arises when you don't get enough vitamins, minerals, and other nutrients you need to be healthy
- listens to sounds in your abdomen using a stethoscope
- taps on your abdomen to check for pain and fullness or swelling

Dental Exam

For some people, a dental visit can be the first step toward discovering celiac disease. Dental enamel defects, such as white, yellow, or brown spots on the teeth, are a pretty common problem in people with celiac disease, especially children. These defects can help dentists and other healthcare professionals identify celiac disease.

What Tests Do Doctors Use to Diagnose Celiac Disease?

Blood Tests

A healthcare professional may take a blood sample from you and send the sample to a lab to test for antibodies common in celiac disease. If blood test results are negative and your doctor still suspects celiac disease, he or she may order more blood tests.

Genetic Tests

If a biopsy and other blood tests do not clearly confirm celiac disease, your doctor may order genetic blood tests to check for certain gene changes, or variants. You are very unlikely to have celiac disease if these gene variants are not present. Having these variants alone is not enough to diagnose celiac disease because they also are common in people without the disease. In fact, most people with these genes will never get celiac disease.

Intestinal Biopsy

If blood tests suggest you have celiac disease, your doctor will perform a biopsy to be sure. During a biopsy, the doctor takes a small piece of tissue from your small intestine during a procedure called an upper gastrointestinal (GI) endoscopy.

Skin Biopsy

If a doctor suspects you have dermatitis herpetiformis (DH), he or she will perform a skin biopsy. For a skin biopsy, the doctor removes tiny pieces of skin tissue to examine with a microscope.

A doctor examines the skin tissue and checks the tissue for antibodies common in celiac disease. If the skin tissue has the antibodies, a doctor will perform blood tests to confirm celiac disease. If the skin biopsy and blood tests both suggest celiac disease, you may not need an intestinal biopsy.

Do Doctors Screen for Celiac Disease?

Screening is testing for diseases when you have no symptoms. Doctors in the United States do not routinely screen people for celiac disease. However, blood relatives of people with celiac disease and those with type 1 diabetes should talk with their doctor about their chances of getting the disease.

Many researchers recommend routine screening of all family members, such as parents and siblings, for celiac disease. However, routine genetic screening for celiac disease is not usually helpful when diagnosing the disease.

Chapter 44

Cystic Fibrosis (CF) Tests

Cystic fibrosis, or CF, is an inherited disease of the secretory glands. Secretory glands include glands that make mucus and sweat. "Inherited" means the disease is passed from parents to children through genes. People who have CF inherit two faulty genes for the disease—one from each parent. The parents likely don't have the disease themselves.

CF mainly affects the lungs, pancreas, liver, intestines, sinuses, and sex organs.

Mucus is a substance made by tissues that line some organs and body cavities, such as the lungs and nose. Normally, mucus is a slippery, watery substance. It keeps the linings of certain organs moist and prevents them from drying out or getting infected.

If you have CF, your mucus becomes thick and sticky. It builds up in your lungs and blocks your airways. (Airways are tubes that carry air in and out of your lungs.) The buildup of mucus makes it easy for bacteria to grow. This leads to repeated, serious lung infections. Over time, these infections can severely damage your lungs.

The thick, sticky mucus also can block tubes, or ducts, in your pancreas (an organ in your abdomen). As a result, the digestive enzymes that your pancreas makes can't reach your small intestine.

These enzymes help break down food. Without them, your intestines can't fully absorb fats and proteins. This can cause vitamin deficiency

This chapter includes text excerpted from "Cystic Fibrosis," National Heart, Lung, and Blood Institute (NHLBI), May 22, 2018.

and malnutrition because nutrients pass through your body without being used. You also may have bulky stools, intestinal gas, a swollen belly from severe constipation, and pain or discomfort.

CF also causes your sweat to become very salty. Thus, when you sweat, you lose large amounts of salt. This can upset the balance of minerals in your blood and cause many health problems. Examples of these problems include dehydration (a lack of fluid in your body), increased heart rate, fatigue (tiredness), weakness, decreased blood pressure, heat stroke, and, rarely, death.

If you or your child has CF, you're also at higher risk for diabetes or two bone-thinning conditions called osteoporosis and osteopenia.

CF also causes infertility in men, and the disease can make it harder for women to get pregnant.

Diagnosis

Doctors diagnose CF based on the results from various tests.

Newborn Screening

All States screen newborns for CF using a genetic test or a blood test. The genetic test shows whether a newborn has faulty cystic fibrosis transmembrane conductance regulator (CFTR) genes. The blood test shows whether a newborn's pancreas is working properly.

Sweat Test

If a genetic test or blood test suggests CF, a doctor will confirm the diagnosis using a sweat test. This test is the most useful test for diagnosing CF. A sweat test measures the amount of salt in sweat.

For this test, the doctor triggers sweating on a small patch of skin on an arm or leg. He or she rubs the skin with a sweat-producing chemical and then uses an electrode to provide a mild electrical current. This may cause a tingling or warm feeling.

Sweat is collected on a pad or paper and then analyzed. The sweat test usually is done twice. High salt levels confirm a diagnosis of CF.

Other Tests

If you or your child has CF, your doctor may recommend other tests, such as:

- **Genetic tests.** Genetic tests to find out what type of CFTR defect is causing your CF

- **A chest X-ray.** This test creates pictures of the structures in your chest, such as your heart, lungs, and blood vessels. A chest X-ray can show whether your lungs are inflamed or scarred, or whether they trap air.

- **A sinus X-ray.** This test may show signs of sinusitis, a complication of CF.

- **Lung function tests.** These tests measure how much air you can breathe in and out, how fast you can breathe air out, and how well your lungs deliver oxygen to your blood.

- **A sputum culture.** For this test, your doctor will take a sample of your sputum (spit) to see whether bacteria are growing in it. If you have bacteria called mucoid Pseudomonas, you may have more advanced CF that needs aggressive treatment.

Prenatal Screening

If you're pregnant, prenatal genetic tests can show whether your fetus has CF. These tests include amniocentesis and chorionic villus sampling (CVS).

In amniocentesis, your doctor inserts a hollow needle through your abdominal wall into your uterus. He or she removes a small amount of fluid from the sac around the baby. The fluid is tested to see whether both of the baby's *CFTR* genes are normal.

In CVS, your doctor threads a thin tube through the vagina and cervix to the placenta. The doctor removes a tissue sample from the placenta using gentle suction. The sample is tested to see whether the baby has CF.

Cystic Fibrosis (CF) Carrier Testing

People who have one normal *CFTR* gene and one faulty *CFTR* gene are CF carriers. CF carriers usually have no symptoms of CF and live normal lives. However, carriers can pass faulty *CFTR* genes on to their children.

If you have a family history of CF or a partner who has CF (or a family history of it) and you're planning a pregnancy, you may want to find out whether you're a CF carrier.

A genetics counselor can test a blood or saliva sample to find out whether you have a faulty CF gene. This type of testing can detect faulty CF genes in 9 out of 10 cases.

Chapter 45

Diabetes Tests

Chapter Contents

Section 45.1

Screening Tests for Diabetes

This section includes text excerpted from "Diabetes Tests and Diagnosis," National Institute of Diabetes and Digestive and Kidney Diseases (NIDDK), November 2016.

Your healthcare professional can diagnose diabetes, prediabetes, and gestational diabetes through blood tests. The blood tests show if your blood glucose, also called blood sugar, is too high.

Do not try to diagnose yourself if you think you might have diabetes. Testing equipment that you can buy over the counter, such as a blood glucose meter, cannot diagnose diabetes.

Who Should Be Tested for Diabetes?

Anyone who has symptoms of diabetes should be tested for the disease. Some people will not have any symptoms but may have risk factors for diabetes and need to be tested. Testing allows healthcare professionals to find diabetes sooner and work with their patients to manage diabetes and prevent complications.

Testing also allows healthcare professionals to find prediabetes. Making lifestyle changes to lose a modest amount of weight if you are overweight may help you delay or prevent type 2 diabetes.

Type 1 Diabetes

Most often, testing for type 1 diabetes occurs in people with diabetes symptoms. Doctors usually diagnose type 1 diabetes in children and young adults. Because type 1 diabetes can run in families, a study called TrialNet offers free testing to family members of people with the disease, even if they don't have symptoms.

Type 2 Diabetes

Experts recommend routine testing for type 2 diabetes if you:

• are age 45 or older

• are between the ages of 19–44, are overweight or obese, and have one or more other diabetes risk factors

• are a woman who had gestational diabetes

Medicare covers the cost of diabetes tests for people with certain risk factors for diabetes. If you have Medicare, find out if you qualify for coverage. If you have different insurance, ask your insurance company if it covers diabetes tests.

Though type 2 diabetes most often develops in adults, children also can develop type 2 diabetes. Experts recommend testing children between the ages of 10–18 who are overweight or obese and have at least two other risk factors for developing diabetes.

Gestational Diabetes

All pregnant women who do not have a prior diabetes diagnosis should be tested for gestational diabetes. If you are pregnant, you will take a glucose challenge test between 24–28 weeks of pregnancy.

What Tests Are Used to Diagnose Diabetes and Prediabetes?

Healthcare professionals most often use the fasting plasma glucose (FPG) test or the A1C test to diagnose diabetes. In some cases, they may use a random plasma glucose (RPG) test.

Fasting Plasma Glucose (FPG) Test

The FPG blood test measures your blood glucose level at a single point in time. For the most reliable results, it is best to have this test in the morning, after you fast for at least 8 hours. Fasting means having nothing to eat or drink except sips of water.

A1C Test

The A1C test is a blood test that provides your average levels of blood glucose over the past 3 months. Other names for the A1C test are hemoglobin A1C, hemoglobin A1c (HbA1C), glycated hemoglobin, and glycosylated hemoglobin test. You can eat and drink before this test. When it comes to using the A1C to diagnose diabetes, your doctor will consider factors such as your age and whether you have anemia or another problem with your blood. The A1C test is not accurate in people with anemia.

Random Plasma Glucose (RPG) Test

Sometimes healthcare professionals use the RPG test to diagnose diabetes when diabetes symptoms are present and they do not want to wait until you have fasted. You do not need to fast overnight for the RPG test. You may have this blood test at any time.

What Tests Are Used to Diagnose Gestational Diabetes?

Pregnant women may have the glucose challenge test, the oral glucose tolerance test, or both. These tests show how well your body handles glucose.

Oral Glucose Tolerance Test (OGTT)

The oral glucose tolerance test (OGTT) measures blood glucose after you fast for at least 8 hours. First, a healthcare professional will draw your blood. Then you will drink the liquid containing glucose. For diagnosing gestational diabetes, you will need your blood drawn every hour for 2–3 hours.

Healthcare professionals also can use the OGTT to diagnose type 2 diabetes and prediabetes in people who are not pregnant. The OGTT helps healthcare professionals detect type 2 diabetes and prediabetes better than the FPG test. However, the OGTT is a more expensive test and is not as easy to give. To diagnose type 2 diabetes and prediabetes, a healthcare professional will need to draw your blood 1 hour after you drink the liquid containing glucose and again after 2 hours.

What Test Numbers Tell You If You Have Diabetes or Prediabetes?

Each test to detect diabetes and prediabetes uses a different measurement. Usually, the same test method needs to be repeated on a second day to diagnose diabetes. Your doctor may also use a second test method to confirm that you have diabetes.

Which Tests Help Your Healthcare Professional Know What Kind of Diabetes You Have?

Even though the tests described here can confirm that you have diabetes, they can't identify what type you have. Sometimes healthcare professionals are unsure if diabetes is type 1 or type 2. A rare type of diabetes that can occur in babies, called monogenic diabetes, can also be mistaken for type 1 diabetes. Treatment depends on the type of diabetes, so knowing which type you have is important.

If you had diabetes while you were pregnant, you should get tested no later than 12 weeks after your baby is born to see if you have type 2 diabetes.

Section 45.2

Continuous Glucose Monitoring

This section includes text excerpted from "Continuous Glucose Monitoring," National Institute of Diabetes and Digestive and Kidney Diseases (NIDDK), June 2017.

What Is Continuous Glucose Monitoring (CGM)?

Continuous glucose monitoring (CGM) automatically tracks blood glucose levels, also called blood sugar, throughout the day and night. You can see your glucose level anytime at a glance. You can also review how your glucose changes over a few hours or days to see trends. Seeing glucose levels in real time can help you make more informed decisions throughout the day about how to balance your food, physical activity, and medicines.

How Does a CGM Work?

A CGM works through a tiny sensor inserted under your skin, usually on your belly or arm. The sensor measures your interstitial glucose level, which is the glucose found in the fluid between the cells. The sensor tests glucose every few minutes. A transmitter wirelessly sends the information to a monitor.

The monitor may be part of an insulin pump or a separate device, which you might carry in a pocket or purse. Some CGMs send information directly to a smartphone or tablet.

Special Features of a CGM

- an alarm can sound when your glucose level goes too low or too high

- you can note your meals, physical activity, and medicines in a CGM device, too, alongside your glucose levels

- you can download data to a computer or smart device to more easily see your glucose trends

Some models can send information right away to a second person's smartphone—perhaps a parent, partner, or caregiver. For example, if a child's glucose drops dangerously low overnight, the CGM could be set to wake a parent in the next room.

Who Can Use a CGM?

Most people who use CGMs have type 1 diabetes. Research is underway to learn how CGMs might help people with type 2 diabetes.

What Are the Benefits of a CGM?

Compared with a standard blood glucose meter, using a CGM system can help you

- better manage your glucose levels every day

- have fewer low blood glucose emergencies

- need fewer finger sticks

A graphic on the CGM screen shows whether your glucose is rising or dropping—and how quickly—so you can choose the best way to reach your target glucose level.

What Are the Limits of a CGM?

Researchers are working to make CGMs more accurate and easier to use. But you still need a finger-stick glucose test twice a day to check the accuracy of your CGM against a standard blood glucose meter.

A CGM system is more expensive than using a standard glucose meter. Check with your health insurance plan or Medicare to see whether the costs will be covered.

What Is an Artificial Pancreas?

A CGM is one part of the "artificial pancreas" systems that are beginning to reach people with diabetes.

In 2016, the U.S. Food and Drug Administration (FDA) approved a type of artificial pancreas system called a hybrid closed-loop system.

This system tests your glucose level every 5 minutes throughout the day and night through a CGM, and automatically gives you the right amount of basal insulin, a long-acting insulin, through a separate insulin pump. You will still need to test your blood with a glucose meter a few times a day. And you'll manually adjust the amount of insulin the pump delivers at mealtimes and when you need a correction dose.

The National Institute of Diabetes and Digestive and Kidney Diseases (NIDDK) has funded—and continues to fund—several important studies on different types of artificial pancreas devices to better help people with type 1 diabetes manage their disease. The devices may also help people with type 2 diabetes and gestational diabetes.

Chapter 46

Eating Disorders: Suggested Medical Tests

Many people with eating disorders either deny that a problem exists or try to hide it from friends, family members, and medical professionals. As a result, diagnosing an eating disorder can be a difficult process, and such conditions as anorexia nervosa, bulimia nervosa, and binge-eating disorder often go undetected for long periods of time. However, doctors have a variety of assessment tools and medical tests available to aid in the diagnosis of eating disorders. If an eating disorder is suspected, the diagnostic process is likely to include the following:

- a full medical history, including information about both physical and emotional health;

- a mental health screening to look for underlying psychological problems, evaluate eating habits, and assess attitudes about food and body image;

- a complete physical examination to check for signs of eating disorders as well as health problems related to malnutrition;

- additional medical tests—including X-rays and chemical analysis of blood and urine—to look for evidence of damage to the heart, kidneys, gastrointestinal tract, and other organs.

"Eating Disorders: Suggested Medical Tests," © 2016 Omnigraphics. Reviewed July 2018.

In the process of diagnosing eating disorders, doctors must rule out other health conditions that may present similar symptoms, such as hyperthyroidism, inflammatory bowel syndrome, immunodeficiency, chronic infection, diabetes, and cancer. In addition, doctors must look for evidence of diseases that often coexist with eating disorders, such as depression, anxiety, obsessive-compulsive disorder, schizophrenia, and substance abuse.

Commonly Used Medical Tests

The initial step in diagnosing eating disorders usually involves administering questionnaires and conducting interviews to gather information about the patient's eating history, body image, and attitudes about food. Interviews are often conducted by a psychologist or psychiatrist in the presence of a supportive friend or family member of the patient. Medical professionals may also administer psychometric tests that are specifically designed to elicit information about eating disorders, such as the Eating Disorders Examination (EDE), the Eating Disorders Examination-Questionnaire (EDE-Q), and the SCOFF questionnaire. The results of these screening assessments help doctors determine whether further testing and evaluation is appropriate.

The next step in diagnosing eating disorders may involve administering a number of different medical tests to detect and rule out physical symptoms and health complications related to eating disorders. Some of the most commonly used tests include:

- a complete blood count, including levels of cholesterol, protein, and electrolytes;

- a urinalysis to evaluate kidney function;

- an oral glucose tolerance test (OGTT) to assess the body's ability to metabolize sugar;

- an enzyme-linked immunosorbent assay (ELISA) to check for antibodies to various viruses and bacteria;

- a secretin-CCK (cholecystokinin) test to evaluate pancreas and gallbladder function;

- a blood urea nitrogen (BUN) test to evaluate protein metabolism and kidney function;

- a BUN-to-creatinine ratio to check for evidence of severe dehydration, kidney failure, congestive heart failure, cirrhosis of the liver, and other serious conditions;

- a serum cholinesterase test to assess liver function and check for signs of malnutrition;

- a luteinizing hormone (Lh) response to gonadotropin-releasing hormone (GnRH) to evaluate pituitary gland function;

- thyroid-stimulating hormone (TSH) and parathyroid hormone (PTH) tests to assess thyroid function;

- a creatine kinase test to evaluate enzyme levels in the heart, brain, and muscles;

- an echocardiogram or electrocardiogram (EKG) to assess heart function;

- an electroencephalogram (EEG) to measure electrical activity in the brain;

- an upper gastrointestinal (GI) series to look for problems in the upper GI tract;

- X-rays or a barium enema to assess issues in the lower GI tract.

Making a Diagnosis

The results of these various medical tests can help medical professionals diagnose an eating disorder as well as pinpoint the specific type of disorder in order to provide effective treatment. To receive a diagnosis of anorexia nervosa, a patient typically has a distorted self-image and an intense fear of gaining weight, which translates into an inability or refusal to maintain a healthy weight for their age, height, and body type. Severely restricting food intake, abusing laxatives or diuretics in an effort to eliminate calories, and exercising excessively are common symptoms of anorexia. In females, the loss of menstrual function for at least three months is another key indicator.

The criteria for diagnosing bulimia nervosa include patterns of purging food from the body through self-induced vomiting or other methods at least twice a week for three months. Bulimia can be difficult to diagnose because patients usually binge and purge secretly and deny that they have a problem. In addition, most people with bulimia fall within their normal weight range. Dental and gum problems, stomach and digestive issues, dehydration, fatigue, and other symptoms related to repeated vomiting are key factors in the diagnosis of bulimia.

The diagnosis of binge-eating disorder often occurs when a patient seeks medical help with losing weight or dealing with an obesity-related health problem. Medical tests aid in the diagnosis by ruling out physical illnesses and detecting health consequences of the eating disorder. With all types of eating disorders, early diagnosis is important to reduce the patient's risk of long-term health problems and improve the chances of successful treatment and recovery.

References

1. "Anorexia Nervosa—Exams and Tests," WebMD, November 14, 2014.

2. "Bulimia Nervosa—Exams and Tests," WebMD, November 14, 2014.

3. "Diagnosing Binge Eating Disorder," WebMD, 2016.

4. Mandal, Ananya. "Eating Disorders Diagnosis," News Medical, 2016.

Chapter 47

Hearing Assessments

Hearing Screening

Hearing screening is a test to tell if people might have hearing loss. Hearing screening is easy and not painful. In fact, babies are often asleep while being screened. It takes a very short time—usually only a few minutes.

Babies

All babies should be screened for hearing loss no later than 1 month of age. It is best if they are screened before leaving the hospital after birth. If a baby does not pass a hearing screening, it's very important to get a full hearing test as soon as possible, but no later than 3 months of age.

Older Babies and Children

If you think a child might have hearing loss, ask the doctor for a hearing screening as soon as possible. Children who are at risk for acquired, progressive, or delayed-onset hearing loss should have at least one hearing test by 2–2 1/2 years of age. Hearing loss that gets

This chapter includes text excerpted from "Hearing Loss in Children—Screening and Diagnosis," Centers for Disease Control and Prevention (CDC), April 11, 2018.

worse over time is known as acquired or progressive hearing loss. Hearing loss that develops after the baby is born is called delayed-onset hearing loss. If a child does not pass a hearing screening, it's very important to get a full hearing test as soon as possible.

Full Hearing Test

All children who do not pass a hearing screening should have a full hearing test. This test is also called an audiology evaluation. An audiologist, who is an expert trained to test hearing, will do the full hearing test. In addition, the audiologist will also ask questions about birth history, ear infection and hearing loss in the family.

There are many kinds of tests an audiologist can do to find out if a person has a hearing loss, how much of a hearing loss there is, and what type it is. The hearing tests are easy and not painful.

Some of the tests the audiologist might use include:

Auditory brainstem response (ABR) test or brainstem auditory evoked response (BAER) test. Auditory brainstem response (ABR) or brainstem auditory evoked response (BAER) is a test that checks the brain's response to sound. Because this test does not rely on a person's response behavior, the person being tested can be sound asleep during the test.

Otoacoustic emissions (OAE). Otoacoustic emissions (OAEs) is a test that checks the inner ear response to sound. Because this test does not rely on a person's response behavior, the person being tested can be sound asleep during the test.

Behavioral audiometry evaluation. Behavioral audiometry evaluation will test how a person responds to sound overall. Behavioral audiometry evaluation tests the function of all parts of the ear. The person being tested must be awake and actively respond to sounds heard during the test.

With the parents' permission, the audiologist will share the results with the child's primary care doctor and other experts, such as:

- an ear, nose and throat doctor, also called an otolaryngologist

- an eye doctor, also called an ophthalmologist

- a professional trained in genetics, also called a clinical geneticist or a genetics counselor

Get Help!

- If a parent or anyone else who knows a child well thinks the child might have hearing loss, ask the doctor for a hearing screening as soon as possible. Don't wait!

- If the child does not pass a hearing screening, ask the doctor for a full hearing test.

- If the child is diagnosed with a hearing loss, talk to the doctor or audiologist about treatment and intervention services.

Hearing loss can affect a child's ability to develop communication, language, and social skills. The earlier children with hearing loss start getting services, the more likely they are to reach their full potential. If you are a parent and you suspect your child has hearing loss, trust your instincts and speak with your doctor.

Chapter 48

Heart and Vascular Disease Screening and Diagnostic Tests

What Is Coronary Heart Disease (CHD)?

Coronary heart disease (CHD) is a disease in which a waxy substance called plaque builds up inside the coronary arteries. These arteries supply oxygen-rich blood to your heart muscle.

When plaque builds up in the arteries, the condition is called atherosclerosis. The buildup of plaque occurs over many years.

Over time, plaque can harden or rupture (break open). Hardened plaque narrows the coronary arteries and reduces the flow of oxygen-rich blood to the heart.

If the plaque ruptures, a blood clot can form on its surface. A large blood clot can mostly or completely block blood flow through a coronary artery. Over time, ruptured plaque also hardens and narrows the coronary arteries.

This section contains text excerpted from the following sources: Text beginning with the heading "What Is Coronary Heart Disease (CHD)?" is excerpted from "Coronary Heart Disease," National Heart, Lung, and Blood Institute (NHLBI), November 9, 2015; Text under the heading "Diagnosis" is excerpted from "Heart Disease in Women," National Heart, Lung, and Blood Institute (NHLBI), March 13, 2017.

If the flow of oxygen-rich blood to your heart muscle is reduced or blocked, angina or a heart attack can occur.

Angina is chest pain or discomfort. It may feel like pressure or squeezing in your chest. The pain also can occur in your shoulders, arms, neck, jaw, or back. Angina pain may even feel like indigestion.

A heart attack occurs if the flow of oxygen-rich blood to a section of heart muscle is cut off. If blood flow isn't restored quickly, the section of heart muscle begins to die. Without quick treatment, a heart attack can lead to serious health problems or death.

Over time, CHD can weaken the heart muscle and lead to heart failure and arrhythmias. Heart failure is a condition in which your heart can't pump enough blood to meet your body's needs. Arrhythmias are problems with the rate or rhythm of the heartbeat.

What Are the Symptoms of CHD?

Some people who have CHD have no signs or symptoms—a condition called silent CHD. The disease might not be diagnosed until a person has signs or symptoms of a heart attack, heart failure, or an arrhythmia (an irregular heartbeat).

Heart Attack

A heart attack occurs if the flow of oxygen-rich blood to a section of heart muscle is cut off. This can happen if an area of plaque in a coronary artery ruptures (breaks open).

Blood cell fragments called platelets stick to the site of the injury and may clump together to form blood clots. If a clot becomes large enough, it can mostly or completely block blood flow through a coronary artery.

If the blockage isn't treated quickly, the portion of heart muscle fed by the artery begins to die. Healthy heart tissue is replaced with scar tissue. This heart damage may not be obvious, or it may cause severe or long-lasting problems.

The most common heart attack symptom is chest pain or discomfort. Most heart attacks involve discomfort in the center or left side of the chest that often lasts for more than a few minutes or goes away and comes back.

The discomfort can feel like uncomfortable pressure, squeezing, fullness, or pain. The feeling can be mild or severe. Heart attack pain sometimes feels like indigestion or heartburn.

The symptoms of angina can be similar to the symptoms of a heart attack. Angina pain usually lasts for only a few minutes and goes away with rest.

Chest pain or discomfort that doesn't go away or changes from its usual pattern (for example, occurs more often or while you're resting) might be a sign of a heart attack. If you don't know whether your chest pain is angina or a heart attack, call 9–1–1.

All chest pain should be checked by a doctor.

Other common signs and symptoms of a heart attack include:

- Upper body discomfort in one or both arms, the back, neck, jaw, or upper part of the stomach

- Shortness of breath, which may occur with or before chest discomfort

- Nausea (feeling sick to your stomach), vomiting, light-headedness or fainting, or breaking out in a cold sweat

- Sleep problems, fatigue (tiredness), or lack of energy

Heart Failure

Heart failure is a condition in which your heart can't pump enough blood to meet your body's needs. Heart failure doesn't mean that your heart has stopped or is about to stop working.

The most common signs and symptoms of heart failure are shortness of breath or trouble breathing; fatigue; and swelling in the ankles, feet, legs, stomach, and veins in the neck.

All of these symptoms are the result of fluid buildup in your body. When symptoms start, you may feel tired and short of breath after routine physical effort, like climbing stairs.

Arrhythmia

An arrhythmia is a problem with the rate or rhythm of the heartbeat. When you have an arrhythmia, you may notice that your heart is skipping beats or beating too fast.

Some people describe arrhythmias as a fluttering feeling in the chest. These feelings are called palpitations.

Some arrhythmias can cause your heart to suddenly stop beating. This condition is called sudden cardiac arrest (SCA). SCA usually causes death if it's not treated within minutes.

537

Diagnosis

Your doctor will diagnose coronary heart disease (CHD) based on your medical and family histories, your risk factors, a physical exam, and the results from tests and procedures.

No single test can diagnose CHD. If your doctor thinks you have CHD, he or she may recommend one or more of the following tests.

Electrocardiogram (EKG)

An EKG is a simple, painless test that detects and records the heart's electrical activity. The test shows how fast the heart is beating and its rhythm (steady or irregular). An EKG also records the strength and timing of electrical signals as they pass through the heart.

An EKG can show signs of heart damage due to CHD and signs of a previous or current heart attack.

Stress Testing

During stress testing, you exercise to make your heart work hard and beat fast while heart tests are done. If you can't exercise, you may be given medicines to increase your heart rate.

When your heart is working hard and beating fast, it needs more blood and oxygen. Plaque-narrowed coronary (heart) arteries can't supply enough oxygen-rich blood to meet your heart's needs.

A stress test can show possible signs and symptoms of CHD, such as:

- Abnormal changes in your heart rate or blood pressure

- Shortness of breath or chest pain

- Abnormal changes in your heart rhythm or your heart's electrical activity

If you can't exercise for as long as what is considered normal for someone your age, your heart may not be getting enough oxygen-rich blood. However, other factors also can prevent you from exercising long enough (for example, lung diseases, anemia, or poor general fitness).

As part of some stress tests, pictures are taken of your heart while you exercise and while you rest. These imaging stress tests can show how well blood is flowing in your heart and how well your heart pumps blood when it beats.

Echocardiography

Echocardiography (echo) uses sound waves to create a moving picture of your heart. The test provides information about the size and shape of your heart and how well your heart chambers and valves are working.

Echo also can show areas of poor blood flow to the heart, areas of heart muscle that aren't contracting normally, and previous injury to the heart muscle caused by poor blood flow.

Chest X-Ray

A chest X-ray creates pictures of the organs and structures inside your chest, such as your heart, lungs, and blood vessels.

A chest X-ray can reveal signs of heart failure, as well as lung disorders and other causes of symptoms not related to CHD.

Blood Tests

Blood tests check the levels of certain fats, cholesterol, sugar, and proteins in your blood. Abnormal levels may be a sign that you're at risk for CHD. Blood tests also help detect anemia, a risk factor for CHD.

During a heart attack, heart muscle cells die and release proteins into the bloodstream. Blood tests can measure the amount of these proteins in the bloodstream. High levels of these proteins are a sign of a recent heart attack.

Coronary Angiography and Cardiac Catheterization

Your doctor may recommend coronary angiography if other tests or factors suggest you have CHD. This test uses dye and special X-rays to look inside your coronary arteries.

To get the dye into your coronary arteries, your doctor will use a procedure called cardiac catheterization.

A thin, flexible tube called a catheter is put into a blood vessel in your arm, groin (upper thigh), or neck. The tube is threaded into your coronary arteries, and the dye is released into your bloodstream.

Special X-rays are taken while the dye is flowing through your coronary arteries. The dye lets your doctor study the flow of blood through your heart and blood vessels.

Coronary angiography detects blockages in the large coronary arteries. However, the test doesn't detect coronary microvascular disease

(MVD). This is because coronary MVD doesn't cause blockages in the large coronary arteries.

Even if the results of your coronary angiography are normal, you may still have chest pain or other CHD symptoms. If so, talk with your doctor about whether you might have coronary MVD.

Your doctor may ask you to fill out a questionnaire called the Duke Activity Status Index (DASI). This questionnaire measures how easily you can do routine tasks. It gives your doctor information about how well blood is flowing through your coronary arteries.

Your doctor also may recommend other tests that measure blood flow in the heart, such as a cardiac MRI (magnetic resonance imaging) stress test.

Cardiac MRI uses radio waves, magnets, and a computer to create pictures of your heart as it beats. The test produces both still and moving pictures of your heart and major blood vessels.

Other tests done during cardiac catheterization can check blood flow in the heart's small arteries and the thickness of the artery walls.

Tests Used to Diagnose Broken Heart Syndrome

If your doctor thinks you have broken heart syndrome, he or she may recommend coronary angiography. Other tests are also used to diagnose this disorder, including blood tests, EKG, echo, and cardiac MRI.

Chapter 49

Infectious Disease Testing

Chapter Contents

Section 49.1

Chlamydia Test

This section includes text excerpted from "Chlamydia Test," MedlinePlus, National Institutes of Health (NIH), September 13, 2017.

What Is a Chlamydia Test?

Chlamydia is one of the most common sexually transmitted diseases (STDs). It is a bacterial infection spread through vaginal, oral, or anal sex with an infected person. Many people with chlamydia have no symptoms, so someone may spread the disease without even knowing they are infected. A chlamydia test looks for the presence of chlamydia bacteria in your body. The disease is easily treated with antibiotics. But if it's not treated, chlamydia can cause serious complications, including infertility in women and swelling of the urethra in men.

Other names: Chlamydia nucleic acid amplification test (NAAT or NAT), Chlamydia/Neisseria gonorrhoeae (GC) STD Panel.

What Is It Used For?

A chlamydia test is used to determine whether or not you have a chlamydia infection.

Why Do I Need a Chlamydia Test?

The Centers for Disease Control and Prevention (CDC) estimates that more than two and a half million Americans are infected with chlamydia every year. Chlamydia is especially common in sexually active people aged 15–24. Many individuals with chlamydia don't have symptoms, so the CDC and other health organizations recommend regular screening for groups at higher risk.

These recommendations include yearly chlamydia tests for:

- Sexually active women under the age of 25

- Women over the age of 25 with certain risk factors, which include:

  - Having new or multiple sex partners

  - Previous chlamydia infections

- Having a sex partner with an STD

- Using condoms inconsistently or incorrectly

- Men who have sex with men

In addition, chlamydia testing is recommended for:

- Pregnant women under the age of 25

- People who are human immunodeficiency virus positive (HIV-positive)

Some people with chlamydia will have symptoms. Your healthcare provider may order a test if you experience symptoms such as:

For women:

- Stomach pain

- Abnormal vaginal bleeding or discharge

- Pain during sex

- Pain when urinating

- Frequent urination

For men:

- Pain or tenderness in the testicles

- Swollen scrotum

- Pus or other discharge from the penis

- Pain when urinating

- Frequent urination

What Happens during a Chlamydia Test?

If you are a woman, your healthcare provider will use a small brush or swab to take a sample of cells from your vagina for testing. You may also be offered the option of testing yourself at home using a test kit. Ask your provider for recommendations on which kit to use. If you do the test at home, be sure to follow all the directions carefully.

If you're a man, your healthcare provider may use a swab to take a sample from your urethra, but it is more likely that a urine test for chlamydia will be recommended. Urine tests can also be used for women. During a urine test, you will be instructed to provide a clean catch sample.

The clean catch method generally includes the following steps:

1. Wash your hands.

2. Clean your genital area with a cleansing pad given to you by your provider. Men should wipe the tip of their penis. Women should open their labia and clean from front to back.

3. Start to urinate into the toilet.

4. Move the collection container under your urine stream.

5. Collect at least an ounce or two of urine into the container, which should have markings to indicate the amounts.

6. Finish urinating into the toilet.

7. Return the sample container as instructed by your healthcare provider.

Will I Need to Do Anything to Prepare for the Test?

If you are a woman, you may need to avoid using douches or vaginal creams for 24 hours before your test. Both men and women may be asked to avoid taking antibiotics for 24 hours before testing. Ask your healthcare provider if there are any special instructions.

Are There Any Risks to the Test?

There are no known risks to having a chlamydia test.

What Do the Results Mean?

A positive result means you have been infected with chlamydia. The infection requires treatment with antibiotics. Your healthcare provider will give you instructions on how to take your medicine. Be sure to take all the required doses. In addition, let your sexual partner know you tested positive for chlamydia, so he or she can be tested and treated promptly.

Is There Anything Else I Need to Know about a Chlamydia Test?

Chlamydia testing enables diagnosis and treatment of the infection before it can cause serious health problems. If you are at risk for chlamydia due to your age and/or lifestyle, talk to your healthcare provider about getting tested.

Section 49.2

Hepatitis Diagnostic Tests

This section includes text excerpted from "Hepatitis Panel," MedlinePlus, National Institutes of Health (NIH), November 7, 2017.

What Is a Hepatitis Panel?

Hepatitis is a type of liver disease. Viruses called hepatitis A, hepatitis B, and hepatitis C are the most common causes of hepatitis. A hepatitis panel is a blood test that checks to see if you have a hepatitis infection caused by one of these viruses.

The viruses are spread in different ways and cause different symptoms:

- **Hepatitis A** is most often spread by contact with contaminated feces (stool) or by eating tainted food. Though uncommon, it can also be spread through sexual contact with an infected person. Most people recover from hepatitis A without any lasting liver damage.

- **Hepatitis B** is spread through contact with infected blood, semen, or other bodily fluids. Some people recover quickly from a hepatitis B infection. For others, the virus can cause long-term, chronic liver disease (CLD).

- **Hepatitis C** is most often spread by contact with infected blood, usually through sharing of hypodermic needles. Though uncommon, it can also be spread through sexual contact with an infected person. Many people with hepatitis C develop CLD and cirrhosis.

A hepatitis panel includes tests for hepatitis antibodies and antigens. Antibodies are proteins that the immune system produces to help fight infections. Antigens are substances that cause an immune

545

response. Antibodies and antigens can be detected before symptoms appear.

Other names: Acute hepatitis panel, viral hepatitis panel, hepatitis screening panel

What Is It Used For?

A hepatitis panel is used to find out if you have a hepatitis virus infection.

Why Do I Need a Hepatitis Panel?

You may need a hepatitis panel if you have symptoms of liver damage. These symptoms include:

- Jaundice, a condition that causes your skin and eyes to turn yellow
- Fever
- Fatigue
- Loss of appetite
- Dark-colored urine
- Pale-colored stool
- Nausea and vomiting

You may also need a hepatitis panel if you have certain risk factors. You may be at a higher risk for a hepatitis infection if you:

- Use illegal, injectable drugs
- Have a sexually transmitted disease (STD)
- Are in close contact with someone infected with hepatitis
- Are on long-term dialysis
- Were born between 1945 and 1965, often referred to as the baby boom years. Though the reasons aren't entirely understood, baby boomers are five times more likely to have hepatitis C than other adults.

What Happens during a Hepatitis Panel?

A healthcare professional will take a blood sample from a vein in your arm, using a small needle. After the needle is inserted, a small amount of blood will be collected into a test tube or vial. You may feel a little sting when the needle goes in or out. This usually takes less than five minutes.

Will I Need to Do Anything to Prepare for the Test?

You don't need any special preparations for a hepatitis panel.

Are There Any Risks to the Test?

There is very little risk to having a blood test. You may have slight pain or bruising at the spot where the needle was put in, but most symptoms go away quickly.

What Do the Results Mean?

A negative result means you probably don't have a hepatitis infection. A positive result may mean you have or previously had an infection from hepatitis A, hepatitis B, or hepatitis C. You may need more tests to confirm a diagnosis. If you have questions about your results, talk to your healthcare provider.

Is There Anything Else I Need to Know about a Hepatitis Panel?

There are vaccines for hepatitis A and hepatitis B. Talk to your healthcare provider to see if you or your children should get vaccinated.

Section 49.3

Human Immunodeficiency Virus (HIV) and Sexually Transmitted Disease (STD) Testing

This section contains text excerpted from the following sources:
Text beginning with the heading "What Is a Rapid Oral Human
Immunodeficiency Virus HIV Test?" is excerpted from "Rapid Oral
Human Immunodeficiency Virus (HIV) Test," U.S. Department of
Veterans Affairs (VA), March 2017; Text under the heading "How
Accurate Is the Rapid Oral HIV Test?" is excerpted from "Frequently
Asked Questions—How Accurate Is the Rapid Oral HIV Test?" U.S.
Department of Veterans Affairs (VA), February 9, 2018.

What Is a Rapid Oral Human Immunodeficiency Virus (HIV) Test?

This is a test for human immunodeficiency virus (HIV), the virus that causes acquired immunodeficiency syndrome (AIDS). With a rapid oral test, results take about 20 minutes. There are also rapid tests that use a blood sample. Rapid tests are usually used when results need to be delivered within a few minutes, like in an outreach center or homeless clinic; otherwise a traditional blood test is used. The rapid oral test is quite good at detecting chronic (longstanding) HIV infection but not so good at detecting very recent HIV infection.

How Does the Rapid Oral HIV Test Work?

When HIV enters the body, antibodies are produced. The test looks for HIV antibodies in your oral fluids. The test uses a swab to collect a sample from the inside of your mouth.

What Happens When You Agree to Be Tested?

- The test is explained to you by a health provider.
- A health provider will ask you to swab your gums with a special swab.
- Results are ready in about 20 minutes.
- You will learn your HIV result and discuss what it means.
- Your provider will give you information about how to protect yourself and others from HIV.

- If your test result is positive, you will do a second, different, test using a blood sample that is sent to the lab.

- Your test result will be confidential (results will only be discussed with you). Your test result will not affect your U.S. Department of Veterans Affairs (VA) benefits.

What Does a Negative Rapid Oral HIV Test Result Mean?

This means that HIV antibodies have not been found in your system. This could mean one of two things:

1. You do not have HIV, or

2. You have HIV but it was not detected by the rapid oral test (this is a false-negative result).

It can take up to 3 months for your system to produce enough antibodies to be detected by the rapid oral test. If you have engaged in activities that might put you at risk of HIV infection in the past 3 months, you should repeat the test in a few weeks, or talk with your VA provider about doing a standard blood test for HIV right away.

What Does a Positive Rapid Oral HIV Test Result Mean?

This means that HIV antibodies may be in your system. Positive results on the rapid test must always be confirmed by doing a second HIV test. This is because sometimes (rarely) the rapid oral test gives a false-positive result. A person is considered to be HIV positive only if two different test results are positive. The second HIV test is a blood test that is sent to the lab; the results may take up to 1–2 weeks to return.

If Your Positive Result Is Confirmed by a Second Test, That Means:

You have HIV and should be evaluated right away for treatment
Your testing site will refer you to a clinic that has expertise in caring for people with HIV. They may also refer you for counseling and other support services.
HIV treatment (medication) greatly improves health, and can prevent transmission (infection) to others

Why Should You Get Tested?

Many HIV-positive people do not know they are infected with HIV, because they have never been tested.

Knowing your HIV status helps you protect yourself and others.

Getting diagnosed early can greatly improve your health. Although there is no cure for HIV, there are many effective medicines that can control it. Most people with HIV who take their medication every day can live long, healthy lives.

If you test negative, you may feel less anxious after testing, and you may be more committed to preventing yourself from becoming infected.

An HIV test is part of routine medical care.

How Accurate Is the Rapid Oral HIV Test?

The rapid oral HIV test detects antibodies made by the immune system in response to HIV infection, just like the standard blood anti-body test. The rapid oral test, however, detects these antibodies in oral fluid, and doesn't require a blood sample.

The rapid oral HIV test is quite accurate (similar to the standard blood antibody test) for persons with chronic, or longstanding, HIV infection, but it is not as accurate for people with new or recent HIV infection. Like any antibody test for HIV, the rapid oral HIV test is not reliable during the "window period" (lasting several weeks to months) between the time a person is infected and the time the body has made enough antibodies for the test to detect. During this window period, someone who is infected might test negative for antibodies (a false-negative result). The "window period" for the rapid oral test is longer than it is for some HIV blood tests, meaning that for someone with acute or new HIV infection certain blood tests can detect HIV earlier than the oral rapid tests can.

It also is possible to have false-positive results (a person may have a positive rapid oral HIV test result but not actually be infected with HIV). That's why anyone who has a positive result with a rapid oral HIV test must have a more specific "confirmatory" blood test before a diagnosis of HIV infection can be made.

Section 49.4

Tuberculosis (TB) Test

This section includes text excerpted from "Testing for
Tuberculosis (TB)," Centers for Disease Control and
Prevention (CDC), September 1, 2016.

Tuberculosis (TB) is a disease that is spread through the air from
one person to another. When someone who is sick with TB coughs,
speaks, laughs, sings, or sneezes, people nearby may breathe TB bacteria into their lungs. TB usually attacks the lungs, but can also attack
other parts of the body, such as the brain, spine, or kidneys.

TB bacteria can live in the body without making a person sick. This
is called **latent TB infection.** People with latent TB infection do not
feel sick, do not have TB symptoms, and cannot spread TB bacteria
to others. Some people with latent TB infection go on to develop **TB
disease**. People with TB disease can spread the bacteria to others,
feel sick, and can have symptoms including fever, night sweats, cough,
and weight loss.

There are two kinds of tests that are used to determine if a person
has been infected with TB bacteria: the tuberculin skin test and TB
blood tests.

Tuberculin Skin Test (TST)

What Is a TST?

The Mantoux tuberculin skin test is a test to check if a person has
been infected with TB bacteria.

How Does the TST Work?

Using a small needle, a healthcare provider injects a liquid (called
tuberculin) into the skin of the lower part of the arm. When injected, a
small, pale bump will appear. This is different from a Bacille Calmette-
Guerin (BCG) shot (a TB vaccine that many people living outside of
the United States receive).

The person given the TST must return within 2 or 3 days to have
a trained healthcare worker look for a reaction on the arm where the
liquid was injected. The healthcare worker will look for a raised, hard
area or swelling, and if present, measure its size using a ruler. Redness
by itself is not considered part of the reaction.

What Does a Positive TST Result Mean?

The TST result depends on the size of the raised, hard area or swelling. It also depends on the person's risk of being infected with TB bacteria and the progression to TB disease if infected.

- **Positive TST:** This means the person's body was infected with TB bacteria. Additional tests are needed to determine if the person has latent TB infection or TB disease. A healthcare worker will then provide treatment as needed.

- **Negative TST:** This means the person's body did not react to the test, and that latent TB infection or TB disease is not likely.

Who Can Receive a TST?

Almost everyone can receive a TST, including infants, children, pregnant women, people living with HIV, and people who have had a BCG shot. People who had a severe reaction to a previous TST should not receive another TST.

How Often Can a TST Be Given?

Usually, there is no problem with repeated TSTs unless a person has had a severe reaction to a previous TST.

Testing for TB in People with a BCG

People who have had a previous BCG shot may receive a TST. In some people, the BCG shot may cause a positive TST when they are not infected with TB bacteria. If a TST is positive, additional tests are needed.

TB Blood Tests

What Is an Interferon Gamma Release Assay (IGRA)?

An IGRA is a blood test that can determine if a person has been infected with TB bacteria. An IGRA measures how strong a person's immune system reacts to TB bacteria by testing the person's blood in a laboratory. Two IGRAs are approved by the U.S. Food and Drug Administration (FDA) and are available in the United States:

1. QuantiFERON®-TB Gold In-Tube test (QFT-GIT)

2. T–SPOT®.TB test (T-Spot)

How Does the IGRA Work?

Blood is collected into special tubes using a needle. The blood is delivered to a laboratory as directed by the IGRA test instructions. The laboratory runs the test and reports the results to the healthcare provider.

What Does a Positive IGRA Result Mean?

Positive IGRA: This means that the person has been infected with TB bacteria. Additional tests are needed to determine if the person has latent TB infection or TB disease. A healthcare worker will then provide treatment as needed.

Negative IGRA: This means that the person's blood did not react to the test and that latent TB infection or TB disease is not likely.

Who Can Receive an IGRA?

Anyone can have an IGRA in place of a TST. This can be for any situation where a TST is recommended. In general, a person should have either a TST or an IGRA, but not both. There are rare exceptions when results from both tests may be useful in deciding whether a person has been infected with TB. IGRAs are the preferred method of TB infection testing for the following:

- People who have received the BCG shot

- People who have a difficult time returning for a second appointment to look at the TST after the test was given

How Often Can an IGRA Be Given?

There is no problem with repeated IGRAs.

Who Should Get Tested for Tuberculosis (TB)?

The Centers for Disease Control and Prevention (CDC) and the U.S. Preventive Services Task Force (USPSTF) recommend testing populations that are at increased risk for TB infection. Certain people should be tested for TB bacteria because they are more likely to get TB disease, including:

- People who have spent time with someone who has TB disease

- People with HIV infection or another medical problem that weakens the immune system

- People who have symptoms of TB disease (fever, night sweats, cough, and weight loss)

- People from a country where TB disease is common (most countries in Latin America, the Caribbean, Africa, Asia, Eastern Europe, and Russia)

- People who live or work somewhere in the United States where TB disease is more common (homeless shelters, prison or jails, or some nursing homes)

- People who use illegal drugs

Choosing a TB Test

Choosing which TB test to use should be done by the person's healthcare provider. Factors in selecting which test to use include the reason for testing, test availability, and cost. Generally, it is not recommended to test a person with both a TST and an IGRA.

Diagnosis of Latent TB Infection or TB Disease

If a person is found to be infected with TB bacteria, other tests are needed to see if the person has TB disease. TB disease can be diagnosed by medical history, physical examination, chest X-ray, and other laboratory tests. TB disease is treated by taking several drugs as recommended by a healthcare provider.

If a person does not have TB disease, but has TB bacteria in the body, then latent TB infection is diagnosed. The decision about taking treatment for latent TB infection will be based on a person's chances of developing TB disease.

Chapter 50

Lung Disease Tests

Chapter Contents

Section 50.1

Understanding Lung Function Tests

This section includes text excerpted from "Lung
Function Tests," National Heart, Lung, and Blood
Institute (NHLBI), June 11, 2014. Reviewed July 2018.

Lung function tests, also called pulmonary function tests, measure
how well your lungs work. These tests are used to look for the cause
of breathing problems.

What Are Lung Function Tests?

Lung function tests, also called pulmonary function tests, measure
how well your lungs work. These tests are used to look for the cause
of breathing problems, such as shortness of breath.

Lung function tests measure:

- How much air you can take into your lungs. This amount is
  compared with that of other people your age, height, and sex.
  This allows your doctor to see whether you're in the normal
  range.

- How much air you can blow out of your lungs and how fast you
  can do it

- How well your lungs deliver oxygen to your blood

- The strength of your breathing muscles

Doctors use lung function tests to help diagnose conditions such
as asthma, pulmonary fibrosis (PF) (scarring of the lung tissue), and
COPD (chronic obstructive pulmonary disease).

Lung function tests also are used to check the extent of damage
caused by conditions such as PF and sarcoidosis. Also, these tests
might be used to check how well treatments, such as asthma medicines, are working.

Lung function tests include breathing tests and tests that measure
the oxygen level in your blood. The breathing tests most often used are:

- **Spirometry.** This test measures how much air you can breathe
  in and out. It also measures how fast you can blow air out.

- **Body plethysmography.** This test measures how much air
  is present in your lungs when you take a deep breath. It also

measures how much air remains in your lungs after you breathe out fully.

- **Lung diffusion capacity.** This test measures how well oxygen passes from your lungs to your bloodstream.

These tests may not show what's causing breathing problems. So, you may have other tests as well, such as an exercise stress test. This test measures how well your lungs and heart work while you exercise on a treadmill or bicycle.

Two tests that measure the oxygen level in your blood are pulse oximetry and arterial blood gas (ABG) tests. These tests also are called blood oxygen tests.

Pulse oximetry measures your blood oxygen level using a special light. For an ABG test, your doctor takes a sample of your blood, usually from an artery in your wrist. The sample is sent to a laboratory, where its oxygen level is measured.

Types of Lung Function Tests

Breathing Tests

Spirometry

Spirometry measures how much air you breathe in and out and how fast you blow it out. This is measured two ways:

1. peak expiratory flow rate (PEFR), and

2. forced expiratory volume in 1 second (FEV1).

PEFR is the fastest rate at which you can blow air out of your lungs. FEV1 refers to the amount of air you can blow out in 1 second.

During the test, a technician will ask you to take a deep breath in. Then, you'll blow as hard as you can into a tube connected to a small machine. The machine is called a spirometer.

Your doctor may have you inhale a medicine that helps open your airways. He or she will want to see whether the medicine changes or improves the test results.

Spirometry helps check for conditions that affect how much air you can breathe in, such as PF (scarring of the lung tissue). The test also helps detect diseases that affect how fast you can breathe air out, like asthma and COPD (chronic obstructive pulmonary disease).

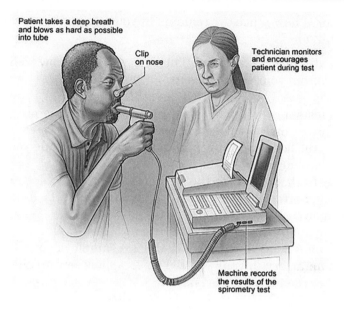

Figure 50.1. *Spirometry*

The image shows how spirometry is done. The patient takes a deep breath and blows as hard as possible into a tube connected to a spirometer. The spirometer measures the amount of air breathed out. It also measures how fast the air was blown out.

Lung Volume Measurement

Body plethysmography is a test that measures how much air is present in your lungs when you take a deep breath. It also measures how much air remains in your lungs after you breathe out fully.

During the test, you sit inside a glass booth and breathe into a tube that's attached to a computer.

For other lung function tests, you might breathe in nitrogen or helium gas and then blow it out. The gas you breathe out is measured to show how much air your lungs can hold.

Lung volume measurement can help diagnose PF or a stiff or weak chest wall.

Lung Diffusion Capacity

This test measures how well oxygen passes from your lungs to your bloodstream. During this test, you breathe in a type of gas through a tube. You hold your breath for a brief moment and then blow out the gas.

Abnormal test results may suggest loss of lung tissue, emphysema (a type of COPD), very bad scarring of the lung tissue, or problems with blood flow through the body's arteries.

Tests to Measure Oxygen Level

Pulse oximetry and ABG tests show how much oxygen is in your blood. During pulse oximetry, a small sensor is attached to your finger or ear. The sensor uses light to estimate how much oxygen is in your blood. This test is painless and no needles are used.

For an ABG test, a blood sample is taken from an artery, usually in your wrist. The sample is sent to a laboratory, where its oxygen level is measured. You may feel some discomfort during an ABG test because a needle is used to take the blood sample.

Testing in Infants and Young Children

Spirometry and other measures of lung function usually can be done for children older than 6 years, if they can follow directions well. Spirometry might be tried in children as young as 5 years. However, technicians who have special training with young children may need to do the testing.

Instead of spirometry, a growing number of medical centers measure respiratory system resistance. This is another way to test lung function in young children.

The child wears nose clips and has his or her cheeks supported with an adult's hands. The child breathes in and out quietly on a mouthpiece, while the technician measures changes in pressure at the mouth. During these lung function tests, parents can help comfort their children and encourage them to cooperate.

Very young children (younger than 2 years) may need an infant lung function test. This requires special equipment and medical staff. This type of test is available only at a few medical centers.

The doctor gives the child medicine to help him or her sleep through the test. A technician places a mask over the child's nose and mouth and a vest around the child's chest.

The mask and vest are attached to a lung function machine. The machine gently pushes air into the child's lungs through the mask. As the child exhales, the vest slightly squeezes his or her chest. This helps push more air out of the lungs. The exhaled air is then measured.

In children younger than 5 years, doctors likely will use signs and symptoms, medical history, and a physical exam to diagnose lung problems.

Doctors can use pulse oximetry and ABG tests for children of all ages.

Who Needs Lung Function Tests?

People who have breathing problems, such as shortness of breath, may need lung function tests. These tests help find the cause of breathing problems.

Doctors use lung function tests to help diagnose conditions such as asthma, pulmonary fibrosis (PF) (scarring of the lung tissue), and COPD (chronic obstructive pulmonary disease).

Lung function tests also are used to check the extent of damage caused by conditions such as PF and sarcoidosis. Also, these tests might be used to check how well treatments, such as asthma medicines, are working.

Diagnosing Lung Conditions

Your doctor will diagnose a lung condition based on your medical and family histories, a physical exam, and test results.

Medical and Family Histories

Your doctor will ask you questions, such as:

- Do you ever feel like you can't get enough air?
- Does your chest feel tight sometimes?
- Do you have periods of coughing or wheezing (a whistling sound when you breathe)?
- Do you ever have chest pain?
- Can you walk or run as fast as other people your age?

Your doctor also will ask whether you or anyone in your family has ever:

- had asthma or allergies
- had heart disease
- smoked
- traveled to places where they may have been exposed to tuberculosis (TB)
- had a job that exposed them to dust, fumes, or particles (like asbestos)

560

Physical Exam

Your doctor will check your heart rate, breathing rate, and blood pressure. He or she also will listen to your heart and lungs with a stethoscope and feel your abdomen and limbs.

Your doctor will look for signs of heart or lung disease, or another disease that might be causing your symptoms.

Lung and Heart Tests

Based on your medical history and physical exam, your doctor will recommend tests. A chest X-ray usually is the first test done to find the cause of a breathing problem. This test takes pictures of the organs and structures inside your chest.

Your doctor may do lung function tests to find out even more about how well your lungs work.

Your doctor also may do tests to check your heart, such as an EKG (electrocardiogram) or an exercise stress test. An EKG detects and records your heart's electrical activity. A stress test shows how well your heart works during physical activity.

What to Expect before Lung Function Tests

If you take breathing medicines, your doctor may ask you to stop them for a short time before spirometry, lung volume measurement, or lung diffusion capacity tests.

No special preparation is needed before pulse oximetry and ABG tests. If you're getting oxygen therapy, your doctor may ask you to stop using it for a short time before the tests. This allows your doctor to check your blood oxygen level without the added oxygen.

What to Expect during Lung Function Tests

Breathing Tests

Spirometry might be done in your doctor's office or in a special lung function laboratory (lab). Lung volume measurement and lung diffusion capacity tests are done in a special lab or clinic. For these tests, you sit in a chair next to a machine that measures your breathing. For spirometry, you sit or stand next to the machine.

Before the tests, a technician places soft clips on your nose. This allows you to breathe only through a tube that's attached to the testing machine. The technician will tell you how to breathe into the tube. For example, you might be asked to breathe normally, slowly, or rapidly.

Some tests require deep breathing, which might make you feel short of breath, dizzy, or light-headed, or it might make you cough.

Spirometry

For this test, you take a deep breath and then exhale as fast and as hard as you can into the tube. With spirometry, your doctor may give you medicine to help open your airways. Your doctor will want to see whether the medicine changes or improves the test results.

Lung Volume Measurement

For body plethysmography, you sit in a clear glass booth and breathe through the tube attached to the testing machine. The changes in pressure inside the booth are measured to show how much air you can breathe into your lungs.

For other tests, you breathe in nitrogen or helium gas and then exhale. The gas that you breathe out is measured.

Lung Diffusion Capacity

During this test, you breathe in gas through the tube, hold your breath for 10 seconds, and then rapidly blow it out. The gas contains a small amount of carbon monoxide, which won't harm you.

Tests to Measure Oxygen Level

Pulse oximetry is done in a doctor's office or hospital. An ABG test is done in a lab or hospital.

Pulse Oximetry

For this test, a small sensor is attached to your finger or ear using a clip or flexible tape. The sensor is then attached to a cable that leads to a small machine called an oximeter. The oximeter shows the amount of oxygen in your blood. This test is painless and no needles are used.

Arterial Blood Gas (ABG)

During this test, your doctor or technician inserts a needle into an artery, usually in your wrist, and takes a sample of blood. You may feel some discomfort when the needle is inserted. The sample is then sent to a lab where its oxygen level is measured.

After the needle is removed, you may feel mild pressure or throbbing at the needle site. Applying pressure to the area for 5–10 minutes should stop the bleeding. You'll be given a small bandage to place on the area.

What to Expect after Lung Function Tests

You can return to your normal activities and restart your medicines after lung function tests. Talk with your doctor about when you'll get the test results.

What Do Lung Function Tests Show?

Breathing Tests

Spirometry

Spirometry can show whether you have:

- A blockage (obstruction) in your airways. This may be a sign of asthma, COPD (chronic obstructive pulmonary disease), or another obstructive lung disorder.

- Smaller than normal lungs (restriction). This may be a sign of heart failure, pulmonary fibrosis (PF) (scarring of the lung tissue), or another restrictive lung disorder.

Lung Volume Measurement

These tests measure how much air your lungs can hold when you breathe in and how much air is left in your lungs when you breathe out. Abnormal test results may show that you have PF or a stiff or weak chest wall.

Lung Diffusion Capacity

This test can show a problem with oxygen moving from your lungs into your bloodstream. This might be a sign of loss of lung tissue, emphysema (a type of COPD), or problems with blood flow through the body's arteries.

Tests to Measure Oxygen Level

Pulse oximetry and ABG tests measure the oxygen level in your blood. These tests show how well your lungs are taking in oxygen and moving it into the bloodstream. A low level of oxygen in the blood might be a sign of a lung or heart disorder.

What Are the Risks of Lung Function Tests?

Spirometry, lung volume measurement tests, and lung diffusion capacity tests usually are safe. These tests rarely cause problems.

Pulse oximetry has no risks. Side effects from ABG tests are rare.

Section 50.2

Chronic Obstructive Pulmonary Disease (COPD)

This section contains text excerpted from the following sources: Text in this section begins with excerpts from "COPD," MedlinePlus, National Institutes of Health (NIH), January 2, 2017; Text under the heading "Getting Tested" is excerpted from "COPD— Getting Tested," National Heart, Lung, and Blood Institute (NHLBI), August 2, 2014. Reviewed July 2018.

Chronic obstructive pulmonary disease (COPD) makes it hard for you to breathe. The two main types are chronic bronchitis (CB) and emphysema. The main cause of COPD is long-term exposure to substances that irritate and damage the lungs. This is usually cigarette smoke. Air pollution, chemical fumes, or dust can also cause it.

At first, COPD may cause no symptoms or only mild symptoms. As the disease gets worse, symptoms usually become more severe. They include:

- A cough that produces a lot of mucus

- Shortness of breath, especially with physical activity

- Wheezing

- Chest tightness

Doctors use lung function tests, imaging tests, and blood tests to diagnose COPD. There is no cure. Treatments may relieve symptoms.

They include medicines, oxygen therapy, surgery, or a lung transplant. Quitting smoking is the most important step you can take to treat COPD.

Getting Tested

Everyone at risk for COPD who has a persistent cough, sputum production, or shortness of breath, should be tested for the disease. The test for COPD is called spirometry.

Spirometry can detect COPD before symptoms become severe. It is a simple, noninvasive breathing test that measures the amount of air a person can blow out of the lungs (volume) and how fast he or she can blow it out (flow). The test helps detect COPD and its severity and can also find out whether other conditions, such as asthma or heart failure, are causing the symptoms. Based on this test, your doctor or healthcare provider can tell if you have COPD, and if so, how severe it is. The spirometry reading can help them to determine the best course of treatment.

Spirometry

Spirometry is one of the best and most common lung function tests. The test is done with a spirometer, a machine that measures how well your lungs function, records the results, and displays them on a graph. You will be asked to take a deep breath, then blow out as hard and as fast as you can using a mouthpiece connected to the machine with tubing. The spirometer then measures the total amount exhaled, called the forced vital capacity or FVC, and how much you exhaled in the first second, called the forced expiratory volume in 1 second or FEV1. Your doctor or healthcare provider will read the results to assess how well your lungs are working and whether or not you have COPD.

Other Tests

Your doctor may recommend other tests, such as:

- **A chest X-ray or chest computed tomography (CT) scan.** These tests create pictures of the structures inside your chest, such as your heart, lungs, and blood vessels. The pictures can show signs of COPD. They also may show whether another condition, such as heart failure, is causing your symptoms.

• **An arterial blood gas (ABG) test.** This blood test measures the oxygen level in your blood using a sample of blood taken from an artery. The results from this test can show how severe your COPD is and whether you need oxygen therapy.

Section 50.3

Pneumonia

This section includes text excerpted from
"Pneumonia," National Heart, Lung, and Blood
Institute (NHLBI), September 27, 2016.

Pneumonia is a bacterial, viral, or fungal infection of one or both sides of the lungs that causes the air sacs, or alveoli, of the lungs to fill up with fluid or pus. Symptoms can be mild or severe and may include a cough with phlegm (a slimy substance), fever, chills, and trouble breathing. Many factors affect how serious pneumonia is, such as the type of germ causing the lung infection, your age, and your overall health. Pneumonia tends to be more serious for children under the age of five, adults over the age of 65, people with certain conditions such as heart failure, diabetes, or COPD (chronic obstructive pulmonary disease), or people who have weak immune systems due to human immunodeficiency virus (HIV)/acquired immunodeficiency syndrome (AIDS), chemotherapy (a treatment for cancer), or organ or blood and marrow stem cell transplant procedures.

Types of Pneumonia

Pneumonia is named for the way in which a person gets the infection or for the germ that causes the infection.

• **Community-acquired pneumonia (CAP).** CAP is the most common type of pneumonia and is usually caused by pneumococcus bacteria. Most cases occur during the winter.

566

CAP occurs outside of hospitals and other healthcare settings. Most people get CAP by breathing in germs (especially while sleeping) that live in the mouth, nose, or throat.

- **Hospital-acquired pneumonia (HAP).** HAP is when people catch pneumonia during a hospital stay for another illness. HAP tends to be more serious than CAP because you're already sick. Also, hospitals tend to have more germs that are resistant to antibiotics that are used to treat bacterial pneumonia.

- **Ventilator-associated pneumonia (VAP).** VAP is when people who are on a ventilator machine to help them breathe get pneumonia.

- **Atypical pneumonia.** Atypical pneumonia is a type of CAP. It is caused by lung infections with less common bacteria than the pneumococcus bacteria that cause CAP. Atypical bacteria include *Legionella pneumophila*, *Mycoplasma pneumoniae*, or *Chlamydia pneumoniae*.

- **Aspiration pneumonia.** This type of pneumonia can occur if you inhale food, drink, vomit, or saliva from your mouth into your lungs. This may happen if something disturbs your normal gag reflex, such as a brain injury, swallowing problem, or excessive use of alcohol or drugs. Aspiration pneumonia can cause lung abscesses.

To diagnose pneumonia, your doctor will review your medical history, perform a physical exam, and order diagnostic tests. This information can help your doctor determine what type of pneumonia you have. If your doctor suspects you got your infection while in a hospital, you may be diagnosed with hospital-acquired pneumonia (HAP). If you have been on a ventilator to help you breathe, you may have ventilator-associated pneumonia (VAP). The most common form of pneumonia is community-acquired pneumonia (CAP), which is when you get an infection outside of a hospital.

Treatment depends on whether bacteria, viruses, or fungi are causing your pneumonia. If bacteria are causing your pneumonia, you usually are treated at home with oral antibiotics. Most people respond quickly to treatment. If your symptoms worsen you should see a doctor right away. If you have severe symptoms or underlying health problems, you may need to be treated in a hospital. It may take several weeks to recover from pneumonia.

Diagnosis of Pneumonia

Sometimes pneumonia is hard to diagnose because it may cause symptoms commonly seen in people with colds or the flu. You may not realize it's more serious until it lasts longer than these other conditions. Your doctor will diagnose pneumonia based on your medical history, a physical exam, and test results. Your doctor may be able to diagnose you with a certain type of pneumonia based on how you got your infection and the type of germ causing your infection.

Medical History

Your doctor will ask about your signs and symptoms and how and when they began. To find out whether you have bacterial, viral, or fungal pneumonia, your doctor also may ask about:

- any recent traveling you've done

- your hobbies

- your exposure to animals

- your exposure to sick people at home, school, or work

- your past and current medical conditions, and whether any have gotten worse recently

- any medicines you take

- whether you smoke

- whether you've had flu or pneumonia vaccinations

Physical Exam

Your doctor will listen to your lungs with a stethoscope. If you have pneumonia, your lungs may make crackling, bubbling, and rumbling sounds when you inhale. Your doctor also may hear wheezing. Your doctor may find it hard to hear sounds of breathing in some areas of your chest.

Diagnostic Tests

If your doctor thinks you have pneumonia, he or she may recommend one or more of the following tests.

- **Chest X-ray** to look for inflammation in your lungs. A chest X-ray is the best test for diagnosing pneumonia. However, this

568

test won't tell your doctor what kind of germ is causing the pneumonia.

- **Blood tests** such as a complete blood count (CBC) to see if your immune system is actively fighting an infection.

- **Blood culture** to find out whether you have a bacterial infection that has spread to your bloodstream. If so, your doctor can decide how to treat the infection.

Your doctor may recommend other tests if you're in the hospital, have serious symptoms, are older, or have other health problems.

- **Sputum test.** Your doctor may collect a sample of sputum (spit) or phlegm (slimy substance from deep in your lungs) that was produced from one of your deep coughs and send the sample to the lab for testing. This may help your doctor find out if bacteria are causing your pneumonia. Then, he or she can plan your treatment.

- **Chest computed tomography (CT) scan** to see how much of your lungs is affected by your condition or to see if you have complications such as lung abscesses or pleural effusions. A CT scan shows more detail than a chest X-ray.

- **Pleural fluid culture.** For this test, a fluid sample is taken from the pleural space (a thin space between two layers of tissue that line the lungs and chest cavity). Doctors use a procedure called thoracentesis to collect the fluid sample. The fluid is studied for bacteria that may cause pneumonia.

- **Pulse oximetry.** For this test, a small sensor is attached to your finger or ear. The sensor uses light to estimate how much oxygen is in your blood. Pneumonia can keep your lungs from moving enough oxygen into your bloodstream. If you're very sick, your doctor may need to measure the level of oxygen in your blood using a blood sample. The sample is taken from an artery, usually in your wrist. This test is called an arterial blood gas (ABG) test.

- **Bronchoscopy** is a procedure used to look inside the lungs' airways. If you're in the hospital and treatment with antibiotics isn't working well, your doctor may use this procedure. Your doctor passes a thin, flexible tube through your nose or mouth, down your throat, and into the airways. The tube has a light and small camera that allow your doctor to see your windpipe and airways and take pictures. Your doctor can see whether something is blocking your airways or whether another factor is contributing to your pneumonia. Your doctor may use this procedure to collect samples of fluid from the site of pneumonia (called bronchoalveolar lavage or BAL) or to take small biopsies of lung tissue to help find the cause of your pneumonia.

Chapter 51

Neurological Diagnostic Tests

Diagnostic tests and procedures are vital tools that help physicians confirm or rule out the presence of a neurological disorder or other medical condition. A century ago, the only way to make a positive diagnosis for many neurological disorders was by performing an autopsy after a patient had died. But decades of basic research into the characteristics of disease, and the development of techniques that allow scientists to see inside the living brain and monitor nervous system activity as it occurs, have given doctors powerful and accurate tools to diagnose disease and to test how well a particular therapy may be working.

Perhaps the most significant changes in diagnostic imaging over the past 20 years are improvements in spatial resolution (size, intensity, and clarity) of anatomical images and reductions in the time needed to send signals to and receive data from the area being imaged. These advances allow physicians to simultaneously see the structure of the brain and the changes in brain activity as they occur. Scientists continue to improve methods that will provide sharper anatomical images and more detailed functional information.

This chapter includes text excerpted from "Neurological Diagnostic Tests and Procedures Fact Sheet," National Institute of Neurological Disorders and Stroke (NINDS), July 6, 2018.

Researchers and physicians use a variety of diagnostic imaging techniques and chemical and metabolic analyses to detect, manage, and treat neurological disease. Some procedures are performed in specialized settings, conducted to determine the presence of a particular disorder or abnormality. Many tests that were previously conducted in a hospital are now performed in a physician's office or at an outpatient testing facility, with little if any risk to the patient. Depending on the type of procedure, results are either immediate or may take several hours to process.

What Are Some of the More Common Screening Tests?

Laboratory screening tests of blood, urine, or other substances are used to help diagnose disease, better understand the disease process, and monitor levels of therapeutic drugs. Certain tests, ordered by the physician as part of a regular check-up, provide general information, while others are used to identify specific health concerns. For example, blood and blood product tests can detect brain and/or spinal cord infection, bone marrow disease, hemorrhage, blood vessel damage, toxins that affect the nervous system, and the presence of antibodies that signal the presence of an autoimmune disease. Blood tests are also used to monitor levels of therapeutic drugs used to treat epilepsy and other neurological disorders. Genetic testing of deoxyribonucleic acid (DNA) extracted from white cells in the blood can help diagnose Huntington disease (HD) and other congenital diseases. Analysis of the fluid that surrounds the brain and spinal cord can detect meningitis, acute and chronic inflammation, rare infections, and some cases of multiple sclerosis (MS). Chemical and metabolic testing of the blood can indicate protein disorders, some forms of muscular dystrophy (MD) and other muscle disorders, and diabetes. Urinalysis can reveal abnormal substances in the urine or the presence or absence of certain proteins that cause diseases including the mucopolysaccharidoses (MPSs).

Genetic testing or counseling can help parents who have a family history of a neurological disease determine if they are carrying one of the known genes that cause the disorder or find out if their child is affected. Genetic testing can identify many neurological disorders, including spina bifida, in utero (while the child is inside the mother's womb). Genetic tests include the following:

- **Amniocentesis**, usually done at 14–16 weeks of pregnancy, tests a sample of the amniotic fluid in the womb for genetic defects (the fluid and the fetus have the same DNA). Under local anesthesia, a thin needle is inserted through the woman's abdomen and into the womb. About 20 milliliters of fluid (roughly 4 teaspoons) is withdrawn and sent to a lab for evaluation. Test results often take 1–2 weeks.

- **Chorionic villus sampling**, or CVS, is performed by removing and testing a very small sample of the placenta during early pregnancy. The sample, which contains the same DNA as the fetus, is removed by catheter or fine needle inserted through the cervix or by a fine needle inserted through the abdomen. It is tested for genetic abnormalities and results are usually available within 2 weeks. CVS should not be performed after the tenth week of pregnancy.

- **Uterine ultrasound** is performed using a surface probe with gel. This noninvasive test can suggest the diagnosis of conditions such as chromosomal disorders.

What Is a Neurological Examination?

A **neurological examination** assesses motor and sensory skills, the functioning of one or more cranial nerves, hearing and speech, vision, coordination and balance, mental status, and changes in mood or behavior, among other abilities. Items including a tuning fork, flashlight, reflex hammer, ophthalmoscope, and needles are used to help diagnose brain tumors, infections such as encephalitis and meningitis, and diseases such as Parkinson disease (PD), Huntington disease (HD), amyotrophic lateral sclerosis (ALS), and epilepsy. Some tests require the services of a specialist to perform and analyze results.

X-rays of the patient's chest and skull are often taken as part of a neurological work-up. X-rays can be used to view any part of the body, such as a joint or major organ system. In a conventional X-ray, also called a radiograph, a technician passes a concentrated burst of low-dose ionized radiation through the body and onto a photographic plate. Since calcium in bones absorbs X-rays more easily than soft tissue or muscle, the bony structure appears white on the film. Any vertebral misalignment or fractures can be seen within minutes. Tissue masses such as injured ligaments or a bulging disc are not visible on conventional X-rays. This fast, noninvasive, painless procedure is usually performed in a doctor's office or at a clinic.

573

Fluoroscopy is a type of X-ray that uses a continuous or pulsed beam of low-dose radiation to produce continuous images of a body part in motion. The fluoroscope (X-ray tube) is focused on the area of interest and pictures are either videotaped or sent to a monitor for viewing. A contrast medium may be used to highlight the images. Fluoroscopy can be used to evaluate the flow of blood through arteries.

What Are Some Diagnostic Tests Used to Diagnose Neurological Disorders?

Based on the result of a neurological exam, physical exam, patient history, X-rays of the patient's chest and skull, and any previous screening or testing, physicians may order one or more of the following diagnostic tests to determine the specific nature of a suspected neurological disorder or injury. These diagnostics generally involve either nuclear medicine imaging, in which very small amounts of radioactive materials are used to study organ function and structure, or diagnostic imaging, which uses magnets and electrical charges to study human anatomy.

The following list of available procedures—in alphabetical rather than sequential order—includes some of the more common tests used to help diagnose a neurological condition.

Angiography is a test used to detect blockages of the arteries or veins. A cerebral angiogram can detect the degree of narrowing or obstruction of an artery or blood vessel in the brain, head, or neck. It is used to diagnose stroke and to determine the location and size of a brain tumor, aneurysm, or vascular malformation. This test is usually performed in a hospital outpatient setting and takes up to 3 hours, followed by a 6- to 8-hour resting period. The patient, wearing a hospital or imaging gown, lies on a table that is wheeled into the imaging area. While the patient is awake, a physician anesthetizes a small area of the leg near the groin and then inserts a catheter into a major artery located there. The catheter is threaded through the body and into an artery in the neck. Once the catheter is in place, the needle is removed and a guide wire is inserted. A small capsule containing a radiopaque dye (one that is highlighted on X-rays) is passed over the guide wire to the site of release. The dye is released and travels through the bloodstream into the head and neck. A series of X-rays is taken and any obstruction is noted. Patients may feel a warm to hot sensation or slight discomfort as the dye is released.

Biopsy involves the removal and examination of a small piece of tissue from the body. Muscle or nerve biopsies are used to diagnose neuromuscular disorders and may also reveal if a person is a carrier of a defective gene that could be passed on to children. A small sample of muscle or nerve is removed under local anesthetic and studied under a microscope. The sample may be removed either surgically, through a slit made in the skin, or by needle biopsy, in which a thin hollow needle is inserted through the skin and into the muscle. A small piece of muscle or nerve remains in the hollow needle when it is removed from the body. The biopsy is usually performed at an outpatient testing facility. A brain biopsy, used to determine tumor type, requires surgery to remove a small piece of the brain or tumor. Performed in a hospital, this operation is riskier than a muscle biopsy and involves a longer recovery period.

Brain scans are imaging techniques used to diagnose tumors, blood vessel malformations, or hemorrhage in the brain. These scans are used to study organ function or injury or disease to tissue or muscle. Types of brain scans include computed tomography (CT), magnetic resonance imaging (MRI), and positron emission tomography (PET).

Cerebrospinal fluid (CSF) analysis involves the removal of a small amount of the fluid that protects the brain and spinal cord. The fluid is tested to detect any bleeding or brain hemorrhage, diagnose infection to the brain and/or spinal cord, identify some cases of MS and other neurological conditions, and measure intracranial pressure.

The procedure is usually done in a hospital. The sample of fluid is commonly removed by a procedure known as a lumbar puncture, or spinal tap. The patient is asked to either lie on one side, in a ball position with knees close to the chest, or lean forward while sitting on a table or bed. The doctor will locate a puncture site in the lower back, between two vertebrate, then clean the area and inject a local anesthetic. The patient may feel a slight stinging sensation from this injection. Once the anesthetic has taken effect, the doctor will insert a special needle into the spinal sac and remove a small amount of fluid (usually about three teaspoons) for testing. Most patients will feel a sensation of pressure only as the needle is inserted.

A common after-effect of a lumbar puncture is headache, which can be lessened by having the patient lie flat. Risk of nerve root injury or infection from the puncture can occur but it is rare. The entire procedure takes about 45 minutes.

575

Computed tomography, also known as a CT scan, is a noninvasive, painless process used to produce rapid, clear two-dimensional images of organs, bones, and tissues. Neurological CT scans are used to view the brain and spine. They can detect bone and vascular irregularities, certain brain tumors and cysts, herniated discs, epilepsy, encephalitis, spinal stenosis (narrowing of the spinal canal), a blood clot or intracranial bleeding in patients with stroke, brain damage from head injury, and other disorders. Many neurological disorders share certain characteristics and a CT scan can aid in proper diagnosis by differentiating the area of the brain affected by the disorder.

Scanning takes about 20 minutes (a CT of the brain or head may take slightly longer) and is usually done at an imaging center or hospital on an outpatient basis. The patient lies on a special table that slides into a narrow chamber. A sound system built into the chamber allows the patient to communicate with the physician or technician. As the patient lies still, X-rays are passed through the body at various angles and are detected by a computerized scanner. The data is processed and displayed as cross-sectional images, or "slices," of the internal structure of the body or organ. A light sedative may be given to patients who are unable to lie still and pillows may be used to support and stabilize the head and body. Persons who are claustrophobic may have difficulty taking this imaging test.

Occasionally a contrast dye is injected into the bloodstream to highlight the different tissues in the brain. Patients may feel a warm or cool sensation as the dye circulates through the bloodstream or they may experience a slight metallic taste.

Although very little radiation is used in CT, pregnant women should avoid the test because of potential harm to the fetus from ionizing radiation.

Discography is often suggested for patients who are considering lumbar surgery or whose lower back pain has not responded to conventional treatments. This outpatient procedure is usually performed at a testing facility or a hospital. The patient is asked to put on a metal-free hospital gown and lie on an imaging table. The physician numbs the skin with anesthetic and inserts a thin needle, using X-ray guidance, into the spinal disc. Once the needle is in place, a small amount of contrast dye is injected and CT scans are taken. The contrast dye outlines any damaged areas. More than one disc may be imaged at the same time. Patient recovery usually takes about an hour. Pain medicine may be prescribed for any resulting discomfort.

An **intrathecal contrast-enhanced CT scan** (also called cisternography) is used to detect problems with the spine and spinal nerve roots. This test is most often performed at an imaging center. The patient is asked to put on a hospital or imaging gown. Following application of a topical anesthetic, the physician removes a small sample of the spinal fluid via lumbar puncture. The sample is mixed with a contrast dye and injected into the spinal sac located at the base of the lower back. The patient is then asked to move to a position that will allow the contrast fluid to travel to the area to be studied. The dye allows the spinal canal and nerve roots to be seen more clearly on a CT scan. The scan may take up to an hour to complete. Following the test, patients may experience some discomfort and/or headache that may be caused by the removal of spinal fluid.

Electroencephalography, or EEG, monitors brain activity through the skull. EEG is used to help diagnose certain seizure disorders, brain tumors, brain damage from head injuries, inflammation of the brain and/or spinal cord, alcoholism, certain psychiatric disorders, and metabolic and degenerative disorders that affect the brain. EEGs are also used to evaluate sleep disorders, monitor brain activity when a patient has been fully anesthetized or loses consciousness, and confirm brain death.

This painless, risk-free test can be performed in a doctor's office or at a hospital or testing facility. Prior to taking an EEG, the person must avoid caffeine intake and prescription drugs that affect the nervous system. A series of cup-like electrodes are attached to the patient's scalp, either with a special conducting paste or with extremely fine needles. The electrodes (also called leads) are small devices that are attached to wires and carry the electrical energy of the brain to a machine for reading. A very low electrical current is sent through the electrodes and the baseline brain energy is recorded. Patients are then exposed to a variety of external stimuli—including bright or flashing light, noise or certain drugs—or are asked to open and close the eyes, or to change breathing patterns. The electrodes transmit the resulting changes in brain wave patterns. Since movement and nervousness can change brain wave patterns, patients usually recline in a chair or on a bed during the test, which takes up to an hour. Testing for certain disorders requires performing an EEG during sleep, which takes at least 3 hours.

In order to learn more about brain wave activity, electrodes may be inserted through a surgical opening in the skull and into the brain to reduce signal interference from the skull.

577

Electromyography, or EMG, is used to diagnose nerve and muscle dysfunction and spinal cord disease. It records the electrical activity from the brain and/or spinal cord to a peripheral nerve root (found in the arms and legs) that controls muscles during contraction and at rest.

During an EMG, very fine wire electrodes are inserted into a muscle to assess changes in electrical voltage that occur during movement and when the muscle is at rest. The electrodes are attached through a series of wires to a recording instrument. Testing usually takes place at a testing facility and lasts about an hour but may take longer, depending on the number of muscles and nerves to be tested. Most patients find this test to be somewhat uncomfortable.

An EMG is usually done in conjunction with a **nerve conduction velocity (NCV)** test, which measures electrical energy by assessing the nerve's ability to send a signal. This two-part test is conducted most often in a hospital. A technician tapes two sets of flat electrodes on the skin over the muscles. The first set of electrodes is used to send small pulses of electricity (similar to the sensation of static electricity) to stimulate the nerve that directs a particular muscle. The second set of electrodes transmits the responding electrical signal to a recording machine. The physician then reviews the response to verify any nerve damage or muscle disease. Patients who are preparing to take an EMG or NCV test may be asked to avoid caffeine and not smoke for 2–3 hours prior to the test, as well as to avoid aspirin and nonsteroidal anti-inflammatory drugs for 24 hours before the EMG. There is no discomfort or risk associated with this test.

Electronystagmography (ENG) describes a group of tests used to diagnose involuntary eye movement, dizziness, and balance disorders, and to evaluate some brain functions. The test is performed at an imaging center. Small electrodes are taped around the eyes to record eye movements. If infrared photography is used in place of electrodes, the patient wears special goggles that help record the information. Both versions of the test are painless and risk-free.

Evoked potentials (also called evoked response) measure the electrical signals to the brain generated by hearing, touch, or sight. These tests are used to assess sensory nerve problems and confirm neurological conditions including multiple sclerosis (MS), brain tumor, acoustic neuroma (small tumors of the inner ear), and spinal cord injury. Evoked potentials are also used to test sight and hearing (especially in infants and young children), monitor brain activity among coma patients, and confirm brain death.

Testing may take place in a doctor's office or hospital setting. It is painless and risk-free. Two sets of needle electrodes are used to test for nerve damage. One set of electrodes, which will be used to measure the electrophysiological response to stimuli, is attached to the patient's scalp using conducting paste. The second set of electrodes is attached to the part of the body to be tested. The physician then records the amount of time it takes for the impulse generated by stimuli to reach the brain. Under normal circumstances, the process of signal transmission is instantaneous.

Auditory evoked potentials (also called brain stem auditory evoked response) are used to assess high-frequency hearing loss, diagnose any damage to the acoustic nerve and auditory pathways in the brainstem, and detect acoustic neuromas. The patient sits in a soundproof room and wears headphones. Clicking sounds are delivered one at a time to one ear while a masking sound is sent to the other ear. Each ear is usually tested twice, and the entire procedure takes about 45 minutes.

Visual evoked potentials detect loss of vision from optic nerve damage (in particular, damage caused by MS). The patient sits close to a screen and is asked to focus on the center of a shifting checkerboard pattern. Only one eye is tested at a time; the other eye is either kept closed or covered with a patch. Each eye is usually tested twice. Testing takes 30–45 minutes.

Somatosensory evoked potentials measure response from stimuli to the peripheral nerves and can detect nerve or spinal cord damage or nerve degeneration from MS and other degenerating diseases. Tiny electrical shocks are delivered by electrode to a nerve in an arm or leg. Responses to the shocks, which may be delivered for more than a minute at a time, are recorded. This test usually lasts less than an hour.

Magnetic resonance imaging (MRI) uses computer-generated radio waves and a powerful magnetic field to produce detailed images of body structures including tissues, organs, bones, and nerves. Neurological uses include the diagnosis of brain and spinal cord tumors, eye disease, inflammation, infection, and vascular irregularities that may lead to stroke. MRI can also detect and monitor degenerative disorders such as MS and can document brain injury from trauma.

The equipment houses a hollow tube that is surrounded by a very large cylindrical magnet. The patient, who must remain still during the test, lies on a special table that is slid into the tube. The patient will be asked to remove jewelry, eyeglasses, removable dental work, or other items that might interfere with the magnetic imaging. The patient should wear a sweatshirt and sweatpants or other clothing free of metal eyelets or buckles. MRI scanning equipment creates a magnetic field around the body strong enough to temporarily realign water molecules in the tissues. Radio waves are then passed through the body to detect the "relaxation" of the molecules back to a random alignment and trigger a resonance signal at different angles within the body. A computer processes this resonance into either a three-dimensional picture or a two-dimensional "slice" of the tissue being scanned, and differentiates between bone, soft tissues and fluid-filled spaces by their water content and structural properties. A contrast dye may be used to enhance visibility of certain areas or tissues. The patient may hear grating or knocking noises when the magnetic field is turned on and off. (Patients may wear special earphones to block out the sounds.) Unlike CT scanning, MRI does not use ionizing radiation to produce images. Depending on the part(s) of the body to be scanned, MRI can take up to an hour to complete. The test is painless and risk-free, although persons who are obese or claustrophobic may find it somewhat uncomfortable. (Some centers also use open MRI machines that do not completely surround the person being tested and are less confining. However, open MRI does not currently provide the same picture quality as standard MRI and some tests may not be available using this equipment). Due to the incredibly strong magnetic field generated by an MRI, patients with implanted medical devices such as a pacemaker should avoid the test.

Functional MRI (fMRI) uses the blood's magnetic properties to produce real-time images of blood flow to particular areas of the brain. An fMRI can pinpoint areas of the brain that become active and note how long they stay active. It can also tell if brain activity within a region occurs simultaneously or sequentially. This imaging process is used to assess brain damage from head injury or degenerative disorders such as Alzheimer disease (AD) and to identify and monitor other neurological disorders, including MS, stroke, and brain tumors.

Myelography involves the injection of a water- or oil-based contrast dye into the spinal canal to enhance X-ray imaging of the spine. *Myelograms* are used to diagnose spinal nerve injury, herniated discs, fractures, back or leg pain, and spinal tumors.

The procedure takes about 30 minutes and is usually performed in a hospital. Following an injection of anesthesia to a site between two vertebrae in the lower back, a small amount of the cerebrospinal fluid is removed by spinal tap and the contrast dye is injected into the spinal canal. After a series of X-rays is taken, most or all of the contrast dye is removed by aspiration. Patients may experience some pain during the spinal tap and when the dye is injected and removed. Patients may also experience headache following the spinal tap. The risk of fluid leakage or allergic reaction to the dye is slight.

Positron emission tomography (PET) scans provide two- and three-dimensional pictures of brain activity by measuring radioactive isotopes that are injected into the bloodstream. PET scans of the brain are used to detect or highlight tumors and diseased tissue, measure cellular and/or tissue metabolism, show blood flow, evaluate patients who have seizure disorders that do not respond to medical therapy and patients with certain memory disorders, and determine brain changes following injury or drug abuse, among other uses. PET may be ordered as a followup to a CT or MRI scan to give the physician a greater understanding of specific areas of the brain that may be involved with certain problems. Scans are conducted in a hospital or at a testing facility, on an outpatient basis. A low-level radioactive isotope, which binds to chemicals that flow to the brain, is injected into the bloodstream and can be traced as the brain performs different functions. The patient lies still while overhead sensors detect gamma rays in the body's tissues. A computer processes the information and displays it on a video monitor or on film. Using different compounds, more than one brain function can be traced simultaneously. PET is painless and relatively risk-free. Length of test time depends on the part of the body to be scanned. PET scans are performed by skilled technicians at highly sophisticated medical facilities.

A **polysomnogram** measures brain and body activity during sleep. It is performed over one or more nights at a sleep center. Electrodes are pasted or taped to the patient's scalp, eyelids, and/or chin. Throughout the night and during the various wake/sleep cycles, the electrodes record brain waves, eye movement, breathing, leg and skeletal muscle activity, blood pressure, and heart rate. The patient may be videotaped to note any movement during sleep. Results are then used to identify any characteristic patterns of sleep disorders, including restless legs syndrome (RLS), periodic limb movement disorder (PLMD), insomnia, and breathing disorders such as obstructive sleep apnea (OSA). Polysomnograms are noninvasive, painless, and risk-free.

Single photon emission computed tomography (SPECT), a nuclear imaging test involving blood flow to tissue, is used to evaluate certain brain functions. The test may be ordered as a follow-up to an MRI to diagnose tumors, infections, degenerative spinal disease, and stress fractures. As with a PET scan, a radioactive isotope, which binds to chemicals that flow to the brain, is injected intravenously into the body. Areas of increased blood flow will collect more of the isotope. As the patient lies on a table, a gamma camera rotates around the head and records where the radioisotope has traveled. That information is converted by computer into cross-sectional slices that are stacked to produce a detailed three-dimensional image of blood flow and activity within the brain. The test is performed at either an imaging center or a hospital.

Thermography uses infrared sensing devices to measure small temperature changes between the two sides of the body or within a specific organ. Also known as digital infrared thermal imaging, thermography may be used to detect vascular disease of the head and neck, soft tissue injury, various neuromusculoskeletal disorders, and the presence or absence of nerve root compression. It is performed at an imaging center, using infrared light recorders to take thousands of pictures of the body from a distance of 5–8 feet. The information is converted into electrical signals which results in a computer-generated two-dimensional picture of abnormally cold or hot areas indicated by color or shades of black and white. Thermography does not use radiation and is safe, risk-free, and noninvasive.

Ultrasound imaging, also called ultrasound scanning or sonography, uses high-frequency sound waves to obtain images inside the body. *Neurosonography* (ultrasound of the brain and spinal column) analyzes blood flow in the brain and can diagnose stroke, brain tumors, hydrocephalus (buildup of cerebrospinal fluid in the brain), and vascular problems. It can also identify or rule out inflammatory processes causing pain. It is more effective than an X-ray in displaying soft tissue masses and can show tears in ligaments, muscles, tendons, and other soft tissue masses in the back. *Transcranial doppler (TCD)* ultrasound is used to view arteries and blood vessels in the neck and determine blood flow and risk of stroke.

During ultrasound, the patient lies on an imaging table and removes clothing around the area of the body to be scanned. A jelly-like lubricant is applied and a transducer, which both sends and receives high-frequency sound waves, is passed over the body. The sound wave echoes are recorded and displayed as a computer-generated real-time visual image of the structure or tissue being examined. Ultrasound is painless, noninvasive, and risk-free. The test is performed on an outpatient basis and takes between 15 and 30 minutes to complete.

Chapter 52

Prenatal and Infertility Tests

Chapter Contents

583

Section 52.1

Prenatal Tests

This section includes text excerpted from "What Tests Might I Need during Pregnancy?" *Eunice Kennedy Shriver* National Institute of Child Health and Human Development (NICHD), January 31, 2017.

What Tests Might I Need during Pregnancy?

Every woman has certain tests during pregnancy. Some women, depending on their age, family history, or ethnicity, may undergo additional testing.

Some tests are screening tests, and others are diagnostic tests. If your healthcare provider orders a screening test, keep in mind that such tests do not diagnose problems. They evaluate risk. So a screening test result that comes back abnormal does not mean there is a problem with your infant. It means that more information is needed. Your healthcare provider can explain what the test results mean and possible next steps.

The types of tests you may have during pregnancy include:

Routine Tests

Glucose challenge screening. Usually given between 24 and 28 weeks of pregnancy, this screening assesses your risk for gestational diabetes. You will consume a sugary drink and get a blood test 1 hour later to measure your blood sugar levels. If you are at high risk—for example, if you have a family history of diabetes, are obese, had a large baby in a previous pregnancy, or are having twins—you should discuss this with your healthcare provider get a test for blood glucose earlier in your pregnancy.

Group B streptococcus (GBS) infection screening. This test is performed between 35 and 37 weeks of pregnancy to look for bacteria (GBS) that can cause pneumonia or other serious infections in your infant. Swabs will be used to take cells from your vagina and rectum. Women who test positive for GBS will need antibiotics when in labor.

Ultrasound exam. You will likely have an ultrasound exam between 18 and 20 weeks of pregnancy to check for any problems with the developing fetus. During an ultrasound exam, gel is spread on your belly and a special tool is moved over it to create a "picture" of the fetus on a monitor.

Urine test. At each prenatal visit, you will give a urine sample, which will be tested for signs of diabetes, urinary tract infections, and preeclampsia.

Screening for Chromosomal and Neural Tube Defects (NTDs) and Other Conditions

Nuchal translucency (NT) screening. This screening test uses ultrasonography to measure the thickness of the back of the fetus's neck between 11 and 14 weeks. This information, combined with the mother's age and the results of the serum screen, helps healthcare providers determine the fetus's potential risk for chromosomal abnormalities and other problems.

First trimester screen. Blood is drawn to test for pregnancy-associated plasma protein A (PAPP-A) and free beta-human chorionic gonadotropin (beta-hCG or hCG) and may be combined with performing a nuchal translucency ultrasound. This test will provide the risk for Down syndrome (DS) as well as other chromosomal problems.

Maternal serum screen (MSS) (also called quad screen, triple test, triple screen, multiple marker screen, or alpha-fetoprotein (AFP)). Blood is drawn to measure the levels of certain substances that determine the risk of the fetus having chromosomal abnormalities and NTDs. This screening test is done between 15 and 20 weeks of pregnancy.

Chorionic villus sampling (CVS). If your fetus is at risk for a chromosomal defect or other genetic disorders, your doctor may recommend this test when you are between 10 and 13 weeks pregnant. In this test, a needle is inserted through the cervix or the abdomen to remove a small sample of cells from the placenta.

Amniocentesis. Given between 15 and 20 weeks of pregnancy, this test is used to diagnose chromosomal disorders, such as Down syndrome (DS) and your infant's risk for neural tube defects (NTDs), such as spina bifida. After a local anesthetic is given, a thin needle is inserted into the abdomen to draw out a small amount of amniotic fluid and cells from the sac surrounding the fetus. The fluid is sent to a lab for testing.

Cell-free fetal deoxyribonucleic acid (cffDNA). A noninvasive test uses the mother's blood to look for increased amounts of material from chromosomes 21, 18, and 13. This test can be given as early as 10 weeks to women whose age, family history, or standard screening results put them at higher risk for having a child with a chromosome disorder. The test is not recommended for women who are at low risk or are carrying multiple fetuses.

Carrier screening for cystic fibrosis (CF). A blood or saliva test determines if you and your partner are carriers for this genetic disease that affects breathing and digestion. Both parents must be a carrier for their child to get CF.

Additional Testing That Your Healthcare Provider May Recommend

Glucose tolerance test (GTT). If the 1-hour glucose challenge screening is above a certain level, your healthcare provider may order this test. You will fast for at least 8 hours before the test. Your blood is drawn to test your "fasting blood glucose level." You will consume a sugary drink, and your blood will be taken every hour for 3 hours to see how your body reacts to the sugar. You may then be diagnosed with gestational diabetes.

Nonstress test (NST). This test is performed in the third trimester (28 weeks or later) to monitor the fetus's health. A belt placed around your belly measures the fetal heart rate while the fetus is at rest and while the fetus is moving or kicking. This test can determine if the fetus is getting enough oxygen.

Biophysical profile (BPP). This test, given in the third trimester of pregnancy, monitors the fetus's breathing, movement, muscle tone, and heart rate as well as the amount of amniotic fluid to determine fetal well-being. The BPP includes an ultrasound test and a nonstress test.

Section 52.2

Infertility Tests

This section includes text excerpted from "Infertility,"
Office on Women's Health (OWH), U.S. Department of
Health and Human Services (HHS), May 22, 2018.

What Is Infertility?

Infertility means not being able to get pregnant after one year of trying (or six months if a woman is 35 or older). Women who can get pregnant but are unable to stay pregnant may also be infertile.

Pregnancy is the result of a process that has many steps. To get pregnant:

- A woman's body must release an egg from one of her ovaries (ovulation).

- The egg must go through a fallopian tube toward the uterus (womb).

- A man's sperm must join with (fertilize) the egg along the way.

- The fertilized egg must attach to the inside of the uterus (implantation).

Infertility can happen if there are problems with any of these steps.

How Will Doctors Find out If a Woman and Her Partner Have Fertility Problems?

Doctors will do an infertility checkup. This involves a physical exam. The doctor will also ask for both partners' health and sexual histories. Sometimes this can find the problem. However, most of the time, the doctor will need to do more tests

In men, doctors usually begin by testing the semen. They look at the number, shape, and movement of the sperm. Sometimes doctors also suggest testing the level of a man's hormones.

In women, the first step is to find out if she is ovulating each month. There are a few ways to do this. A woman can track her ovulation at home by:

- Writing down changes in her morning body temperature for several months

- Writing down how her cervical mucus looks for several months

- Using a home ovulation test kit (available at drug or grocery stores)

Doctors can also check ovulation with blood tests. Or they can do an ultrasound of the ovaries. If ovulation is normal, there are other fertility tests available.

Some common tests of fertility in women include:

- **Hysterosalpingography (HSG):** This is an X-ray of the uterus and fallopian tubes. Doctors inject a special dye into the uterus through the vagina. This dye shows up in the X-ray. Doctors can then watch to see if the dye moves freely through the uterus and fallopian tubes. This can help them find physical blocks that may be causing infertility. Blocks in the system can keep the egg from moving from the fallopian tube to the uterus. A block could also keep the sperm from reaching the egg.

- **Laparoscopy:** A minor surgery to see inside the abdomen. The doctor does this with a small tool with a light called a laparoscope. She or he makes a small cut in the lower abdomen and inserts the laparoscope. With the laparoscope, the doctor can check the ovaries, fallopian tubes, and uterus for disease and physical problems. Doctors can usually find scarring and endometriosis by laparoscopy.

Finding the cause of infertility can be a long and emotional process. It may take time to complete all the needed tests. So don't worry if the problem is not found right away.

Chapter 53

Sleep Disorder Tests

Research has uncovered many of the nuts and bolts that link the need for sleep to the chemistry of life in the brain and virtually every part of our body. Insufficient sleep damages areas of the brain involved in managing stress, learning, and memory. Individuals who experience excessive sleepiness are often unable to perform at school or in the workplace. Sleep problems also contribute to the risk of serious medical conditions and the management of mental health illnesses.

The challenge with sleep disorders is that unlike many other medical conditions, your healthcare provider depends on you to explain the problem, which occurs in the privacy of your bedroom while you are sleeping. There is no pain associated with sleep disorders. Instead, people often have daytime symptoms, such as a morning headache or daytime sleepiness. There is no blood test to help diagnose a sleep disorder. Instead, successful diagnosis depends on the patient. It is important to discuss your symptoms with your physician so he or she can help you determine if you have sleep apnea or another sleep disorder.

Diagnosing Sleep Disorders

Depending on your symptoms, it may help you to gather information on your sleep behaviors. Your healthcare provider will review

This chapter includes text excerpted from "Advances in Sleep Studies," MedlinePlus, National Institutes of Health (NIH), 2015.

this information and consider several possible tests when trying to diagnose a sleep disorder.

Sleep History and Sleep Log

If you believe you have a sleep problem, consider keeping a sleep diary and bringing it to your next medical appointment. Your physician will ask you how many hours you sleep each night, how often you awaken during the night and for how long, how long it takes you to fall asleep, how well rested you feel upon awakening, and how sleepy you feel during the day. If you don't already keep a sleep diary, your health professional may ask you to keep one for a few weeks. Your provider also may ask you whether you have any symptoms of a sleep disorder, such as loud snoring, snorting or gasping, morning headaches, tingling or unpleasant sensations in the limbs that are relieved by moving them, and jerking of the limbs during sleep. You may want to ask your sleeping partner if you have these symptoms, since you may not be aware of them yourself.

Sleep Recording in a Sleep Laboratory

A sleep recording or polysomnogram (PSG) may be done while you stay overnight at a sleep center or at home. Your doctor will suggest the appropriate location for the PSG based on your symptoms and health. Electrodes and other monitors are placed on your scalp, face, chest, limbs, and finger. While you sleep, these devices measure your brain activity, eye movements, muscle activity, heart rate and rhythm, blood pressure, and how much air moves in and out of your lungs. This test also checks the amount of oxygen in your blood. A PSG test is painless. In certain circumstances, the PSG can be done at home. A home monitor can be used to record heart rate, how air moves in and out of your lungs, the amount of oxygen in your blood, and your breathing effort.

Multiple Sleep Latency Test (MSLT)

This daytime sleep study measures how sleepy you are and is particularly useful for diagnosing problems staying awake during the day. The multiple sleep latency test (MSLT) is conducted in a sleep laboratory and typically done after an overnight sleep recording (PSG). In this test, monitoring devices for sleep stage are placed on your scalp and face. You are asked to nap four or five times for 20 minutes every two hours during the day. Technicians note how quickly you fall asleep

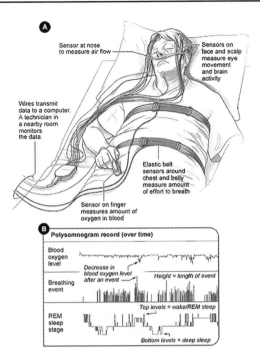

Figure 53.1. *Polysomnogram* (Source: "Sleep Studies—What to Expect during a Sleep Study," National Heart, Lung, and Blood Institute (NHLBI).)

The image shows the standard setup for a polysomnogram. In figure A, the patient lies in a bed with sensors attached to the body. In figure B, the polysomnogram recording shows the blood oxygen level, breathing event, and rapid eye movement (REM) sleep stage over time.

and how long it takes you to reach various stages of sleep, especially REM (rapid eye movement) sleep, during your naps. Normal individuals either do not fall asleep during these short-designated naptimes or take a long time to fall asleep. People who fall asleep in less than five minutes are likely to require treatment for a sleep disorder, as are those who quickly reach REM sleep during their naps.

Chapter 54

Thyroid Tests

Chapter Contents

Section 54.1

Graves Disease Testing

This section includes text excerpted from "Graves' Disease,"
National Institute of Diabetes and Digestive and Kidney
Diseases (NIDDK), September 2017.

What Is Graves Disease?

Graves disease is an autoimmune disorder that causes hyperthyroidism, or overactive thyroid. With this disease, your immune system
attacks the thyroid and causes it to make more thyroid hormone than
your body needs. The thyroid is a small, butterfly-shaped gland in
the front of your neck. Thyroid hormones control how your body uses
energy, so they affect nearly every organ in your body—even the way
your heart beats.

If left untreated, hyperthyroidism can cause serious problems with
the heart, bones, muscles, menstrual cycle, and fertility. During pregnancy, untreated hyperthyroidism can lead to health problems for the
mother and baby. Graves disease also can affect your eyes and skin.

How Do Healthcare Professionals Diagnose Graves Disease?

Your healthcare provider may suspect Graves disease based on
your symptoms and findings during a physical exam. One or more
blood tests can confirm that you have hyperthyroidism and may point
to Graves disease as the cause.

Other clues that hyperthyroidism is caused by Graves disease are:

- An enlarged thyroid

- Signs of Graves eye disease, present in about one out of three
  people with Graves disease

- A history of other family members with thyroid or autoimmune
  problems

If the diagnosis is uncertain, your doctor may order further blood
or imaging tests to confirm Graves disease as the cause.

A blood test can detect thyroid-stimulating immunoglobulin (TSI).
However, in mild cases of Graves disease, TSI may not show up in
your blood. The next step may be one of two imaging tests that use

small, safe doses of radioactive iodine. Your thyroid collects iodine from your bloodstream and uses it to make thyroid hormones; it will collect radioactive iodine in the same way.

- **Radioactive iodine uptake test.** This test measures the amount of iodine the thyroid collects from the bloodstream. If your thyroid collects large amounts of iodine, you may have Graves disease.

- **Thyroid scan.** This scan shows how and where iodine is distributed in the thyroid. With Graves disease, the entire thyroid is involved, so the iodine shows up throughout the gland. With other causes of hyperthyroidism such as nodules— small lumps in the gland—the iodine shows up in a different pattern.

Section 54.2

Hashimoto Disease Testing

This section includes text excerpted from "Hashimoto's Disease," Office on Women's Health (OWH), U.S. Department of Health and Human Services (HHS), April 25, 2018.

What Is Hashimoto Disease?

Hashimoto disease is an autoimmune disease that affects the thyroid gland. Your thyroid is a small gland at the base of your neck. Your thyroid gland makes hormones that control many activities in your body, including how fast your heart beats and how fast you burn calories.

In people with Hashimoto disease, the immune system makes antibodies that attack the thyroid gland. This damages your thyroid gland, so it does not make enough thyroid hormone. Hashimoto disease often leads to hypothyroidism. Hypothyroidism, when severe, can cause your metabolism to slow down, which can lead to weight gain, fatigue, and other symptoms.

Hashimoto disease affects more women than men. It can happen in teens and young women, but it most often appears between ages 40–60. Hashimoto disease often runs in families.

Your risk of getting Hashimoto disease is higher if you have another autoimmune disease, such as rheumatoid arthritis (RA), celiac disease, type 1 diabetes, pernicious anemia (vitamin B_{12} deficiency anemia), or lupus.

How Do Doctors Diagnose Hashimoto Disease?

If you have symptoms of hypothyroidism, your doctor or nurse will do an exam and order one or more tests. Tests used to find out whether you have hypothyroidism and Hashimoto disease include:

Thyroid function test. This blood test tells whether your body has the right amounts of thyroid stimulating hormone (TSH) and thyroid hormone. A high level of TSH is a sign of an underactive thyroid. When the thyroid begins to fail, the pituitary gland makes more TSH to trigger the thyroid to make more thyroid hormone. When the damaged thyroid can no longer keep up, your thyroid hormone levels drop below normal.

Antibody test. This blood test tells whether you have the antibodies that suggest Hashimoto disease. More than one in 10 people have the antibodies but have normal thyroid function. Having only the antibodies does not cause hypothyroidism.

Section 54.3

Thyroid Function and Disease Tests

This section includes text excerpted from "Thyroid Tests,"
National Institute of Diabetes and Digestive and Kidney
Diseases (NIDDK), May 2017.

Healthcare professionals use thyroid tests to check how well your thyroid is working and to find the cause of problems such as hyperthyroidism or hypothyroidism. The thyroid is a small, butterfly-shaped gland in the front of your neck that makes two thyroid hormones: thyroxine (T_4) and triiodothyronine (T_3). Thyroid hormones control how the body uses energy, so they affect nearly every organ in your body, even your heart.

Thyroid tests help healthcare professionals diagnose thyroid diseases such as:

- Hyperthyroidism—when thyroid hormone levels are too high

- Graves disease, the most common cause of hyperthyroidism

- Hypothyroidism—when thyroid hormones levels are too low

- Hashimoto disease, of the most common cause of hypothyroidism

- Thyroid nodules and thyroid cancer

Your doctor will start with blood tests and may also order imaging tests.

What Blood Tests Do Doctors Use to Check Thyroid Function?

Doctors may order one or more blood tests to check your thyroid function. Tests may include thyroid stimulating hormone (TSH), T_4, T_3, and thyroid antibody tests.

For these tests, a healthcare professional will draw blood from your arm and send it to a lab for testing. Your doctor will talk to you about your test results.

Thyroid Stimulating Hormone (TSH) Test

Healthcare professionals usually check the amount of TSH in your blood first. TSH is a hormone made in the pituitary gland that tells the thyroid how much T_4 and T_3 to make.

A high TSH level most often means you have hypothyroidism, or an underactive thyroid. This means that your thyroid isn't making enough hormone. As a result, the pituitary keeps making and releasing TSH into your blood.

A low TSH level usually means you have hyperthyroidism, or an overactive thyroid. This means that your thyroid is making too much hormone, so the pituitary stops making and releasing TSH into your blood.

If the TSH test results are not normal, you will need at least one other test to help find the cause of the problem.

T_4 Tests

A high blood level of T_4 may mean you have hyperthyroidism. A low level of T_4 may mean you have hypothyroidism. In some cases, high or low T_4 levels may not mean you have thyroid problems. If you are pregnant or are taking oral contraceptives, your thyroid hormone levels will be higher. Severe illness or using corticosteroids—medicines to treat asthma, arthritis, skin conditions, and other health problems—can lower T_4 levels. These conditions and medicines change the amount of proteins in your blood that "bind," or attach, to T_4. Bound T_4 is kept in reserve in the blood until it's needed. "Free" T_4 is not bound to these proteins and is available to enter body tissues. Because changes in binding protein levels don't affect free T_4 levels, many healthcare professionals prefer to measure free T_4.

T_3 Test

If your healthcare professional thinks you may have hyperthyroidism even though your T_4 level is normal, you may have a T_3 test to confirm the diagnosis. Sometimes T_4 is normal yet T_3 is high, so measuring both T_4 and T_3 levels can be useful in diagnosing hyperthyroidism.

Thyroid Antibody Tests

Measuring levels of thyroid antibodies may help diagnose an autoimmune thyroid disorder such as Graves disease—the most common cause of hyperthyroidism—and Hashimoto disease—the most common cause of hypothyroidism. Thyroid antibodies are made when your immune system attacks the thyroid gland by mistake. Your healthcare professional may order thyroid antibody tests if the results of other blood tests suggest thyroid disease.

What Imaging Tests Do Doctors Use to Diagnose and Find the Cause of Thyroid Disease?

Your healthcare professional may order one or more imaging tests to diagnose and find the cause of thyroid disease. A trained technician usually does these tests in your doctor's office, outpatient center, or hospital. A radiologist, a doctor who specializes in medical imaging, reviews the images and sends a report for your healthcare professional to discuss with you.

Ultrasound

Ultrasound of the thyroid is most often used to look for, or more closely at, thyroid nodules. Thyroid nodules are lumps in your neck. Ultrasound can help your doctor tell if the nodules are more likely to be cancerous.

For an ultrasound, you will lie on an exam table and a technician will run a device called a transducer over your neck. The transducer bounces safe, painless sound waves off your neck to make pictures of your thyroid. The ultrasound usually takes around 30 minutes.

Thyroid Scan

Healthcare professionals use a thyroid scan to look at the size, shape, and position of the thyroid gland. This test uses a small amount of radioactive iodine to help find the cause of hyperthyroidism and check for thyroid nodules. Your healthcare professional may ask you to avoid foods high in iodine, such as kelp, or medicines containing iodine for a week before the test.

For the scan, a technician injects a small amount of radioactive iodine or a similar substance into your vein. You also may swallow the substance in liquid or capsule form. The scan takes place 30 minutes after an injection, or up to 24 hours after you swallow the substance, so your thyroid has enough time to absorb it.

During the scan, you will lie on an exam table while a special camera takes pictures of your thyroid. The scan usually takes 30 minutes or less. Thyroid nodules that make too much thyroid hormone show up clearly in the pictures. Radioactive iodine that shows up over the whole thyroid could mean you have Graves disease.

Even though only a small amount of radiation is needed for a thyroid scan and it is thought to be safe, you should not have this test if you are pregnant or breastfeeding.

Radioactive Iodine Uptake (RAIU) Test

A radioactive iodine uptake (RAIU) test, also called a thyroid uptake test, can help check thyroid function and find the cause of hyperthyroidism. The thyroid "takes up" iodine from the blood to make thyroid hormones, which is why this is called an uptake test. Your healthcare professional may ask you to avoid foods high in iodine, such as kelp, or medicines containing iodine for a week before the test.

For this test, you will swallow a small amount of radioactive iodine in liquid or capsule form. During the test, you will sit in a chair while a technician places a device called a gamma probe in front of your neck, near your thyroid gland. The probe measures how much radioactive iodine your thyroid takes up from your blood. Measurements are often taken 4–6 hours after you swallow the radioactive iodine and again at 24 hours. The test takes only a few minutes.

If your thyroid collects a large amount of radioactive iodine, you may have Graves disease, or one or more nodules that make too much thyroid hormone. You may have this test at the same time as a thyroid scan.

Even though the test uses a small amount of radiation and is thought to be safe, you should not have this test if you are pregnant or breastfeeding.

What Tests Do Doctors Use If for Diagnosing a Thyroid Nodule?

If your healthcare professional finds a nodule or lump in your neck during a physical exam or on thyroid imaging tests, you may have a fine needle aspiration biopsy to see if the lump is cancerous or noncancerous.

For this test, you will lie on an exam table and slightly bend your neck backward. A technician will clean your neck with an antiseptic and may use medicine to numb the area. An endocrinologist who treats people with endocrine gland problems like thyroid disease, or a specially trained radiologist, will place a needle through the skin and use ultrasound to guide the needle to the nodule. Small samples of tissue from the nodule will be sent to a lab for testing. This procedure usually takes less than 30 minutes. Your healthcare professional will talk with you about the test result when it is available.

Section 54.4

Thyroid-Stimulating Hormone (TSH) Test

This section includes text excerpted from "TSH (Thyroid-Stimulating Hormone) Test," MedlinePlus, National Institutes of Health (NIH), November 6, 2017.

What Is a Thyroid-Stimulating Hormone (TSH) Test?

TSH stands for thyroid stimulating hormone. A TSH test is a blood test that measures this hormone. The thyroid is a small, butterfly-shaped gland located near your throat. Your thyroid makes hormones that regulate the way your body uses energy. It also plays an important role in regulating your weight, body temperature, muscle strength, and even your mood. TSH is made in a gland in the brain called the pituitary. When thyroid levels in your body are low, the pituitary gland makes more TSH. When thyroid levels are high, the pituitary gland makes less TSH. TSH levels that are too high or too low can indicate your thyroid isn't working correctly.

This test is also known as thyrotropin test.

What Is It Used for and Who May Need to Take It?

A TSH test is used to find out how well the thyroid is working. You may need a TSH test if you have symptoms of too much thyroid hormone in your blood (hyperthyroidism), or too little thyroid hormone (hypothyroidism).

Symptoms of hyperthyroidism, also known as overactive thyroid, include:

- Anxiety

- Weight loss

- Tremors in the hands

- Increased heart rate

- Puffiness

- Bulging of the eyes

- Difficulty sleeping

Symptoms of hypothyroidism, also known as underactive thyroid, include:

- Weight gain

- Tiredness

- Hair loss

- Low tolerance for cold temperatures

- Irregular menstrual periods

- Constipation

What Happens during a TSH Test?

A healthcare professional will take a blood sample from a vein in your arm, using a small needle. After the needle is inserted, a small amount of blood will be collected into a test tube or vial. You may feel a little sting when the needle goes in or out. This usually takes less than five minutes.

What Preparations You Need to Do before Undergoing the Test?

You don't need any special preparations for a TSH blood test. If your healthcare provider has ordered other blood tests, you may need to fast (not eat or drink) for several hours before the test. Your healthcare provider will let you know if there are any special instructions to follow.

What Do the Results Mean?

High TSH levels can mean your thyroid is not making enough thyroid hormones, a condition called hypothyroidism. Low TSH levels can mean your thyroid is making too much of the hormones, a condition called hyperthyroidism. A TSH test does not explain why TSH levels are too high or too low. If your test results are abnormal, your healthcare provider will probably order additional tests to determine the cause of your thyroid problem. These tests may include:

- Thyroxine (T_4) thyroid hormone tests

- Triiodothyronine (T_3) thyroid hormone tests

- Tests to diagnose Graves disease, an autoimmune disease that causes hyperthyroidism

- Tests to diagnose Hashimoto thyroiditis, an autoimmune disease that causes hypothyroidism

What Else You Should Know about a TSH Test?

Thyroid changes can happen during pregnancy. These changes are usually not significant, but some women can develop thyroid disease during pregnancy. Hyperthyroidism occurs in about one in every 500 pregnancies, while hypothyroidism occurs in approximately one in every 250 pregnancies. Hyperthyroidism, and less often, hypothyroidism, may remain after pregnancy. If you develop a thyroid condition during pregnancy, your healthcare provider will monitor your condition after your baby is born. If you have a history of thyroid disease, be sure to talk with your healthcare provider if you are pregnant or are thinking of becoming pregnant.

Are There Any Risks to the Test?

There is very little risk to having a blood test. You may have slight pain or bruising at the spot where the needle was put in, but most symptoms go away quickly.

Chapter 55

Vision Tests

Chapter Contents

605

Section 55.1

Routine Eye Exam

This section includes text excerpted from "Get Your Eyes Tested," Office of Disease Prevention and Health Promotion (ODPHP), U.S. Department of Health and Human Services (HHS), December 21, 2017.

The Basics

Have your eyes tested (examined) regularly to help find problems early, when they may be easier to treat. The doctor will also do tests to make sure you are seeing as clearly as possible.

How Often Do I Need an Eye Exam?

How often you need an eye exam depends on your risk for eye disease. Talk to your doctor about how often to get your eyes tested.
Get an eye exam every 1–2 years if you:

- Are over age 60

- Are African American and over age 40

- Have a family history of glaucoma

People with diabetes may need eye exams more often.
If you have diabetes, it's important to get your eyes tested at least once a year. Talk to your doctor about what's right for you.

What Happens during an Eye Exam?

- The doctor will ask you questions about your health and vision.

- You will read charts with letters and numbers so the doctor can check your vision.

- The doctor will do tests to look for problems with your eyes, including glaucoma.

- The doctor will put drops in your eyes to dilate (enlarge) your pupils. A dilated eye exam is the only way to find some types of eye disease.

What's the Difference between a Vision Screening and an Eye Exam?

A vision screening is a short checkup for your eyes. It usually takes place during a regular doctor visit. Vision screenings can only find certain eye problems.

An eye exam takes more time than a vision screening, and it's the only way to find some types of eye disease.

These 2 kinds of doctors can perform eye exams:

* Optometrist

* Ophthalmologist

Take Action

Protect your vision. Get regular eye exams so you can find problems early, when they may be easier to treat.

Schedule an Eye Exam

Ask your doctor or health center for the name of an eye care professional. Or use these tips for finding an eye doctor.

When you go for your exam, be sure to:

* Ask the doctor for a dilated eye exam.

* Tell the doctor if anyone in your family has eye problems or diabetes.

What about Cost?

Check with your insurance plan about costs and copayments. Medicare covers eye exams for:

* People with diabetes

* People who are at high risk for glaucoma

* Some people who have age-related macular degeneration (AMD)

If you don't have insurance, look for free or low-cost eye care programs where you live.

Tell a Doctor about Problems

See an eye doctor right away if you have any of these problems:

* Sudden loss of vision

- Flashes of light

- Tiny spots that float across your eye

- Eye pain

- Redness or swelling

Section 55.2

Color Blindness Testing

This section includes text excerpted from "Facts about Color Blindness," National Eye Institute (NEI), February 2015.

What Is Color Blindness?

Most of us share a common color vision sensory experience. Some people, however, have a color vision deficiency, which means their perception of colors is different from what most of us see. The most severe forms of these deficiencies are referred to as color blindness. People with color blindness aren't aware of differences among colors that are obvious to the rest of us. People who don't have the more severe types of color blindness may not even be aware of their condition unless they're tested in a clinic or laboratory.

Inherited color blindness is caused by abnormal photopigments. These color-detecting molecules are located in cone-shaped cells within the retina, called cone cells. In humans, several genes are needed for the body to make photopigments, and defects in these genes can lead to color blindness.

There are three main kinds of color blindness, based on photopigment defects in the three different kinds of cones that respond to blue, green, and red light. Red-green color blindness is the most common, followed by blue-yellow color blindness. A complete absence of color vision—total color blindness—is rare.

Sometimes color blindness can be caused by physical or chemical damage to the eye, the optic nerve, or parts of the brain that process color information. Color vision can also decline with age, most often because of cataract—a clouding and yellowing of the eye's lens.

What Are the Different Types of Color Blindness?

The most common types of color blindness are inherited. They are the result of defects in the genes that contain the instructions for making the photopigments found in cones. Some defects alter the photopigment's sensitivity to color, for example, it might be slightly more sensitive to deeper red and less sensitive to green. Other defects can result in the total loss of a photopigment. Depending on the type of defect and the cone that is affected problems can arise with red, green, or blue color vision.

Red-Green Color Blindness

The most common types of hereditary color blindness are due to the loss or limited function of red cone (known as protan) or green cone (deutan) photopigments. This kind of color blindness is commonly referred to as red-green color blindness.

- **Protanomaly:** In males with protanomaly, the red cone photopigment is abnormal. Red, orange, and yellow appear greener and colors are not as bright. This condition is mild and doesn't usually interfere with daily living. Protanomaly is an X-linked disorder estimated to affect 1 percent of males.

- **Protanopia:** In males with protanopia, there are no working red cone cells. Red appears as black. Certain shades of orange, yellow, and green all appear as yellow. Protanopia is an X-linked disorder that is estimated to affect 1 percent of males.

- **Deuteranomaly:** In males with deuteranomaly, the green cone photopigment is abnormal. Yellow and green appear redder and it is difficult to tell violet from blue. This condition is mild and doesn't interfere with daily living. Deuteranomaly is the most common form of color blindness and is an X-linked disorder affecting 5 percent of males.

- **Deuteranopia:** In males with deuteranopia, there are no working green cone cells. They tend to see reds as brownish-yellow and greens as beige. Deuteranopia is an X-linked disorder that affects about 1 percent of males.

Blue-Yellow Color Blindness

Blue-yellow color blindness is rarer than red-green color blindness. Blue-cone (tritan) photopigments are either missing or have limited function.

609

- **Tritanomaly:** People with tritanomaly have functionally limited blue cone cells. Blue appears greener and it can be difficult to tell yellow and red from pink. Tritanomaly is extremely rare. It is an autosomal dominant disorder affecting males and females equally.

- **Tritanopia:** People with tritanopia, also known as blue-yellow color blindness, lack blue cone cells. Blue appears green and yellow appears violet or light grey. Tritanopia is an extremely rare autosomal recessive disorder affecting males and females equally.

Complete Color Blindness

People with complete color blindness (monochromacy) don't experience color at all and the clearness of their vision (visual acuity) may also be affected.

There are two types of monochromacy:

- **Cone monochromacy (CM):** This rare form of color blindness results from a failure of two of the three cone cell photopigments to work. There is red cone monochromacy, green cone monochromacy, and blue cone monochromacy. People with cone monochromacy have trouble distinguishing colors because the brain needs to compare the signals from different types of cones in order to see color. When only one type of cone works, this comparison isn't possible. People with blue cone monochromacy, may also have reduced visual acuity, near-sightedness, and uncontrollable eye movements, a condition known as nystagmus. Cone monochromacy is an autosomal recessive disorder.

- **Rod monochromacy (RM) or achromatopsia (ACHM):** This type of monochromacy is rare and is the most severe form of color blindness. It is present at birth. None of the cone cells have functional photopigments. Lacking all cone vision, people with rod monochromacy see the world in black, white, and gray. And since rods respond to dim light, people with rod monochromacy tend to be photophobic—very uncomfortable in bright environments. They also experience nystagmus. Rod monochromacy is an autosomal recessive disorder.

How Is Color Blindness Diagnosed?

Eye care professionals use a variety of tests to diagnose color blindness. These tests can quickly diagnose specific types of color blindness.

The Ishihara Color Test is the most common test for red-green color blindness. The test consists of a series of colored circles, called Ishihara plates, each of which contains a collection of dots in different colors and sizes. Within the circle are dots that form a shape clearly visible to those with normal color vision, but invisible or difficult to see for those with red-green color blindness.

The newer Cambridge Color Test uses a visual array similar to the Ishihara plates, except displayed on a computer monitor. The goal is to identify a C shape that is different in color from the background. The "C" is presented randomly in one of four orientations. When test-takers see the "C," they are asked to press one of four keys that correspond to the orientation.

The anomaloscope uses a test in which two different light sources have to be matched in color. Looking through the eyepiece, the viewer sees a circle. The upper half is a yellow light that can be adjusted in brightness. The lower half is a combination of red and green lights that can be mixed in variable proportions. The viewer uses one knob to adjust the brightness of the top half, and another to adjust the color of the lower half. The goal is to make the upper and lower halves the same brightness and color.

The Hardy-Rand-Rittler (HRR) Pseudoisochromatic Color Test is another red-green color blindness test that uses color plates to test for color blindness.

The Farnsworth-Munsell 100 (FM100) Hue Test uses a set of blocks or pegs that are roughly the same color but in different hues (shades of the color). The goal is to arrange them in a line in order of hue. This test measures the ability to discriminate subtle color changes. It is used by industries that depend on the accurate color perception of its employees, such as graphic design, photography, and food quality inspection.

The Farnsworth Lantern Test (FALANT) is used by the U.S. military to determine the severity of color blindness. Those with mild forms pass the test and are allowed to serve in the armed forces.

Section 55.3

Comprehensive Dilated Eye Exam

This section includes text excerpted from "What Is a Comprehensive Dilated Eye Exam?" National Eye Institute (NEI), December 23, 2014. Reviewed July 2018.

You may think your eyes are healthy, but visiting an eye care professional for a comprehensive dilated eye exam is the only way to really be sure. During the exam, each eye is closely inspected for signs of common vision problems and eye diseases, many of which have no early warning signs. Annual comprehensive dilated eye exams are generally recommended starting at age 60. However, African Americans are advised to start having comprehensive dilated eye exams starting at age 40 because of their higher risk of glaucoma. It's also especially important for people with diabetes to have a comprehensive dilated exam at least once a year.

Key elements of a comprehensive dilated eye examination include dilation, tonometry, visual field test and a visual acuity test.

Dilation is an important part of a comprehensive eye exam because it enables your eye care professional to view the inside of the eye. Drops placed in each eye widen the pupil, which is the opening in the center of the iris (the colored part of the eye). Dilating the pupil allows more light to enter the eye the same way opening a door allows light into a dark room. Once dilated, each eye is examined using a special magnifying lens that provides a clear view of important tissues at the back of the eye, including the retina, the macula, and the optic nerve.

In a person with **diabetic retinopathy**, the most common diabetic eye disease and a leading cause of blindness in the United States, the exam may show swelling or leaking of blood vessels in the retina, the light-sensitive layers of tissue at the back of the eye. The eye care professional may also see abnormal growth of blood vessels in the retina associated with diabetic retinopathy.

In **age-related macular degeneration (AMD)**, a common cause of vision loss and blindness in people over the age of 50, the exam may show yellow deposits called drusen or clumps of pigment beneath the retina. In some cases, the exam may also show abnormal growth of blood vessels beneath the retina. These AMD-related changes tend to cause deterioration of a small area of the retina called the macula, which is needed for sharp, central vision.

A comprehensive dilated eye exam is also critical for detecting **glaucoma**, a disease that damages the optic nerve, which carries information from the eyes to the brain. In a person with glaucoma, the dilated exam may show changes in the shape and color of the optic nerve fibers. The exam may also show excessive cupping of the optic disc, the place where the optic nerve fibers exit the eye and enter the brain.

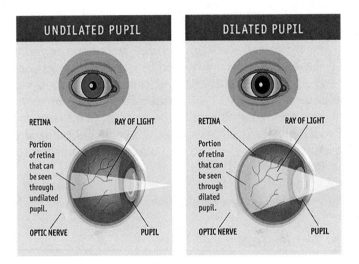

Figure 55.1. *Undilated Eyes and Dilated Eyes*

Tonometry is a test that helps detect glaucoma. By directing a quick puff of air onto the eye, or gently applying a pressure-sensitive tip near or against the eye, your eye care professional can detect elevated eye pressure, which can be a risk factor for glaucoma. Numbing drops may be applied to your eye for this test.

A **Visual field test** measures your side (peripheral) vision. A loss of peripheral vision may be a sign of glaucoma.

A **Visual acuity test** will require you to read an eye chart, which allows your eye care professional to gauge how well you see at various distances.

Section 55.4

Common Vision Tests

"Common Vision Tests," © 2017 Omnigraphics.
Reviewed July 2018.

Experts recommend that people undergo regular, comprehensive eye examinations to check the clarity of their vision and the health of their eyes. A typical eye examination includes a number of tests designed to evaluate the structure and function of the eye and measure different aspects of eyesight. Some of the most common vision tests check the patient's ability to see details from a distance or close up, see colors, track moving objects, and see objects on the periphery of the field of vision. All of these tests help the ophthalmologist or optometrist determine whether corrective measures are needed to improve the quality of the patient's vision.

Some of the vision tests that are most likely to be performed during an eye examination include the following:

Visual Acuity Test

The visual acuity test measures the sharpness or clarity of the patient's near vision and distance vision. Both tests are usually conducted by asking the patient to read rows of letters on an eye chart. The test of distance vision, known as a Snellen test after the Dutch ophthalmologist who created it, uses a wall chart with rows of letters that gradually decrease in size from top to bottom. The patient typically stands about 20 feet (6 meters) away from the chart, covers one eye, and tries to read the letters on each line. The size of the letters on one of the lines corresponds to normal visual acuity, or what a person with normal eyesight can read from a distance of 20 feet.

Using the Snellen measurement system, a person with normal visual acuity is said to have 20/20 vision. The numerator (top number) of the Snellen fraction refers to the patient's distance from the eye chart, while the denominator (bottom number) refers to the distance at which a person with normal visual acuity can read that line. About 35 percent of adults have 20/20 vision without corrective lenses. A person with 20/40 vision would have visual acuity that is worse than normal, while a person with 20/10 vision would have visual acuity that is better than normal. The goal of corrective measures like eyeglasses, contact lenses, and laser surgery is to bring a patient's vision to 20/20, and about 75 percent of adults can reach that goal with correction.

Most states require people to demonstrate visual acuity of 20/40 or better in order to qualify for a driver's license. People whose visual acuity is measured at 20/200 or worse, even with corrective lenses, are considered legally blind.

The test of close-up vision is conducted using a Jaeger chart, which is a small card containing a few lines of printed text that get smaller moving from top to bottom. The patient holds the card about 14 inches from their face to determine the smallest print they can read comfortably. In the test of near vision, both eyes are tested at the same time. Many people experience a deterioration of their near vision as part of the normal aging process, so they require reading glasses or bifocals in middle age.

Refraction

The most common problems affecting visual acuity—nearsightedness (myopia) and farsightedness (hyperopia)—occur when the lens and cornea in the eye do not focus light on the retina accurately. Instead, the light is bent or refracted so that it is focused in front of or behind the retina, causing blurry vision when the patient looks at objects far away (myopia) or up close (hyperopia). The refraction test is used to determine the exact amount of the refraction error in each eye so that it can be corrected with an eyeglass prescription.

To perform a refraction, an eye doctor uses an instrument called a phoropter to show the patient a series of lenses. The patient must decide which lens option provides greater clarity in their vision. The lens power is fine-tuned through this interactive process until the eye doctor determines the final prescription for corrective lenses.

Retinoscopy

Retinoscopy is a test that can be used to approximate the results of a refraction. The patient looks through a series of lenses in a phoropter while the eye doctor shines a light into their eyes. When the light reflects onto the correct spot on the retina in the back of the patient's eye, the doctor can determine the lens power needed to correct the refraction error. This test can be used to speed up the refraction process or to determine the corrective lens prescription for young children and other people who may have trouble providing accurate feedback during other vision tests.

Machines called autorefractors and aberrometers can also be used to estimate the results of a refraction test. The autorefractor works the same way as a manual retinoscopy. The machine shines a light into the patient's eyes and determines the corrective lens power needed to focus the light accurately on the retina. An aberrometer is a sophisticated machine that uses wavefront technology to detect abnormalities in the way light travels through a patient's eye. It is usually used to determine the precise corrections to be made during surgical vision correction procedures.

Color Vision Test

Another test commonly performed in a comprehensive eye examination is designed to test the patient's ability to distinguish between colors. About 8 percent of men and 0.5 percent of women worldwide have a color vision deficiency or color blindness. Although most cases are hereditary, deficiencies in color vision can sometimes indicate problems with eye health. The typical color vision test asks patients to find colored numbers or symbols hidden within a pattern of different-colored dots. People with normal color vision are able to identify the numbers or symbols, while those with color vision deficiencies will have difficulty distinguishing one or more colors. Color vision tests are sometimes used to screen people for employment in jobs that require good color perception, such as electricians, pilots, and truck drivers.

Cover Test

A comprehensive eye examination also includes a simple test designed to check the patient's binocular vision, or how well their eyes work together. The cover test is performed by asking the patient to stare at an object while the doctor alternately covers one eye, then the other. The doctor watches to make sure that each eye is able to maintain its focus on the fixed object while it is covered and then uncovered.

Ocular Motility Test

Ocular motility is the eyes' ability to follow a moving object or shift focus quickly between two separate objects. To test ocular motility, an eye doctor will typically ask the patient to follow the movement of a small light with their eyes while keeping their head still.

Ideally, the patient's eyes should move smoothly and in tandem. To test quick eye movements, an eye doctor may hold two objects some distance apart and ask the patient to move their eyes back and forth between them.

Stereopsis Test

Stereopsis, also known as depth perception, is the eyes' ability to discern the three-dimensional nature of objects. The two eyes must work together as a team to perceive depth. In the most common stereopsis test, the patient wears special 3D (three-dimensional) glasses while viewing a series of test patterns. For each pattern, the patient is asked to identify which letter or symbol appears closer.

Slit Lamp Exam

A slit lamp is a microscope that an eye doctor uses to examine the structures of the eye under magnification. This type of test can detect a variety of eye conditions and diseases, such as cataracts, macular degeneration, or corneal ulcers. It is often performed with the patient's pupils dilated in order to provide the best possible view of the internal structures of the eye. Pupil dilation is achieved by placing special drops in the patient's eyes. The effects can last for several hours, during which time the patient will likely be sensitive to light and have trouble focusing on close objects. If the patient will be exposed to bright light during this time, it is important for them to wear sunglasses to minimize glare and avoid damaging the eyes.

Glaucoma Test

Glaucoma is a serious eye condition caused by a buildup of pressure inside the eye when the fluid does not circulate properly. This interocular pressure can cause progressive damage to the optic nerve that carries visual signals to the brain, resulting in permanent, total blindness. Since people with glaucoma rarely experience any early symptoms or warning signs, it is important to get tested regularly. The most common glaucoma test, known as noncontact tonometry (NCT), involves a small puff of air being blown into the patient's open eye. The tonometer measures the eye's resistance to the puff of air in order to calculate its internal pressure. NCT is quick and painless, and the machine never touches the patient's eye.

Visual Field Test

A visual field test is used to detect gaps or blind spots in the patient's peripheral or side vision. Blind spots, known as scotomas, in the normal field of vision can indicate the presence of certain eye diseases or brain damage from a stroke or tumor. There are several different methods of testing a patient's field of vision. In a confrontation test, the patient covers one eye and stares at the doctor's eye or nose. The doctor slowly moves their hand from the edge of the patient's visual field toward the center, and the patient indicates the point at which they are able to see the hand. In a perimetry test, the patient stares at a dot inside a machine called a perimeter. The machine flashes lights at various points around the visual field, and the patient pushes a button each time they see a flash. At the end of the test, the machine prints a report showing any gaps or blind spots within the patient's field of vision.

If any of the above tests indicate problems with the patient's eye health or vision, the patient may be referred to a specialist for further testing.

References

1. Heiting, Gary, and Jennifer Palombi. "What to Expect during a Comprehensive Eye Exam," All About Vision, September 2016.

2. "Vision Tests," WebMD, 2017.

Chapter 56

Vestibular (Balance) Problem Tests

What Is a Balance Disorder?

A balance disorder is a condition that makes you feel unsteady or dizzy. If you are standing, sitting, or lying down, you might feel as if you are moving, spinning, or floating. If you are walking, you might suddenly feel as if you are tipping over.

Everyone has a dizzy spell now and then, but the term "dizziness" can mean different things to different people. For one person, dizziness might mean a fleeting feeling of faintness, while for another it could be an intense sensation of spinning (vertigo) that lasts a long time.

About 15 percent of American adults (33 million) had a balance or dizziness problem. Balance disorders can be caused by certain health conditions, medications, or a problem in the inner ear or the brain. A balance disorder can profoundly affect daily activities and cause psychological and emotional hardship.

If you have a balance disorder, your symptoms might include:

- Dizziness or vertigo (a spinning sensation)

- Falling or feeling as if you are going to fall

- Staggering when you try to walk

This chapter includes text excerpted from "Balance Disorders," National Institute on Deafness and Other Communication Disorders (NIDCD), March 6, 2018.

- Lightheadedness, faintness, or a floating sensation

- Blurred vision

- Confusion or disorientation

Other symptoms might include nausea and vomiting; diarrhea; changes in heart rate and blood pressure; and fear, anxiety, or panic. Symptoms may come and go over short time periods or last for a long time and can lead to fatigue and depression.

How Does My Body Keep Its Balance?

Your sense of balance relies on a series of signals to your brain from several organs and structures in your body, specifically your eyes, ears, and the muscles and touch sensors in your legs. The part of the ear that assists in balance is known as the vestibular system, or the labyrinth, a maze-like structure in your inner ear made of bone and soft tissue.

Within the labyrinth are structures known as semicircular canals. The semicircular canals contain three fluid-filled ducts, which form loops arranged roughly at right angles to one another. They tell your brain when your head rotates. Inside each canal is a gelatin-like structure called the cupula, stretched like a thick sail that blocks off one end of each canal. The cupula sits on a cluster of sensory hair cells. Each hair cell has tiny, thin extensions called stereocilia that protrude into the cupula.

When you turn your head, fluid inside the semicircular canals moves, causing the cupulae to flex or billow like sails in the wind, which in turn bends the stereocilia. This bending creates a nerve signal that is sent to your brain to tell it which way your head has turned.

Between the semicircular canals and the cochlea (a snail-shaped, fluid-filled structure in the inner ear) lie two otolithic organs: fluid-filled pouches called the utricle and the saccule. These organs tell your brain the position of your head with respect to gravity, such as whether you are sitting up, leaning back, or lying down, as well as any direction your head might be moving, such as side to side, up or down, forward or backward.

The utricle and the saccule also have sensory hair cells lining the floor or wall of each organ, with stereocilia extending into an overlying gel-like layer. Here, the gel contains tiny, dense grains of calcium carbonate called otoconia. Whatever the position of your head, gravity pulls on these grains, which then move the stereocilia to signal your head's position to your brain. Any head movement creates a signal that tells your brain about the change in head position.

When you move, your vestibular system detects mechanical forces, including gravity, that stimulate the semicircular canals and the otolithic organs. These organs work with other sensory systems in your body, such as your vision and your musculoskeletal sensory system, to control the position of your body at rest or in motion. This helps you maintain stable posture and keep your balance when you're walking or running. It also helps you keep a stable visual focus on objects when your body changes position.

When the signals from any of these sensory systems malfunction, you can have problems with your sense of balance, including dizziness or vertigo. If you have additional problems with motor control, such as weakness, slowness, tremor, or rigidity, you can lose your ability to recover properly from imbalance. This raises the risk of falling and injury.

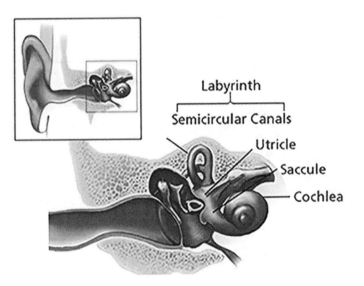

Figure 56.1. *Structures of the Balance System Inside the Inner Ear*

How Are Balance Disorders Diagnosed?

Diagnosis of a balance disorder is difficult. To find out if you have a balance problem, your primary doctor may suggest that you see an otolaryngologist and an audiologist. An otolaryngologist is a physician and surgeon who specializes in diseases and disorders of the ear, nose, neck, and throat. An audiologist is a clinician who specializes in the function of the hearing and vestibular systems.

You may be asked to participate in a hearing examination, blood tests, a video nystagmogram (a test that measures eye movements and the muscles that control them), or imaging studies of your head and brain. Another possible test is called posturography. For this test, you stand on a special movable platform in front of a patterned screen.

Posturography measures how well you can maintain steady balance during different platform conditions, such as standing on an unfixed, movable surface. Other tests, such as rotational chair testing, brisk head-shaking testing, or even tests that measure eye or neck muscle responses to brief clicks of sound, may also be performed. The vestibular system is complex, so multiple tests may be needed to best evaluate the cause of your balance problem.

Part Six

Home and Self-Ordered Tests

Chapter 57

An Introduction to Home-Use Medical Tests

Home-use tests allow you to test for some diseases or conditions at home. These tests are cost effective, quick, and confidential. Home-use tests can help:

- detect possible health conditions when you have no symptoms, so that you can get early treatment and lower your chance of developing later complications (i.e., cholesterol testing, hepatitis testing)

- detect specific conditions when there are no signs so that you can take immediate action (i.e., pregnancy testing)

- monitor conditions to allow frequent changes in treatment (i.e., glucose testing to monitor blood sugar levels in diabetes)

Despite the benefits of home testing, you should take precautions when using home-use tests. Home-use tests are intended to help you with your healthcare, but they should not replace periodic visits to your doctor. Many times, you should talk to your doctor

This chapter contains text excerpted from the following sources: Text in this chapter begins with excerpts from "Home Use Tests," U.S. Food and Drug Administration (FDA), March 26, 2018; Text under the heading "How You Can Get the Best Results with Home-Use Tests" is excerpted from "How You Can Get the Best Results with Home Use Tests," U.S. Food and Drug Administration (FDA), December 28, 2017.

even if you get normal test results. Most tests are best evaluated together with your medical history, a physical exam, and other testing. Always see your doctor if you are feeling sick, are worried about a possible medical condition, or if the test instructions recommend you do so.

How You Can Get the Best Results with Home-Use Tests

Follow the tips listed here to use home-use tests as safely and effectively as possible.

- **Read the label and instructions carefully.** Review all instructions and pictures carefully to make sure you understand how to perform the test. Be sure you know:

  - what the test is for and what it is not for

  - how to store the test before you use it

  - how to collect and store the sample

  - when and how to run the test, including timing instructions

  - how to interpret the test

  - what might interfere with the test

  - the manufacturer's phone number if you have questions

- **Use only tests regulated by U.S. Food and Drug Administration (FDA).** There are several ways to find out if FDA regulates a home-use test. You can ask your pharmacist or the vendor selling the test. If FDA does not regulate the test, the U.S. government has not determined that the test is reasonably safe or effective, or substantially equivalent to another legally marketed device.

- **Follow all instructions.** You must follow all test instructions to get an accurate result. Most home tests require specific timing, materials, and sample amounts. You should also check the expiration dates and storage conditions before performing a test to make sure the components still work correctly.

- **Keep good records of your testing.**

- **Call the "800" telephone number listed on your home-use test if you have any questions.**

- **When in doubt, contact your doctor.** All tests can give false results. You should see your doctor if you believe your test results are wrong.

- **Don't change medications or dosages based on a home-use test without talking to your doctor.**

Chapter 58

Cholesterol Home-Use Test

What Cholesterol Is

Cholesterol is a fat (lipid) in your blood. High-density lipoprotein (HDL) ("good" cholesterol) helps protect your heart, but low-density lipoprotein (LDL) ("bad" cholesterol) can clog the arteries of your heart. Some cholesterol tests also measure triglycerides, another type of fat in the blood.

What Cholesterol Home-Use Test Does

This is a home-use test kit to measure total cholesterol.

What Type of Test This Is

This is a quantitative test—you find out the amount of total cholesterol present in your sample.

Why You Should Do This Test

You should do this test to find out if you have high total cholesterol. High cholesterol increases your risk of heart disease. When the blood vessels of your heart become clogged by cholesterol, your heart does not receive enough oxygen. This can cause heart disease.

This chapter includes text excerpted from "Home Use Tests—Cholesterol," U.S. Food and Drug Administration (FDA), February 6, 2018.

How Often You Should Do This Test

If you are more than 20 years old, you should test your cholesterol about every 5 years. If your doctor has you on a special diet or drugs to control your cholesterol, you may need to check your cholesterol more frequently. Follow your doctor's recommendations about how often you test your cholesterol.

What Your Cholesterol Levels Should Be

Your total cholesterol level should be 200 mg/dL or less, according to recommendations in the National Cholesterol Education Program (NCEP) Third Adult Treatment Panel (ATP III). You should try to keep your LDL values less than 100 mg/dL, your HDL values greater or equal to 40 mg/dL, and your triglyceride values less than 150 mg/dL.

How Accurate This Test Is

This test is about as accurate as the test your doctor uses, but you must follow the directions carefully.

Total cholesterol tests vary in accuracy from brand to brand. Information about the test's accuracy is printed on its package. Tests that say they are "traceable" to a program of the Centers for Disease Control and Prevention (CDC) may be more accurate than others.

What to Do You If Your Test Shows High Cholesterol

Talk to your doctor if your test shows that your cholesterol is higher than 200 mg/dL. Many things can cause high cholesterol levels including diet, exercise, and other factors. Your doctor may want you to test your cholesterol again.

How You Do This Test

You prick your finger with a lancet to get a drop of blood. Then you put the drop of blood on a special piece of paper that contains special chemicals. The paper will change color depending on how much cholesterol is in your blood. Some testing kits use a small machine to tell you how much cholesterol there is in the sample.

Chapter 59

Direct-to-Consumer Genetic Testing

Most of the time, genetic testing is done through healthcare providers such as physicians, nurse practitioners, and genetic counselors. Healthcare providers determine which test is needed, order the test from a laboratory, collect and send the deoxyribonucleic acid (DNA) sample, interpret the test results, and share the results with the patient. Often, a health insurance company covers part or all of the cost of testing.

Direct-to-consumer (DTC) genetic testing is different: these genetic tests are marketed directly to customers via television, print advertisements, or the Internet, and the tests can be bought online or in stores. Customers send the company a DNA sample and receive their results directly from a secure website or in a written report. Direct-to-consumer genetic testing provides people access to their genetic information without necessarily involving a healthcare provider or health insurance company in the process.

Dozens of companies offer DTC genetic tests for a variety of purposes. The most popular tests use genetic variations to make predictions about health, provide information about common traits, and offer clues about a person's ancestry. The number of companies providing DTC genetic testing is growing, along with the range of health

This chapter includes text excerpted from "Direct-To-Consumer Genetic Testing," Genetics Home Reference (GHR), National Institutes of Health (NIH), May 2018.

conditions and traits covered by these tests. Because there is little regulation of DTC genetic testing services, it is important to assess the quality of available services before pursuing any testing.

Other names for DTC genetic testing include DTC genetic testing, direct-access genetic testing, at-home genetic testing, and home DNA testing. Ancestry testing (also called genealogy testing) is also considered a form of DTC genetic testing.

Kinds of Direct-to-Consumer (DTC) Genetic Tests

With so many companies offering direct-to-consumer (DTC) genetic testing, it can be challenging to determine which tests will be most informative and helpful to you. When considering testing, think about what you hope to get out of the test. Some DTC genetic tests are very specific (such as paternity tests), while other services provide a broad range of health, ancestry, and lifestyle information.

Some of the major types of DTC genetic tests are described below.

Disease Risk and Health

The results of these tests estimate your genetic risk of developing several common diseases, such as celiac disease, Parkinson disease (PD), and Alzheimer disease (AD). Some companies also include a person's carrier status for less common conditions, including cystic fibrosis (CF) and sickle cell disease (SCD). A carrier is someone who has one copy of a gene mutation that, when present in two copies, causes a genetic disorder. The tests may also look for genetic variations related to other health-related traits, such as weight and metabolism (how a person's body converts the nutrients from food into energy).

Ancestry or Genealogy

The results of these tests provide clues about where a person's ancestors might have come from, their ethnicity, and genetic connections between families.

Kinship

The results of these tests can indicate whether tested individuals are biologically related to one another. For example, kinship testing can establish whether one person is the biological father of another (paternity testing). The results of DTC kinship tests, including paternity tests, are usually not admissible in a court of law.

Lifestyle

The results of these tests claim to provide information about lifestyle factors, such as nutrition, fitness, weight loss, skincare, sleep, and even your wine preferences, based on variations in your DNA. Many of the companies that offer this kind of testing also sell services, products, or programs that they customize on the basis of your test results.

Before choosing a DTC genetic test, find out what kinds of health, ancestry, or other information will be reported to you. Think about whether there is any information you would rather not know. In some cases, you can decline to find out specific information if you tell the company before it delivers your results.

Genetic Ancestry Testing

Genetic ancestry testing, or genetic genealogy, is a way for people interested in family history (genealogy) to go beyond what they can learn from relatives or from historical documentation. Examination of DNA variations can provide clues about where a person's ancestors might have come from and about relationships between families. Certain patterns of genetic variation are often shared among people of particular backgrounds. The more closely related two individuals, families, or populations are, the more patterns of variation they typically share.

Three types of genetic ancestry testing are commonly used for genealogy and they are described below.

Y Chromosome Testing

Variations in the Y chromosome, passed exclusively from father to son, can be used to explore ancestry in the direct male line. Y chromosome testing can only be done on males, because females do not have a Y chromosome. However, women interested in this type of genetic testing sometimes recruit a male relative to have the test done. Because the Y chromosome is passed on in the same pattern as are family names in many cultures, Y chromosome testing is often used to investigate questions such as whether two families with the same surname are related.

Mitochondrial Deoxyribonucleic Acid (mDNA) Testing

This type of testing identifies genetic variations in mitochondrial DNA (mDNA). Although most DNA is packaged in chromosomes within the cell nucleus, cell structures called mitochondria also have a small amount of their own DNA (known as mitochondrial DNA). Both males and females have mitochondrial DNA, which is passed on from their mothers, so this type of testing can be used by either sex. It provides information about the direct female ancestral line. Mitochondrial DNA testing can be useful for genealogy because it preserves information about female ancestors that may be lost from the historical record because of the way surnames are often passed down.

Single Nucleotide Polymorphism (SNP) Testing

These tests evaluate large numbers of variations (single nucleotide polymorphisms or SNPs) across a person's entire genome. The results are compared with those of others who have taken the tests to provide an estimate of a person's ethnic background. For example, the pattern of SNPs might indicate that a person's ancestry is approximately 50 percent African, 25 percent European, 20 percent Asian, and 5 percent unknown. Genealogists use this type of test because Y chromosome and mitochondrial DNA test results, which represent only single ancestral lines, do not capture the overall ethnic background of an individual.

Genetic ancestry testing has a number of limitations. Test providers compare individuals' test results to different databases of previous tests, so ethnicity estimates may not be consistent from one provider to another. Also, because most human populations have migrated many times throughout their history and mixed with nearby groups, ethnicity estimates based on genetic testing may differ from an individual's expectations. In ethnic groups with a smaller range of genetic variation due to the group's size and history, most members share many SNPs, and it may be difficult to distinguish people who have a relatively recent common ancestor, such as fourth cousins, from the group as a whole.

Genetic ancestry testing is offered by several companies and organizations. Most companies provide online forums and other services to allow people who have been tested to share and discuss their results with others, which may allow them to discover previously unknown relationships. On a larger scale, combined genetic ancestry test results from many people can be used by scientists to explore the history of populations as they arose, migrated, and mixed with other groups.

Benefits and Risks of DTC Genetic Testing

Direct-to-consumer (DTC) genetic testing has both benefits and limitations, although they are somewhat different than those of genetic testing ordered by a healthcare provider.

Benefits

- DTC genetic testing promotes awareness of genetic diseases.

- It provides personalized information about your health, disease risk, and other traits.

- It may help you be more proactive about your health.

- It does not require approval from a healthcare provider or health insurance company.

- It is often less expensive than genetic testing obtained through a healthcare provider.

- DNA sample collection is usually simple and noninvasive, and results are available quickly.

- Your data is added to a large database that can be used to further medical research. Depending on the company, the database may represent up to several million participants.

Risks and Limitations

- Tests may not be available for the health conditions or traits that interest you.

- This type of testing cannot tell definitively whether you will or will not get a particular disease.

- Unexpected information that you receive about your health, family relationships, or ancestry may be stressful or upsetting.

- People may make important decisions about disease treatment or prevention based on inaccurate, incomplete, or misunderstood information from their test results.

- There is little oversight or regulation of testing companies as of now.

- Unproven or invalid tests can be misleading. There may not be enough scientific evidence to link a particular genetic variation with a given disease or trait.

- Genetic privacy may be compromised if testing companies use your genetic information in an unauthorized way or if your data is stolen.

- The results of genetic testing may impact your ability to obtain life, disability, or long-term care insurance.

DTC genetic testing provides only partial information about your health. Other genetic and environmental factors, lifestyle choices, and family medical history also affect the likelihood of developing many disorders. These factors would be discussed during a consultation with a doctor or genetic counselor, but in many cases they are not addressed when using at-home genetic tests.

Choosing a DTC Genetic Testing Company

If you are interested in DTC genetic testing, do some research into the companies that offer these services. Questions that can help you assess the quality and credibility of a testing company include:

- Does the company's website appear professional? Does the company provide adequate information about the services it offers, including sample reports, pricing, and methodology?

- Does the company have experienced genetics professionals, such as medical geneticists and genetic counselors, on its staff? Does the company offer consultation with a genetics professional if you have questions about your test results?

- Does the company explain which genetic variations it is testing for? Does it include the scientific evidence linking those variations with a particular disease or trait? Are the limitations of the test and the interpretation of results made clear?

- What kind of laboratory does the genetic testing, and is the laboratory inside or outside the United States? Is the laboratory certified or accredited? For example, does the laboratory meet U.S. federal regulatory standards called the Clinical Laboratory Improvement Amendments (CLIA)? Is the test approved by the U.S. Food and Drug Administration (FDA)?

- Does the company indicate how it will protect your privacy and keep your genetic data safe? Does that information include both current privacy practices and what may happen to your genetic data in the future?

- Does the company indicate who will have access to your data and how it may be shared? Does it share or sell their customers' genetic data for research or other purposes? For some companies, much of their profit comes from selling large amounts of participant data for research and drug development, not from selling individual test kits.

Be sure to read and understand the "fine print" on the company's website before purchasing a DTC genetic test. This detailed information, which is often called the "terms of use" or "terms of service," is a legally binding agreement between you and the company providing the testing. It spells out what is included and excluded in the service and details your rights and the company's responsibilities. If you still have questions, contact the company to get more information before you make a decision about testing.

How DTC Genetic Testing Is Done

For most types of DTC genetic testing, the process involves:

1. **Purchasing a test.** Test kits can be purchased online (and are shipped to your home) or at a store. The price of some test kits includes the analysis and interpretation, while in other cases this information is purchased separately.

2. **Collecting the sample.** Collection of the DNA sample usually involves spitting saliva into a tube or swabbing the inside of your cheek. You then mail the sample as directed by the company. In some cases, you will need to visit a health clinic to have blood drawn.

3. **Analyzing the sample.** A laboratory will analyze the sample to look for particular genetic variations. The variations included in the test depend on the purpose of the test.

4. **Receiving results.** In most cases, you will be able to access your results on a secure website. Other test companies share results in the mail or over the phone. The results usually include interpretation of what specific genetic variations may mean for your health or ancestry. In some cases, a genetic counselor or other healthcare provider is available to explain the results and answer questions.

The test kit will include step-by-step instructions, so be sure you understand them before you begin. If you have questions, contact the company before collecting your sample.

What the Results of DTC Genetic Testing Mean

Direct-to-consumer (DTC) genetic testing can provide interesting information about your health, traits, and ancestry. However, the results may not be as clear-cut as many people assume. Companies that provide these tests often tell their customers that the results are for information, education, and research purposes only—they are not meant to diagnose, prevent, or treat any disease or health condition. It is useful to keep this distinction in mind when interpreting your own test results.

Health and Disease Risk

The results of these genetic tests provide information about your chance of developing certain diseases and the likelihood that you have particular traits (such as dimples or lactose intolerance). These results are usually based on an analysis of one or more genetic variations that are known or suspected to be associated with the disease or trait.

The results of tests to predict disease risk do not provide a "yes or no" answer about whether a person will develop a given disease. Other factors, including genetic variations that were not tested, environmental factors, and lifestyle choices (such as diet and exercise) also contribute to disease risk in ways that may not be fully understood. Therefore, a result showing an increased risk does not mean you will definitely develop the disease, and a result showing a reduced risk does not mean you will never develop the disease.

Ancestry

The results of these tests give clues about major geographic areas that are your family's origins. These results are calculated on the basis of genetic variations that are more common in people from certain areas of the world than in others. You may also choose to receive information about individuals who are likely related to you. (These individuals have also undergone testing, and the predictions are based on similarities among DNA sequences.)

Sometimes the results of ancestry testing are unexpected or inconsistent with what a person understands about his or her family history. These tests can uncover previously unknown information about biological relationships among people (such as paternity). People who are closely related, such as siblings, may receive slightly different information about their ancestry because results are limited by the number and diversity of people who have submitted DNA samples to a given DTC genetic testing company. It is important to be aware that receiving unexpected or ambiguous information about your background or family is a potential risk with this type of testing.

Lifestyle

In most cases, DTC lifestyle tests assess genetic variations related to very specific traits, such as how your body converts the nutrients from food into energy (metabolism), day/night (circadian) rhythm, or the senses of taste and smell. The company may recommend specific diet or fitness programs, dietary supplements, skincare products, or other products and services on the basis of your results. However, in most cases the link between a given genetic variation and a complex trait like weight, athletic performance, or sleep is indirect or unknown. Therefore, the results of these tests can be challenging to interpret, and it can be difficult to predict whether a recommended product or service will be helpful to you.

If you have questions about the meaning of your test results, professional support (such as guidance from a genetic counselor) may be available from the company that provided the test. You can also share questions about your results with your own healthcare provider. Talk to your doctor before making any major changes in managing your health, diet, or fitness after you receive results of a DTC genetic test.

Chapter 60

Drugs of Abuse Home Tests

Drugs of Abuse

Drugs of abuse are illegal or prescription medicines (for example, Oxycodone or Valium) that are taken for a nonmedical purpose. Nonmedical purposes for a prescription drug include taking the medication for longer than your doctor prescribed it for or for a purpose other than what the doctor prescribed it for. Medications are not drugs of abuse if they are taken according to your doctor's instructions.

What These Tests Do

These tests indicate if one or more prescription or illegal drugs are present in urine. These tests detect the presence of drugs such as:

- Marijuana
- Cocaine
- Opiates
- Methamphetamine
- Amphetamines
- Phencyclidine (PCP)

This chapter includes text excerpted from "Drugs of Abuse Tests—Drugs of Abuse Home Use Test," U.S. Food and Drug Administration (FDA), December 28, 2017.

- Benzodiazepine

- Barbiturates

- Methadone

- Tricyclic antidepressants (TCAs)

- Ecstasy

- Oxycodone

The testing is done in two steps. First, you do a quick at-home test. Second, if the test suggests that drugs may be present, you send the sample to a laboratory for additional testing.

What Type of Test These Are

They are qualitative tests—you find out if a particular drug may be in the urine, but not how much is present.

When You Should Do These Tests

You should use these tests when you think someone might be abusing prescription or illegal drugs. If you are worried about a specific drug, make sure to check the label to confirm that this test is designed to detect the drug you are looking for.

How Accurate These Tests Are

The at-home testing part of this test is fairly sensitive to the presence of drugs in the urine. This means that if drugs are present, you will usually get a preliminary (or presumptive) positive test result. If you get a preliminary positive result, you should send the urine sample to the laboratory for a second test.

It is very important to send the urine sample to the laboratory to confirm a positive at-home result because certain foods, food supplements, beverages, or medicines can affect the results of at-home tests. Laboratory tests are the most reliable way to confirm drugs of abuse.

Many things can affect the accuracy of these tests, including (but not limited to):

- the way you did the test

- the way you stored the test or urine

- what the person ate or drank before taking the test

any other prescription or over-the-counter (OTC) drugs the person may have taken before the test

Note that a result showing the presence of an amphetamine should be considered carefully, even when this result is confirmed in the laboratory testing. Some OTC medications will produce the same test results as illegally-abused amphetamines.

What a Positive Test Result Means

Take no serious actions until you get the laboratory's result. Remember that many factors may cause a false positive result in the home test. Also remember that a positive test for a prescription drug does not mean that a person is abusing the drug, because there is no way for the test to indicate acceptable levels compared to abusive levels of prescribed drugs.

What a Negative Test Result Means

No drug test of this type is 100 percent accurate. There are several factors that can make the test results negative even though the person is abusing drugs. First, you may have tested for the wrong drugs. Or, you may not have tested the urine when it contained drugs. It takes time for drugs to appear in the urine after a person takes them, and they do not stay in the urine indefinitely; you may have collected the urine too late or too soon. It is also possible that the chemicals in the test went bad because they were stored incorrectly or they passed their expiration date.

If you get a negative test result, but still suspect that someone is abusing drugs, you can test again at a later time. Talk to your doctor if you need more help deciding what steps to take next.

When Drug Intake Shows up in a Drug Test

The drug clearance rate tells how soon a person may have a positive test after taking a particular drug. It also tells how long the person may continue to test positive after the last time he or she took the drug. Clearance rates for common drugs of abuse are given below. These are only guidelines, however, and the times can vary significantly from these estimates based on how long the person has been taking the drug, the amount of drug they use, or the person's metabolism.

Table 60.1. Drug Result Timing Chart

Drug	How Soon after Taking Drug Will There Be a Positive Drug Test?	How Long after Taking Drug Will There Continue to Be a Positive Drug Test?
Marijuana/Pot	1–3 hours	1–7 days
Crack (Cocaine)	2–6 hours	2–3 days
Heroin (Opiates)	2–6 hours	1–3 days
Speed/Uppers (Amphetamine, methamphetamine)	4–6 hours	2–3 days
Angel Dust/Phencyclidine (PCP)	4–6 hours	7–14 days
Ecstacy	2–7 hours	2–4 days
Benzodiazepine	2–7 hours	1–4 days
Barbiturates	2–4 hours	1–3 weeks
Methadone	3–8 hours	1–3 days
Tricyclic Antidepressants (TCAs)	8–12 hours	2–7 days
Oxycodone	1–3 hours	1–2 days

How a Drugs of Abuse Test Can Be Done by You

These tests usually contain a sample collection cup, the drug test (it may be test strips, a test card, a test cassette, or other method for testing the urine), and an instruction leaflet or booklet. It is very important that the person doing the test reads and understands the instructions first, before even collecting the sample. This is important because with most test kits, the result must be visually read within a certain number of minutes after the test is started.

You collect urine in the sample collection cup and test it according to the instructions. If the test indicates the preliminary presence of one or more drugs, the sample should be sent to a laboratory where a more specific chemical test will be used order to obtain a final result. Some home-use kits have a shipping container and preaddressed mailer in them. If you have questions about using these tests, or the results that you are getting, you should contact your healthcare provider.

Chapter 61

Gynecological Concerns Home Tests

Chapter Contents

Section 61.1

Ovulation (Saliva Test)

This section includes text excerpted from "Home Use Tests—Ovulation (Saliva Test)," U.S. Food and Drug Administration (FDA), February 6, 2018.

What Ovulation Test Does

This is a home-use test kit to predict ovulation by looking at patterns formed by your saliva. When your estrogen increases near your time of ovulation, your dried saliva may form a fern-shaped pattern. This is a qualitative test—you find out whether or not you may be near your ovulation time, not if you will definitely become pregnant.

Why You Should You Do Ovulation Test

You should do this test if you want to know when you expect to ovulate and be in the most fertile part of your menstrual cycle. This test can be used to help you plan to become pregnant. You should not use this test to help prevent pregnancy, because it is not reliable for that purpose.

How Accurate This Test Is

This test may not work well for you. Some of the reasons are:

- not all women fern
- you may not be able to see the fern
- women who fern on some days of their fertile period don't necessarily fern on all of their fertile days
- ferning may be disrupted by:
  - smoking
  - eating
  - drinking
  - brushing your teeth
  - how you put your saliva on the slide
  - where you were when you did the test

How You Can Do This Test

In this test, you get a small microscope with built-in or removable slides. You put some of your saliva on a glass slide, allow it to dry, and look at the pattern it makes. You will see dots and circles, a fern (full or partial), or a combination depending on where you are in your monthly cycle.

You will get your best results when you use the test within the 5-day period around your expected ovulation. This period includes the 2 days before and the 2 days after your expected day of ovulation. The test is not perfect, though, and you might fern outside of this time period or when you are pregnant. Even some men will fern.

How This Test Differs from the One Performed by the Doctor

The fertility tests your doctor uses are automated, and they may give more consistent results. Your doctor may use other tests that are not yet available for home use (i.e., blood and urine laboratory tests) and information about your history to get a better view of your fertility status.

Test Results and What They Mean

A positive test indicates that you may be near ovulation. It does not mean that you will definitely become pregnant. The negative test results does not mean that you are not ovulating.

There may be many reasons why you did not detect your time of ovulation. You should not use this test to help prevent pregnancy, because it is not reliable for that purpose.

Section 61.2

Ovulation (Urine Test)

This section includes text excerpted from "Home Use
Tests—Ovulation (Urine Test)," U.S. Food and Drug
Administration (FDA), February 4, 2018.

What Ovulation (Urine Test) Does

The ovulation (urine test) is a home-use test kit to measure luteinizing hormone (LH) in your urine. This helps detect the LH surge that happens in the middle of your menstrual cycle, about 1–1½ days before ovulation. Some tests also measure another hormone—estrone-3-glucuronide (E3G).

This is a qualitative test—you find out whether or not you have elevated LH or E3G levels, not if you will definitely become pregnant.

Luteinizing Hormone (LH)

Luteinizing hormone (LH) is a hormone produced by your pituitary gland. Your body always makes a small amount of LH, but just before you ovulate, you make much more LH. This test can detect this LH surge, which usually happens 1–1½ days before you ovulate.

Estrone-3-Glucuronide (E3G)

Estrone-3-glucuronide (E3G) is produced when estrogen breaks down in your body. It accumulates in your urine around the time of ovulation and causes your cervical mucus to become thin and slippery. Sperm may swim more easily in your thin and slippery cervical mucus, increasing your chances of getting pregnant.

Why You Should Do This Test

You should do this test if you want to know when you expect to ovulate and be in the most fertile part of your menstrual cycle. This test can be used to help you plan to become pregnant. You should not use this test to help prevent pregnancy, because it is not reliable for that purpose.

Accuracy of This Test

How well this test will predict your fertile period depends on how well you follow the instructions. These tests can detect LH and E3G reliably about 9 times out of 10, but you must do the test carefully.

How You Can Do This Test

You add a few drops of your urine to the test, hold the tip of the test in your urine stream, or dip the test in a cup of your urine. You either read the test by looking for colored lines on the test or you put the test device into a monitor. You can get results in about 5 minutes. The details of what the color looks like, or how to use the monitor varies among the different brands.

Most kits come with multiple tests to allow you to take measurements over several days. This can help you find your most fertile period, the time during your cycle when you can expect to ovulate based on your hormone levels. Follow the instructions carefully to get good results. You will need to start your testing at the proper time during your cycle, otherwise the test will be unreliable, and you will not find your hormonal surges or your fertile period.

How This Test Differs from the One Performed by the Doctor

The fertility tests your doctor uses are automated, and they may give more consistent results. Your doctor may use other tests that are not yet available for home use (i.e., blood and urine laboratory tests) and information about your history to get a better view of your fertility status.

Section 61.3

Home Pregnancy Test

This section includes text excerpted from "Home Use
Tests—Pregnancy," U.S. Food and Drug
Administration (FDA), December 28, 2018.

What the Home Pregnancy Test Does

You should use this test to find out if you are pregnant. This is a
qualitative test—you find out whether or not you have elevated hCG
levels indicating that you are pregnant. This test kit is used to measure
human chorionic gonadotropin (hCG) in your urine. You produce this
hormone only when you are pregnant.

The hCG is a hormone produced by your placenta when you are
pregnant. It appears shortly after the embryo attaches to the wall of
the uterus. If you are pregnant, this hormone increases very rapidly. If
you have a 28-day menstrual cycle, you can detect hCG in your urine
12–15 days after ovulation.

How Accurate This Test Is

The accuracy of this test depends on how well you follow the instructions and interpret the results. If you mishandle or misunderstand the
test kit, you may get poor results.

Most pregnancy tests have about the same ability to detect hCG,
but their ability to show whether or not you are pregnant depends on
how much hCG you are producing. If you test too early in your cycle
or too close to the time you became pregnant, your placenta may not
have had enough time to produce hCG. This would mean that you are
pregnant but you got a negative test result.

Because many women have irregular periods, and women may
miscalculate when their period is due, 10–20 pregnant women out
of every 100 will not detect their pregnancy on the first day of their
missed period.

How You Can Do This Test

For most home pregnancy tests, you either hold a test strip in
your urine stream or you collect your urine in a cup and dip your test
strip into the cup. If you are pregnant, most test strips produce a colored line, but this will depend on the brand you purchased. Read the

650

instructions for the test you bought and follow them carefully. Make sure you know how to get good results. The test usually takes only about 5 minutes.

The different tests for sale vary in their abilities to detect low levels of hCG. For the most reliable results, test 1–2 weeks after you miss your period. There are some tests for sale that are sensitive enough to show you are pregnant before you miss your period.

You can improve your chances for an accurate result by using your first-morning urine for the test. If you are pregnant, it will have more hCG in it than later urines. If you think you are pregnant, but your first test was negative, you can take the test again after several days. Since the amount of hCG increases rapidly when you are pregnant, you may get a positive test on later days. Some test kits come with more than one test in them to allow you to repeat the test.

How This Test Differs from the One Performed by the Doctor

The home pregnancy test and the test your doctor uses are similar in their abilities to detect hCG, however, your doctor is probably more experienced in running the test. If you produce only a small amount of hCG, your doctor may not be able to detect it any better than you could. Your doctor may also use a blood test to see if you are pregnant. Finally, your doctor may have more information about you from your history, physical exam, and other tests that may give a more reliable result.

Test Results and What They Mean

Usually, a positive test mean you are pregnant. But you must be sure to read and interpret the results correctly. At the same time negative test results does not mean that you are not pregnant. There are several reasons why you could receive false negative test results. If you tested too early in your cycle, your placenta may not have had time to produce enough hCG for the test to detect. Or, you may not have waited long enough before you took this test.

If you have a negative result, you would be wise to consider this a tentative finding. You should not use medications and should consider avoiding potentially harmful behaviors, such as smoking or drinking alcohol, until you have greater certainty that you are not pregnant.

You will probably recognize incorrect results with the passage of time. You may detect false negatives by the unexpected onset of menses (regular vaginal bleeding associated with "periods"). Repeat testing and/or other investigations such as ultrasound may provide corrected results.

Section 61.4

Home Vaginal pH Test

This section includes text excerpted from "Home Use Tests—Vaginal pH," U.S. Food and Drug Administration (FDA), December 28, 2017.

What Home Vaginal pH (Potential of Hydrogen) Test Is

Potential of hydrogen (pH) is a way to describe how acidic a substance is. It is given by a number on a scale of 1–14. The lower the number, the more acidic the substance.

The vaginal pH is a home-use test kit to measure the pH of your vaginal secretions. It is a quantitative test—you find out how acidic your vaginal secretions are.

Why You Should Do This Test

You should do this test to help evaluate if your vaginal symptoms (i.e., itching, burning, unpleasant odor, or unusual discharge) are likely caused by an infection that needs medical treatment. The test is not intended for human immunodeficiency virus (HIV), chlamydia, herpes, gonorrhea, syphilis, or group B streptococcus (GBS).

How Accurate This Test Is

Home vaginal pH tests showed good agreement with a doctor's diagnosis. However, just because you find changes in your vaginal pH, doesn't always mean that you have a vaginal infection. pH changes also do not help or differentiate one type of infection from another. Your doctor diagnoses a vaginal infection by using a combination of pH, microscopic examination of the vaginal discharge, amine odor, culture, wet preparation, and gram stain.

Test Results and What They Mean

A positive test does not mean you have a vaginal infection. At the same time a positive test (elevated pH) could occur for other reasons. If you detect elevated pH, you should see your doctor for further testing and treatment. There are no over-the-counter (OTC) medications for treatment of an elevated vaginal pH.

If test results are negative, can you be sure that you do not have a vaginal infection? No, you may have an infection that does not show up in these tests. If you have no symptoms, your negative test could suggest the possibility of chemical, allergic, or other noninfectious irritation of the vagina. Or, a negative test could indicate the possibility of a yeast infection. You should see your doctor if you find changes in your vaginal pH or if you continue to have symptoms.

How You Can Do This Test

You hold a piece of pH paper against the wall of your vagina for a few seconds, then compare the color of the pH paper to the color on the chart provided with the test kit. The number on the chart for the color that best matches the color on the pH paper is the vaginal pH number.

How This Test Differs from the One Performed by the Doctor

The home vaginal pH tests are practically identical to the ones sold to doctors. But your doctor can provide a more thorough assessment of your vaginal status through your history, physical exam, and other laboratory tests than you can using a single pH test in your home.

Chapter 62

Menopause Home Test

Menopause

Menopause is the stage in your life when menstruation stops for at least 12 months. The time before this is called perimenopause and could last for several years. You may reach menopause in your early 40s or as late as your 60s.

What Menopause Home Test Is

The menopause home test is a home-use test kit to measure follicle stimulating hormone (FSH) in your urine. FSH is a hormone produced by your pituitary gland. FSH levels increase temporarily each month to stimulate your ovaries to produce eggs. When you enter menopause and your ovaries stop working, your FSH levels also increase. This is a qualitative test—you find out whether or not you have elevated FSH levels, not if you definitely are in menopause or perimenopause.

Why You Should Do This Test

You should use this test if you want to know if your symptoms, such as irregular periods, hot flashes, vaginal dryness, or sleep

This chapter includes text excerpted from "Home Use Tests—Menopause," U.S. Food and Drug Administration (FDA), December 28, 2017.

problems are part of menopause. While many women may have little or no trouble when going through the stages of menopause, others may have moderate to severe discomfort and may want treatment to alleviate their symptoms. This test may help you be better informed about your current condition when you see your doctor.

How Accurate This Test Is

These tests will accurately detect FSH about 9 out of 10 times. This test does not detect menopause or perimenopause. As you grow older, your FSH levels may rise and fall during your menstrual cycle. While your hormone levels are changing, your ovaries continue to release eggs and you can still become pregnant.

Your test will depend on whether you:

- used your first-morning urine

- drank large amounts of water before the test

- use, or recently stopped using, oral or patch contraceptives, hormone replacement therapy (HRT), or estrogen supplements

How This Test Is Done

In this test, you put a few drops of your urine on a test device, put the end of the testing device in your urine stream, or dip the test device into a cup of urine. Chemicals in the test device react with FSH and produce a color. Read the instructions with the test you buy to learn exactly what to look for in this test.

Some home menopause tests are identical to the one your doctor uses. However, doctors would not use this test by itself.

Test Results and What They Mean

A positive test indicates that you may be in a stage of menopause. If you have a positive test, or if you have any symptoms of menopause, you should see your doctor. Do not stop taking contraceptives based on the results of these tests because they are not foolproof and you could become pregnant.

If you have a negative test result, but you have symptoms of menopause, you may be in perimenopause or menopause. You should not assume that a negative test means you have not reached menopause, there could be other reasons for the negative result. You should always discuss your symptoms and your test results with your doctor. Do not use these tests to determine if you are fertile or can become pregnant. These tests will not give you a reliable answer on your ability to become pregnant.

Chapter 63

Hepatitis C Home Test

Hepatitis C Infection and Hepatitis C Home Test

Hepatitis C infection is caused by the hepatitis C virus (HCV). Untreated, hepatitis C can cause liver disease. The Hepatitis C Home Test is a home-use collection kit to determine if you may have a hepatitis C infection now or had one in the past. You collect a blood sample and send it to a testing laboratory for analysis.

Why You Should Do Hepatitis C Home Test

You should do this test if you think you may have been infected with HCV. If you are infected with HCV, you should take steps to avoid spreading the disease to others. At least 8 out of 10 people with acute hepatitis C develop chronic liver infection, and 2–3 out of 10 develop cirrhosis. A small number of people may also develop liver cancer. Hepatitis C infection is the number 1 cause for liver transplantation in the United States.

When You Should You Do Hepatitis C Home Test

The Centers for Disease Control and Prevention (CDC) recommends that you do this test if you have any of the following:

- Have ever injected illegal drugs

This chapter includes text excerpted from "Home Use Tests—Hepatitis C," U.S. Food and Drug Administration (FDA), February 4, 2018.

- Received clotting factor concentrates produced before 1987

- Were ever on long-term dialysis

- Received a blood transfusion before July 1992

- Received an organ transplant before July 1992

- Are a healthcare, emergency medicine, or public safety worker who contacted HCV-positive blood through needle sticks, sharps, or mucosal exposure

How Accurate Hepatitis C Home Test Is

This test is about as accurate as the test your doctor uses, but you must carefully follow the directions about getting the sample and sending it to the testing laboratory. Proper sample collection is important for obtaining accurate results. Researchers found that about 90 of 100 home users were able to obtain acceptable samples to send to the laboratory. After the laboratory received these 90 samples, it could get results for about 81 of them. Of these 81 samples, the laboratory got correct results in 77 and incorrect results in 4.

Test Results and What They Mean

If you have a positive test, you either are infected with HCV now or you have been infected with HCV in the past. You need to see your doctor to find out if you have an active infection and what therapy you should have. Some people who become infected with HCV develop antibodies and then are no longer infected.

A negative test does not guarantee that you don't have HCV infection since it takes some time for you to develop antibodies after you are infected with this virus. If you think you were exposed to the virus and might be infected, you should see your doctor for a more accurate laboratory test.

How You Can Do Hepatitis C Home Test

The test kit comes with a small piece of filter paper, a lancet, and instructions for obtaining a blood sample and placing it on the filter paper. You first prick your finger with the lancet to get a drop of blood. Then, you put your drop of blood on a piece of filter paper and send it in a special container to the testing laboratory. You get the results of your test by phone from the laboratory. The laboratory does a preliminary (screening) test that separates the samples into three groups:

1. Samples that are clearly positive

2. Samples that *might* be positive, and

3. Samples that are negative

All samples that "**might** be positive" receive a more specific (confirmatory) test to find those that are truly positive. All the "clearly positives" from the preliminary test and the "truly positives" from the more specific test are reported to you as positive.

You should note that a positive result does not mean that you are infected with HCV. If you receive a positive result from this test, you should see your doctor for further testing and information.

Chapter 64

HIV Home Test

What Is Human Immunodeficiency Virus (HIV)?

Human immunodeficiency virus (HIV) is the virus that causes acquired immunodeficiency syndrome (AIDS).

What Does This Test Do?

This is a home-use collection kit to detect whether or not you have antibodies to HIV.

What Type of Test Is This?

This is a qualitative test—you find out whether or not you have this infection, not how advanced your disease is.

Why Should You Do This Test?

You should do this test to find out if you have an HIV infection. If you know that you have an HIV infection,

- You can obtain medical treatment that helps slow the course of the disease, and

- You can take precautions to keep from infecting others.

This chapter includes text excerpted from "Home Use Tests—Human Immunodeficiency Virus (HIV)," U.S. Food and Drug Administration (FDA), February 4, 2018.

Untreated, HIV destroys your immune system. The most advanced stage of HIV infection is AIDS, an often-fatal disease.

When Should You Do This Test?

You should do this test if you believe there is a chance you may have an HIV infection. You are at greatest risk for HIV if you:

- Have ever shared injection drug needles and syringes or "works"

- Have ever had sex without a condom with someone who had HIV

- Have ever had a sexually transmitted disease, like chlamydia or gonorrhea

- Received a blood transfusion or a blood-clotting factor between 1978 and 1985

- Have ever had sex with someone who has done any of those things

If you use this test, no one but you will know you were tested for HIV or what the results showed.

How Accurate Is This Test?

This test is similar to the test your doctor would use. Researchers have found that about 90 of 100 home users were able to obtain acceptable samples for sending to the laboratory. After the laboratory got these 90 samples, they could get results for about 81 of 100 of them. Of these 81 samples, the laboratory almost always shows whether or not the person tested had HIV infection.

Does a Positive Test Mean You Have HIV?

If you test positive in this test, you are infected with the HIV virus. You should take precautions so you do not spread this infection to your sexual partners or others who might be at risk. You should not donate blood because this infection could spread to others. Having HIV infection does not necessarily mean you have AIDS. You should see your doctor so you can learn the status of your disease and decide what therapy, if any, you need.

If Your Results Are Negative, Can You Be Sure That You Do Not Have HIV Infection?

If you test negative for HIV, it means you did not have antibodies to HIV at the time of the test. However, if you are newly infected, it will take time for you to make antibodies. It is uncertain how long it may take you to develop antibodies—it may take more than 3 months. So, although you may be infected, the results of your testing will not verify that you are infected for several months. If you think you were exposed to the virus and might be infected, you should test yourself again in a few months.

How Do You Do This Test?

The test comes with sterile lancets, an alcohol pad, gauze pads, a blood specimen collection card, a bandage, a lancet disposal container, a shipping pouch, and instructions. To do the test, you

- Call a specified telephone number.
- Register a code number that is included with the specimen collection kit.
- Prick your finger with a lancet to get a drop of blood.
- Place drops of blood on the card.
- Send the shipping pouch by express courier service to the central testing laboratory.
- Receive results by phone after 3–7 business days later
- If you test positive for HIV, you get counseling on what to do about your infection.

Chapter 65

Prothrombin Home Test

Prothrombin Time[1]

Prothrombin is a protein made by the liver. Prothrombin helps blood to make normal clots. The "prothrombin time" (PT) is one way of measuring how long it takes blood to form a clot, and it is measured in seconds (such as 13.2 seconds). A normal PT indicates that a normal amount of blood-clotting protein is available.

What Does Prothrombin Home Test Do?[2]

This is a home-use test kit to measure how long it takes for your blood to clot.

What Type of Test Is This?[2]

This is a quantitative test—you find out the length of time it takes your blood to clot.

This chapter includes text excerpted from documents published by two public domain sources. Text under the headings marked 1 are excerpted from "Viral Hepatitis," U.S. Department of Veterans Affairs (VA), February 14, 2018; Text under the headings marked 2 are excerpted from "Medical Devices—Prothrombin," U.S. Food and Drug Administration (FDA), December 28, 2017.

Why Should You Do This Test?[2]

If you take blood-thinning drugs such as Coumadin or Warfarin, you may need to test your blood regularly to make sure it clots properly. Doctors often prescribe these drugs to prevent blood clots in patients who have artificial heart valves, irregular heart beats or inherited clotting tendencies. Your doctor will prescribe this test for you if you need to do it.

How Often Should You Do This Test?[2]

You should follow your doctor's instructions about how often you do this test. Your doctor may ask you to use the results to adjust the amount of drugs you to take to control your blood clotting. Never change the drugs you take without your doctor's permission.

How Do You Do This Test?[2]

You prick your finger with a lancet to get a drop of blood. Place the drop of blood on a test strip or cartridge, and insert it into your test meter. Your meter will measure how long it takes for the blood to form a clot and how much anticoagulant effect there is.

How Can You Make Sure Your Meter Works Properly?[2]

Your meter has some built-in features that allow it to test itself and detect problems in its operation. Your meter comes with sample solutions to use instead of your blood to assure that it is working properly. Look in your meter operator manual to see how to check on its accuracy.

Take your meter with you to your doctor's office. Have your doctor watch you do your testing. Your doctor may want to take a sample of your blood and compare the clotting time of that sample with the time your meter gives. If the value you get matches your doctor's value, that you will know your meter is working well and that you are doing the test correctly.

Explanation of Test Results[1]

When the PT is high, it takes longer for the blood to clot (17 seconds, for example). This usually happens because the liver is not making the right amount of blood clotting proteins, so the clotting process takes longer. A high PT usually means that there is serious liver damage or cirrhosis.

Part Seven

Additional Help and Information

Chapter 66

Glossary of Terms Related to Medical Tests

angiography: A procedure to X-ray blood vessels. The blood vessels can be seen because of an injection of a dye that shows up in the X-ray.

assessment: In healthcare, a process used to learn about a patient's condition. This may include a complete medical history, medical tests, a physical exam, a test of learning skills, tests to find out if the patient is able to carry out the tasks of daily living, a mental health evaluation, and a review of social support and community resources available to the patient.

biopsy: The removal of cells or tissues for examination by a pathologist. The pathologist may study the tissue under a microscope or perform other tests on the cells or tissue. There are many different types of biopsy procedures. The most common types include: (1) incisional biopsy, in which only a sample of tissue is removed; (2) excisional biopsy, in which an entire lump or suspicious area is removed; and (3) needle biopsy, in which a sample of tissue or fluid is removed with a needle.

body mass index (BMI): A measure that relates body weight to height. BMI is sometimes used to measure total body fat and whether

---

This glossary contains terms excerpted from documents produced by several sources deemed reliable.

a person is a healthy weight. Excess body fat is linked to an increased risk of some diseases including heart disease and some cancers.

bronchoscopy: A procedure that uses a bronchoscope to examine the inside of the trachea, bronchi (air passages that lead to the lungs), and lungs. A bronchoscope is a thin, tube-like instrument with a light and a lens for viewing. It may also have a tool to remove tissue to be checked under a microscope for signs of disease.

cardiovascular: Having to do with the heart and blood vessels.

colonoscopy: Examination of the inside of the colon using a colonoscope, inserted into the rectum. A colonoscope is a thin, tube-like instrument with a light and a lens for viewing. It may also have a tool to remove tissue to be checked under a microscope for signs of disease.

complete blood count (CBC): A test to check the number of red blood cells (RBCs), white blood cells (WBCs), and platelets in a sample of blood.

computed tomography (CT) scan: A series of detailed pictures of areas inside the body taken from different angles. The pictures are created by a computer linked to an X-ray machine. Also called computerized axial tomography (CAT) scan.

contrast material: A dye or other substance that helps show abnormal areas inside the body. It is given by injection into a vein, by enema, or by mouth. Contrast material may be used with X-rays, CT scans, magnetic resonance imaging (MRI), or other imaging tests.

core biopsy: The removal of tissue or fluid with a wide needle for examination under a microscope.

cystoscopy: Examination of the bladder and urethra using a cystoscope, inserted into the urethra. A cystoscope is a thin, tube-like instrument with a light and a lens for viewing. It may also have a tool to remove tissue to be checked under a microscope for signs of disease.

deoxyribonucleic acid (DNA): The molecules inside cells that carry genetic information and pass it from one generation to the next.

DEXA scan: An imaging test that measures bone density (the amount of bone mineral contained in a certain volume of bone) by passing X-rays with two different energy levels through the bone. It is used to diagnose osteoporosis (decrease in bone mass and density). Also, called bone mineral density (BMD) scan, dual energy X-ray absorptiometric (DEXA) scan, dual X-ray absorptiometry (DXA).

electrocardiogram (EKG): A line graph that shows changes in the electrical activity of the heart over time. It is made by an instrument called an electrocardiograph (ECG or EKG). The graph can show that there are abnormal conditions, such as blocked arteries, changes in electrolytes (particles with electrical charges), and changes in the way electrical currents pass through the heart tissue.

endoscopic retrograde cholangiopancreatography (ERCP): A procedure that uses an endoscope to examine and X-ray the pancreatic duct, hepatic duct, common bile duct, duodenal papilla, and gallbladder. An endoscope is a thin, tube-like instrument with a light and a lens for viewing.

endoscopy: A procedure that uses an endoscope to examine the inside of the body. An endoscope is a thin, tube-like instrument with a light and a lens for viewing. It may also have a tool to remove tissue to be checked under a microscope for signs of disease.

false-positive test result: A test result that indicates that a person has a specific disease or condition when the person actually does not have the disease or condition.

fine-needle aspiration (FNA) biopsy: The removal of tissue or fluid with a thin needle for examination under a microscope.

fluoroscopy: An X-ray procedure that makes it possible to see internal organs in motion.

genetic counseling: A communication process between a specially trained health professional and a person concerned about the genetic risk of disease. The person's family and personal medical history may be discussed, and counseling may lead to genetic testing.

genetic testing: Analyzing deoxyribonucleic acid (DNA) to look for a genetic alteration that may indicate an increased risk for developing a specific disease or disorder.

imaging: In medicine, a process that makes pictures of areas inside the body. Imaging uses methods such as X-rays (high-energy radiation), ultrasound (high-energy sound waves), and radio waves.

laboratory test: A medical procedure that involves testing a sample of blood, urine, or other substance from the body. Tests can help determine a diagnosis, plan treatment, check to see if treatment is working, or monitor the disease over time.

lower gastrointestinal (GI) series: X-rays of the colon and rectum that are taken after a person is given a barium enema.

673

lumbar puncture: A procedure in which a thin needle called a spinal needle is put into the lower part of the spinal column to collect cerebrospinal fluid (CSF) or to give drugs. Also, called spinal tap.

magnetic resonance imaging (MRI): A procedure in which radio waves and a powerful magnet linked to a computer are used to create detailed pictures of areas inside the body. These pictures can show the difference between normal and diseased tissue. MRI makes better images of organs and soft tissue than other scanning techniques, such as computed tomography (CT) or X-ray. MRI is especially useful for imaging the brain, the spine, the soft tissue of joints, and the inside of bones. Also, called nuclear magnetic resonance imaging (NMRI).

monitor: In medicine, to regularly watch and check a person or condition to see if there is any change. Also refers to a device that records and or displays patient data, such as for an electrocardiogram (EKG).

myelogram: An X-ray of the spinal cord after an injection of dye into the space between the lining of the spinal cord and brain.

nuclear magnetic resonance imaging (NMRI): A procedure in which radio waves and a powerful magnet linked to a computer are used to create detailed pictures of areas inside the body. These pictures can show the difference between normal and diseased tissue. NMRI is especially useful for imaging the brain, the spine, the soft tissue of joints, and the inside of bones.

optical coherence tomography (OCT): A procedure that uses infrared light waves to give three-dimensional (3D) pictures of structures inside tissues and organs. The pictures are made by a computer linked to the light source.

Papanicolaou test (Pap test): A procedure in which cells are scraped from the cervix for examination under a microscope. It is used to detect cancer and changes that may lead to cancer. Also, called Pap smear test.

pelvic exam: A physical examination in which the healthcare professional will feel for lumps or changes in the shape of the vagina, cervix, uterus, fallopian tubes, ovaries, and rectum. The healthcare professional will also use a speculum to open the vagina to look at the cervix and take samples for a Pap test. Also, called internal examination.

positive test result: A test result that reveals the presence of a specific disease or condition for which the test is being done.

positron emission tomography (PET) scan: A procedure in which a small amount of radioactive glucose (sugar) is injected into a vein, and a scanner is used to make detailed, computerized pictures of areas inside the body where the glucose is used. Because cancer cells often use more glucose than normal cells, the pictures can be used to find cancer cells in the body.

radiology: The use of radiation (such as X-rays) or other imaging technologies (such as ultrasound and magnetic resonance imaging (MRI)) to diagnose or treat disease.

screening: Checking for disease when there are no symptoms. Since screening may find diseases at an early stage, there may be a better chance of curing the disease. Examples of cancer screening tests are the mammogram (breast), colonoscopy (colon), Pap smear (cervix), and prostate-specific antigen (PSA) blood level and digital rectal exam (DRE) (prostate). Screening can also include checking for a person's risk of developing an inherited disease by doing a genetic test.

sentinel lymph node biopsy (SLNB): Removal and examination of the sentinel node(s) (the first lymph node(s) to which cancer cells are likely to spread from a primary tumor).

sigmoidoscopy: Examination of the lower colon using a sigmoidoscope, inserted into the rectum. A sigmoidoscope is a thin, tube-like instrument with a light and a lens for viewing. It may also have a tool to remove tissue to be checked under a microscope for signs of disease.

single photon emission computed tomography (SPECT): A special type of computed tomography (CT) scan in which a small amount of a radioactive drug is injected into a vein and a scanner is used to make detailed images of areas inside the body where the radioactive material is taken up by the cells. Single photon emission computed tomography (SPECT) can give information about blood flow to tissues and chemical reactions (metabolism) in the body.

skin test: A test for an immune response to a compound by placing it on or under the skin. slit-lamp eye exam: An eye exam using an instrument that combines a low-power microscope with a light source that makes a narrow beam of light. The instrument may be used to examine the retina, optic nerve, and other parts of the eye. Also, called slit-lamp biomicroscopy.

spiral computed tomography (CT) scan: Detailed picture of areas inside the body. The pictures are created by a computer linked to an X-ray machine that scans the body in a spiral path. Also, called helical computed tomography (CT).

symptom: An indication that a person has a condition or disease. Some examples of symptoms are headache, fever, fatigue, nausea, vomiting, and pain.

ultrasound: A procedure in which high-energy sound waves are bounced off internal tissues or organs and make echoes. The echo patterns are shown on the screen of an ultrasound machine, forming a picture of body tissues called a sonogram. Also, called ultrasonography.

upper endoscopy: Examination of the inside of the stomach using an endoscope, passed through the mouth and esophagus. An endoscope is a thin, tube-like instrument with a light and a lens for viewing. It may also have a tool to remove tissue to be checked under a microscope for signs of disease. Also, called gastroscopy.

upper gastrointestinal (GI) series: A series of X-ray pictures of the esophagus, stomach, and duodenum (the first part of the small intestine). The X-ray pictures are taken after the patient drinks a liquid containing barium sulfate (a form of the silver-white metallic element barium). The barium sulfate coats and outlines the inner walls of the upper gastrointestinal tract so that they can be seen on the X-ray pictures.

ureteroscopy: Examination of the inside of the kidney and ureter, using a ureteroscope. A ureteroscope is a thin, tube-like instrument with a light and a lens for viewing. It may also have a tool to remove tissue to be checked under a microscope for signs of disease. The ureteroscope is passed through the urethra into the bladder, ureter, and renal pelvis (part of the kidney that collects, holds, and drains urine).

urinalysis: A test that determines the content of the urine.

virtual colonoscopy (VC): A method to examine the inside of the colon by taking a series of X-rays. A computer is used to make two-dimensional (2D) and three-dimensional (3D) pictures of the colon from these X-rays. The pictures can be saved, changed to give better viewing angles, and reviewed after the procedure, even years later. Also, called computed tomographic colonography (CTC).

X-ray: A type of high-energy radiation. In low doses, X-rays are used to diagnose diseases by making pictures of the inside of the body. In high doses, X-rays are used to treat cancer.

Chapter 67

Online Health Screening Tools

Web-Based Online Information for Medical Tests

Alcoholism, Drug Dependence, and Addictions

Alcohol and Drug Assessments and Evaluation
Hazelden Betty Ford Foundation (HBFF)
Website: www.aboutmydrinking.org

Food Addiction
Addiction.com
Website: www.addiction.com/addiction-a-to-z/food-addiction

Nicotine Addiction
Addiction.com
Website: www.addiction.com/addiction-a-to-z/drug-addiction/
nicotine-addiction

The mobile apps listed in this chapter were excerpted from "FDA-Cleared Mobile Medical Applications," U.S. Food and Drug Administration (FDA), January 9, 2017. Inclusion does not constitute endorsement, and there is no implication associated with omission. All website information was verified and updated in July 2018.

Auditory

Auditory Sensitivity Toolkit
The Watson Institute
Website: www.thewatsoninstitute.org/watson-life-resources/
situation/auditory-sensitivity-toolkit

What Hearing Loss Sounds Like
Starkey
Website: www.starkey.com/hearing-loss-simulator

Autism

Autistic Disorder Test
Iautistic
Website: iautistic.com/free-autism-tests.php

Developmental Milestones
Centers for Disease Control and Prevention (CDC)
Website: www.cdc.gov/ncbddd/actearly/milestones

Bone and Joint Risk Assessments

Health Risk Assessments
Kaweah Delta Medical Center
Website: www.kaweahdelta.org/Health-Risk-Assessments.aspx

JointAware Risk Assessment
Kaweah Delta Medical Center
Website: www.kaweahdelta.org/Our-Services/Orthopedics/
JointAware-Risk-Assessment.aspx

Orthopedic Health Risk Assessments
HealthAware
Website: healthaware.com/health-risk-assessment-orthopedic

Cancer Risk Assessments

Breast Cancer Risk Assessment Tool
National Cancer Institute (NCI)
Website: www.cancer.gov/bcrisktool/Default.aspx

Lung Cancer Screening Decision Tool
Memorial Sloan-Kettering Cancer Center (MSKCC)
Website: www.mskcc.org/cancer-care/types/lung/screening/
lung-screening-decision-tool

Ovarian Cancer Risk Assessment
University of Rochester Medical Center (URMC)
Website: www.urmc.rochester.edu/encyclopedia/content.
aspx?contenttypeid=42&contentid=OvarianCancerRisk

Prostate Cancer Prevention Trial Risk Calculator (PCPTRC)
CCF Risk Calculator
Website: riskcalc.org/PCPTRC

Risk Assessment Test
Pancreatic Cancer Action Network (PanCAN)
Website: www.pancan.org/facing-pancreatic-cancer/
about-pancreatic-cancer/risk-factors/risk-assessment-test

Stomach Cancer Risk Factors
American Cancer Society (ACS)
Website: www.cancer.org/cancer/stomach-cancer/causes-risks-
prevention/risk-factors.html

Uterine Cancer Risk
Foundation for Women's Cancer (FWC)
Website: www.foundationforwomenscancer.org/risk-awareness/
uterine-cancer-risk

Your Disease Risk
Siteman Cancer Center, Washington University in St. Louis
Website: siteman.wustl.edu/prevention/
ydr/?lang=english&func=home&quiz=osteoporosis

Diabetes and Kidney Disease Risk

Diabetes Risk Assessment
Harold Hamm Diabetes Center
Website: haroldhamm.org/diabetesprevention/risk.aspx

Diabetes Risk Score
Diabetes UK
Website: riskscore.diabetes.org.uk/start

Glomerular Filtration Rate (GFR) Calculators
National Institute of Diabetes and Digestive and Kidney Diseases
(NIDDK)
Website: www.niddk.nih.gov/health-information/
communication-programs/nkdep/laboratory-evaluation/
glomerular-filtration-rate-calculators

Type 2 Diabetes Risk Test
American Diabetes Association (ADA)
Website: www.diabetes.org/diabetes-basics/prevention/
diabetes-risk-test

Heart Attack Risk, Heart Disease Risk, and Arterial Age Risk

Heart Disease Risk Assessment
American College of Cardiology (ACC)
Website: www.cardiosmart.org/Tools/Heart-Disease-Risk-Assessment

My Life Check—Life's Simple 7
American Heart Association (AHA)
Website: mylifecheck.heart.org/PledgePage.
aspx?NavID=5&CultureCode=en-US

MESA Risk Score Calculator
MESA Coordinating Center
Website: www.mesa-nhlbi.org/CACReference.aspx

Warning Signs of a Heart Attack
American Heart Association (AHA)
Website: www.heart.org/HEARTORG/Conditions/HeartAttack/
WarningSignsofaHeartAttack/Warning-Signs-of-a-Heart-Attack_
UCM_002039_Article.jsp#.W1A64R9fg8o

Infectious Disease Risk Assessment

Are You at Risk for HIV?
TheBody.com
Website: www.thebody.com/surveys/sexsurvey.html

Malaria Risk Assessment for Travelers
Centers for Disease Control and Prevention (CDC)
Website: www.cdc.gov/malaria/travelers/risk_assessment.html

Mental Health Risk Assessments

**Adult ADHD Self-Report Scale (ASRS-v1.1) Symptom Checklist
Instructions**
Attention Deficit Disorder Association (ADDA)
Website: add.org/wp-content/uploads/2015/03/adhd-questionnaire-
ASRS111.pdf

Adult ADHD Self-Report Scale-V1.1 (ASRS-V1.1) Symptoms Checklist from WHO Composite International Diagnostic Interview
Harvard Medical School
Website: www.hcp.med.harvard.edu/ncs/ftpdir/adhd/18Q_ASRS_English.pdf

Bipolar Disorder Test
Psych Central
Website: psychcentral.com/quizzes/bipolar-quiz

Diagnosing Anxiety Disorders in Adults
NYU Langone Hospitals
Website: www.med.nyu.edu/psych/patient-care/screening-tests/anxiety-screening-test

Stress Screener
Mental Health America (MHA)
Website: www.mentalhealthamerica.net/stress-screener

Pregnancy

Online Pregnancy Test
BabyMed.com
Website: www.babymed.com/online-pregnancy-test

Ovulation Calendar
American Pregnancy Association
Website: americanpregnancy.org/ovulation-calendar

Pregnancy Due Date Calculator
BabyMed.com
Website: www.babycenter.com/pregnancy-due-date-calculator

Radiation Exposure Risk

RADAR Medical Procedure Radiation Dose Calculator and Consent Language Generator
RADAR
Website: www.doseinfo-radar.com/RADARDoseRiskCalc.html

Sexual Health

Sexual Addiction Screening Test (Women)
Healthy Place
Website: www.healthyplace.com/psychological-tests/sexual-addiction-screening-test-women

Sexual Addiction Screening Test (Men)
Healthy Place
Website: www.healthyplace.com/psychological-tests/
sexual-addiction-screening-test-men

Sleep

Sleep Risk Assessment
Austin Medical Group
Website: www.austinmedicalgroup.com/contents/
sleep-risk-assessment

Stroke

Stroke Risk Assessment Tool (SRAT)
National Stroke Association
Website: www.stroke.org/we-can-help/healthcare-professionals/
improve-your-skills/tools-training-and-resources/tools/stroke

Visual Tests

Color Vision Testing
ColorVisionTesting
Website: www.colorvisiontesting.com

Distance Vision Test for Adults
Prevent Blindness America (PBA)
Website: www.preventblindness.org/distance-vision-test-adults

Near Vision Test for Adults
Prevent Blindness America (PBA)
Website: www.preventblindness.org/near-vision-test-adults

Weight Risk

Body Mass Index Calculator
National, Heart, Lung, and Blood Institute (NHLBI)
Website: www.nhlbi.nih.gov/health/educational/lose_wt/BMI/
bmicalc.htm

Weight Assessment Tools
Capital District Physicians' Health Plan (CDPHP)
Website: www.cdphp.com/weight-management/
weight-assessment-tools

Mobile Apps for Medical Tests

ACCU-CHEK® Connect App

The Accu-Chek® Connect diabetes management app is intended as an aid in the treatment of diabetes. The Accu-Chek® Connect diabetes management app provides for electronic download of blood glucose meters, manual data entry, storage, display, transfer, and self-managing of blood glucose and other related health indicators that can be shown in report and graphical format.
Website: play.google.com/store/apps/details?id=com.roche. acconnect&hl=en_IN

AirStrip ONE®

AirStrip ONE® is the complete enterprise solution that provides the architecture and interactive user experience that fully delivers on the promise of clinical mobility. Since all relevant capabilities are built into the system, AirStrip ONE® can dramatically accelerate enterprise-wide implementation, time-to-benefit, and return on investment (ROI).
Website: play.google.com/store/apps/details?id=com.airstrip. one&hl=en_IN

aycan mobile

The aycan mobile is an iPad app that allows to display Digital Imaging and Communications in Medicine (DICOM) images.
Website: itunes.apple.com/sg/app/aycan-mobile/id419601797?mt=8

BlueStar Diabetes

BlueStar® is an in-app diabetes coach. You can lower your A1C and achieve your diabetes health goals using this app.
Website: play.google.com/store/apps/details?id=com.welldoc. platform.android&hl=en_IN

Change Healthcare ECG Mobile

Change Healthcare Cardiology ECG Mobile is much more than an electrocardiography (ECG) viewing application. ECG Mobile is a full-featured reporting platform designed with a robust set of clinical tools to easily and intuitively diagnose 12-lead resting ECGs anytime anywhere.
Website: itunes.apple.com/th/app/mckesson-ecg-mobile/ id869262739?mt=8

683

Gmate® SMART

Gmate® SMART is designed to help diabetics measure their blood glucose. You would need an additional device that is connected to Galaxy S3 to test your blood glucose as Gmate® SMART will show you. Your glucose level will be displayed on the screen after the test and you can e-mail the test result with additional memo.

Website: play.google.com/store/apps/details?id=com.philosys. gmatesmart&hl=en

Jack Imaging Medical

Jack Imaging Medical Image Viewer is a medical image viewer for the iPad that supports reading the Digital Imaging and Communications in Medicine (DICOM) format. Jack Imaging Medical Image Viewer supports fast-user interaction for the most common actions, including zoom, pan, windowing (brightness and contrast adjustment) using multitouch gestures.

Website: itunes.apple.com/us/app/jack-imaging-medical/ id431495135?mt=8

Kardia

The Kardia app, paired with Kardia Mobile, is used for accurate electrocardiogram (ECG or EKG) recordings.

Website: itunes.apple.com/in/app/kardia/id579769143?mt=8

Mobile MIM

The Mobile MIM software program is used for the viewing, registration, fusion, and/or display for diagnosis of medical images from the following modalities: Single-photon emission computed tomography (SPECT), positron emission tomography (PET), computed tomography (CT), magnetic resonance imaging (MRI), X-ray, and Ultrasound. Mobile MIM can be used to review images, contours, DVH, and isodose curves from radiation treatment plans. Mobile MIM can be used to approve these plans. Mobile MIM provides wireless and portable access to medical images. This app is not to be used for mammography.

Website: itunes.apple.com/in/app/mobile-mim/id281922769?mt=8

NIH's BMI Calculator

The National Heart, Lung, and Blood Institute's (NHLBI) body mass index (BMI) calculator is tool to screen for weight categories that may lead to health problems. The downloadable phone application puts the

fully functioning calculator right on your phone, along with links to resources on the NHLBI site.
Website: itunes.apple.com/us/app/nhlbi-bmi-calculator/ id446441346?mt=8

Optum TeleHealth

The Optum TeleHealth Solution delivers that knowledge wirelessly through scales, blood pressure monitors, pulse oxymeters, thermometers, and user-friendly health questions. The information collected through these devices is shared securely with both patients and their providers, arming both with vital data to help people stay healthy, get healthy or live with a condition.
Website: play.google.com/store/apps/details?id=com.optum. telehealth&hl=en_IN

Chapter 68

Directory of Breast and Cervical Cancer Early Detection Programs

Alabama

Breast and Cervical Cancer Early Detection Program, Alabama Department of Public Health (ADPH)
P.O. Box 303017
Montgomery, AL 36130
Toll-Free: 877-252-3324
Website: www.alabamapublichealth.gov/bandc

Alaska

Breast and Cervical Health Check (BCHC), Division of Public Health Section of Women's, Children's, and Family Health
3601 C St.
Ste. 902
Anchorage, AK 99503
Toll-Free: 800-410-6266
Phone: 907-269-3476
Website: dhss.alaska.gov/dph/wcfh/Pages/bchc/default.aspx

Resources in this chapter were compiled from several sources deemed reliable; all contact information was verified and updated in July 2018.

Arizona

Well Woman HealthCheck Program (WWHP)
150 N., 18th Ave.
Phoenix, AZ 85007
Phone: 602-542-1025
Fax: 602-542-0883
Website: azdhs.gov/hsd/
healthcheck/wellwoman

California

Cancer Detection Programs: Every Woman Counts (EWC), California Department of Health Care Services (DHCS)
MS 4600, P.O. Box 997417
Sacramento, CA 95899-7417
Toll-Free: 800-511-2300
Phone: 916-449-5300
Fax: 916-440-5310
Website: www.dhcs.ca.gov/services/
Cancer/ewc/Pages/default.aspx
E-mail: cancerdetection@dhcs.
ca.gov

Colorado

Women's Wellness Connection (WWC), Colorado Department of Public Health and Environment (CDPHE)
4300 Cherry Creek Dr. S.
Denver, CO 80246
Toll-Free: 800-886-7689
Phone: 303-692-2200
Website: www.
colorado.gov/cdphe/
womens-wellness-connection
E-mail: cdphe.information@
state.co.us

Connecticut

Breast and Cervical Cancer Program (BCCP), Connecticut Department of Public Health (DPH)
410 Capitol Ave.
Hartford, CT 06134
Phone: 860-509-8000
Website: portal.ct.gov/DPH/
Comprehensive-Cancer/
Comprehensive-Cancer/
The-Connecticut-Breast-
and-Cervical-Cancer-Early-
Detection-Program

Delaware

Screening for Life, Division of Public Health (DPH)
417 Federal St.
Dover, DE 19901
Phone: 302-744-4704
Website: dhss.delaware.gov/dph/
dpc/sfl.html

District of Columbia

Breast and Cervical Cancer Early Detection Program, District of Columbia Department of Health
899 N. Capitol St. N.E.
Washington, DC 20002
Phone: 202-442-5900
Website: dchealth.dc.gov/vi/
service/breast-and-cervical-
cancer-program-project-wish

Florida

Breast and Cervical Cancer Early Detection Program, Florida Department of Health (DOH)
4052 Bald Cypress Way Bin A18
Tallahassee, FL 32399
Phone: 850-245-4330
Website: www.floridahealth.gov/
diseases-and-conditions/cancer/
breast-cancer/bccedp.html
E-mail: cancer@flhealth.gov

Georgia

Breast and Cervical Cancer Program (BCCP), Georgia Department of Public Health (DPH)
2 Peachtree St. N.W.
15th Fl.
Atlanta, GA 30303-3186
Toll-Free: 866-782-4584
Phone: 404-657-2700
Website: dph.georgia.gov/BCCP

Hawaii

Breast and Cervical Cancer Control Program (BCCCP), Hawaii Department of Health (DOH)
601 Kamokila Blvd.
Ste. 344
Kapolei, HI 96707
Phone: 808-692-7460
Fax: 808-692-7478
Website: health.hawaii.gov/
cancer/home/bcccp/
E-mail: webmail@doh.hawaii.gov

Illinois

Breast and Cervical Cancer Program (BCCP), Illinois Department of Public Health (IDPH)
525-535 W. Jefferson St.
Springfield, IL 62761
Toll-Free: 888-522-1282
Phone: 217-782-4977
Website: dph.illinois.gov/topics-
services/life-stages-populations/
womens-health-services/ibccp

Indiana

Breast and Cervical Cancer Early Detection Program, Indiana State Department of Health (ISDH)
2 N. Meridian St.
Indianapolis, IN 46204
Phone: 317-233-1325
Website: www.in.gov/isdh/24967.
htm

Iowa

Care for Yourself, Breast and Cervical Cancer Early Detection Program, Iowa Department of Public Health (IDPH)
Lucas State Office Bldg.
321 E. 12th St.
Des Moines, IA 50319
Toll-Free: 800-735-2942
Phone: 515-281-7689
Website: www.idph.state .ia.us/
careforyourself

Kansas

Early Detection Works (EDW), Kansas Department of Health and Environment (KDHE)
State Office Bldg., 1000 S.W.
Jackson, Ste. 230
Topeka, KS 66612-1274
Toll-Free: 877-277-1368
Phone: 785-296-1207
Fax: 785-559-4235
Website: www.kdheks.gov/edw/
E-mail: kdhe.edw@ks.gov

Kentucky

Women's Cancer Screening Program
275 E. Main St., HS1WF
Frankfort, KY 40621
Toll-Free: 844-249-0708
Phone: 502-564-3236
Fax: 502-564-1552
Website: chfs.ky.gov/agencies/
dph/dwh/Pages/cancer-screening.
aspx

Maine

Maine Breast and Cervical Health Program (MBCHP), Maine Department of Health and Human Services (DHHS)
11 State House Stn
Augusta, ME 04333
Toll-Free: 800-350-5180
Phone: 207-287-4348
Website: www.maine.gov/dhhs/
mecdc/population-health/bcp/
index.htm

Maryland

Breast and Cervical Cancer Screening Program, Center for Cancer Surveillance and Control (CCSC), Maryland Department of Health and Mental Hygiene (DHMH)
P.O. Box 13528
Baltimore, MD 21203
Toll-Free: 800-477-9774
Phone: 410-767-6787
Website: phpa.health.maryland.
gov/cancer/Pages/bccdt_home.aspx

Massachusetts

Women's Health Network, Massachusetts Department of Public Health (DPH)
250 Washington St.
Boston, MA 02108
Toll-Free: 877-414-4447
Phone: 617-624-6000
TTY: 617-624-6001
Fax: 617-624-5206
Website: www.mass.gov/eohhs/
gov/departments/dph

Michigan

Breast and Cervical Cancer Control Program (BCCCP), Michigan Department of Community Health (MDCH)
Capitol View Bldg., 333 S.
Grand Ave.
P.O. Box 30195
Lansing, MI 48913
Phone: 517-373-3740
Toll-Free TTY: 800-649-3777
Website: www.michigan.gov/
mdch/1,1607,7-132-2940_2955-
13487--,00.html

690

Minnesota

*SAGE Screening Program,
Minnesota Department of
Health*
85 E. Seventh Pl.,
P.O. Box 64882
St. Paul, MN 55164
Toll-Free: 888-643-2584
Phone: 651-201-5600
Fax: 651-201-5601
Website: www.health.state.
mn.us/divs/healthimprovement/
working-together/who-we-are/
sage.html

Mississippi

*Breast and Cervical Cancer
Early Detection Program,
Mississippi State Department
of Health (MSDH)*
570 E. Woodrow Wilson Dr.
Jackson, MS 39215
Toll-Free: 866-458-4948
Phone: 601-576-7400
Website: msdh.ms.gov/
msdhsite/_static/41,0,103.html

Missouri

*Show Me Healthy Women
(SMHW) Program, Missouri
Department of Health and
Senior Services*
P.O. Box 570
Jefferson City, MO 65102-0570
Toll-Free: 866-726-9926
Phone: 573-522-2845
Fax: 573-522-2898
Website: health.mo.gov/living/
healthcondiseases/chronic/
showmehealthywomen
E-mail: info@health.mo.gov

Montana

*Cancer Screening Services,
Montana Department of
Public Health and Human
Services (DPHHS)*
1400 Bdwy. Rm. C317
P.O. Box 202951
Helena, MT 59620-2951
Toll-Free: 888-803-9343
Phone: 406-444-0063
Toll-Free Fax: 877-764-7575
Website: dphhs.mt.gov/
publichealth/Cancer/
CancerScreening
E-mail: mwamsley@mt.gov

Nebraska

*Every Woman Matters
(EWM) Program, Nebraska
Department of Health and
Human Services*
301 Centennial Mall S. Third Fl.
P.O. Box 94817
Lincoln, NE 68509
Toll-Free: 800-532-2227
Phone: 402-471-0314
Fax: 402-471-0913
Website: dhhs.ne.gov/
publichealth/Pages/
womenshealth_ewm.aspx

Nevada

Women's Health Connection (WHC), Nevada Division of Public and Behavioral Health (DPBH)
4150 Technology Way
Carson City, NV 89706
Toll-Free: 877-385-2345
Phone: 775-684-2200
Fax: 775-684-4245
Website: dpbh.nv.gov/Programs/
WHC/Women_s_Health_
Connection_-_Home

New Hampshire

Breast and Cervical Cancer Program (BCCP), New Hampshire Department of Health and Human Services (DHHS)
129 Pleasant St.
Concord, NH 03301-3852
Toll-Free: 800-852-3345
Phone: 603-271-4931
Website: www.dhhs.nh.gov/dphs/
cdpc/bccp

New Jersey

New Jersey Cancer Education and Early Detection (NJCEED) Program, New Jersey Department of Health and Senior Services
P.O. Box 360
Trenton, NJ 08625-0360
Toll-Free: 800-328-3838
Website: www.state.nj.us/health/
ces/public/resources/njceed.shtml

New Mexico

Breast and Cervical Cancer Early Detection Program, New Mexico Department of Health
5301 Central Ave. N.E.
Ste. 800
Albuquerque, NM 87108
Toll-Free: 877-852-2585
Phone: 505-841-5840
Website: nmhealth.org/about/
phd/cdb/bcc

New York

Cancer Services Program (CSP), New York State Department of Health (NYSDOH)
Corning Tower, Empire State Plaza
Albany, NY 12237
Toll-Free: 866-442-CANCER
(866-442-2262)
Phone: 518-474-1222
Website: www.health.ny.gov/
contact
E-mail: dohweb@health.ny.gov

North Carolina

Breast and Cervical Cancer Control Program (BCCCP)
1922 Mail Service Center
Raleigh, NC 27699-1922
Phone: 919-707-5300
Fax: 919-870-4812
Website: bcccp.ncdhhs.gov/
contact.htm

North Dakota

Women's Way, North Dakota Department of Health
600 E. Blvd. Ave.
Dept. 301
Bismarck, ND 58505-0200
Toll-Free: 800-44-WOMEN
(800-449-6636)
Phone: 701-328-2306
Fax: 701-328-2036
Website: www.ndhealth.gov/womensway
E-mail: womensway@nd.gov

Oklahoma

Breast and Cervical Cancer Early Detection Program, Oklahoma State Department of Health (OSDH)
1000 N.E. 10th St.
Oklahoma City, OK 73117
Toll-Free: 888-669-5934
Phone: 405-271-4072
Fax: 405-271-6315
Website: www.ok.gov/health/Wellness/Chronic_Disease_Service/Cancer/Take_Charge,_Oklahomas_Breast_&_Cervical_Cancer_Early_Detection_Program

Oregon

Breast and Cervical Cancer Screening, Oregon Department of Human Services (ODHS)
800 N.E. Oregon St., Ste. 370
Portland, OR 97232
Toll-Free: 877-255-7070
Phone: 971-673-0581
Fax: 971-673-0997
Website: www.oregon.gov/oha/PH/HEALTHYPEOPLEFAMILIES/WOMEN/HEALTHSCREENING/Pages/Program-Information.aspx
E-mail: screenwise.info@dhsoha.state.or.us

Pennsylvania

HealthyWoman Program, Pennsylvania Department of Health
508 Main Capitol Bldg.
Harrisburg, PA 17120
Toll-Free: 800-215-7494
Fax: 717-772-0608
Website: www.health.pa.gov/My%20Health/Womens%20Health/HealthyWomen/Pages/Healthy%20Woman.aspx#.W024mnVuY8o

Rhode Island

Women's Cancer Screening Program, Rhode Island Department of Health
3 Capitol Hill
Providence, RI 02908
Phone: 401-222-4324
Website: www.health.ri.gov/programs/womenscancerscreening

South Dakota

*All Women Count! (AWC!)
Program, South Dakota
Department of Health (DOH)*
Robert Hayes Bldg., 600 E.
Capitol Ave.
Pierre, SD 57501-2536
Toll-Free: 800-738-2301
Phone: 605-773-3361
Fax: 605-773-5683
Website: doh.sd.gov/prevention/
all-women-count.aspx

Tennessee

*Breast and Cervical Cancer
Early Detection Program,
Tennessee Department of
Health*
Cordell Hull Bldg., 425 Fifth
Ave. N., Third Fl.
Nashville, TN 37247
Toll-Free: 877-969-6636
Phone: 615-532-6762
Fax: 615-253-5187
Website: www.tn.gov/health/
health-program-areas/fhw/mch-
cancer.html
E-mail: hit.health@state.tn.us

Texas

*Breast and Cervical Cancer
Services (BCCS), Texas
Health and Human Services
Commission (HHSC)*
1100 W. 49th St.
MC 1913, P.O. Box 149347
Austin, TX 78714-9347
Phone: 512-776-7796
Fax: 512-776-7203
Website: www.dshs.state.tx.us/
contact.shtm
E-mail: BCCSProgram@hhsc.
state.tx.us.

Utah

*Utah Cancer Control
Program (UCCP), Bureau
of Health Promotion, Utah
Department of Health
(UDOH)*
P.O. Box 142107
Salt Lake City, UT 84117-2107
Toll-Free: 800-717-1811
Fax: 801-536-0172
Website: cancerutah.org/
contact-us
E-mail: cyhealth@utah.gov

Vermont

*Ladies First, Vermont
Department of Health*
108 Cherry St.
Burlington, VT 05402
Toll-Free: 800-508-2222
Phone: 802-863-7330
Website: www.
healthvermont.gov/wellness/
ladies-first-members

Virginia

Breast and Cervical Cancer Screening, Virginia Department of Health (VDH)
109 Governor St.
P.O. Box 2448
Richmond, VA 23218-2448
Toll-Free: 866-395-4968
Website: www.vdh.virginia.gov/contact-us
E-mail: Free_screens@vdh.virginia.gov

West Virginia

Breast and Cervical Cancer Screening Program, Bureau for Public Health, West Virginia Department of Health and Human Resources (DHHR)
350 Capitol St., Rm. 427
Charleston, WV 25301
Toll-Free: 800-642-8522
Phone: 304-558-5388
Website: www.wvdhhr.org

Wisconsin

Wisconsin Well Woman Program (WWWP), Department of Health Services (DHS)
One W. Wilson St.
Madison, WI 53703
Phone: 608-266-1865
TTY: 711-947-3529
Toll-Free TTY: 800-947-3529
Website: www.dhs.wisconsin.gov/contacts.htm
E-mail: DHSwebmaster@dhs.wisconsin.gov

Wyoming

Wyoming Cancer Program, Wyoming Department of Health (WDH)
401 Hathaway Bldg.
Cheyenne, WY 82002
Toll-Free: 866-571-0944
Phone: 307-777-7656
Fax: 307-777-7439
Website: www.health.wyo.gov/publichealth/prevention/cancer

Chapter 69

Organizations with Resources for People Undergoing Medical Tests

Government Organizations Providing Information about Medical Tests

Agency for Healthcare Research and Quality (AHRQ)
Office of Communications and Knowledge Transfer (OCKT)
5600 Fishers Ln.
Seventh Fl.
Rockville, MD 20857
Phone: 301-427-1364 (For public inquiries: 301-427-1104)
Website: www.ahrq.gov

Centers for Disease Control and Prevention (CDC)
1600 Clifton Rd.
Atlanta, GA 30329-4027
Toll-Free: 800-CDC-INFO (800-232-4636)
Phone: 404-639-3311
Toll-Free TTY: 888-232-6348
Website: www.cdc.gov
E-mail: cdcinfo@cdc.gov

Resources in this chapter were compiled from several sources deemed reliable; all contact information was verified and updated in July 2018.

Centers for Medicare & Medicaid Services (CMS)
7500 Security Blvd.
Baltimore, MD 21244
Toll-Free: 800-MEDICARE
(800-633-4227)
Toll-Free TTY: 877-486-2048
Website: www.cms.gov

FDA Center for Devices and Radiological Health (CDRH)
U.S. Food and Drug Administration (FDA)
Website: www.fda.gov/
AboutFDA/CentersOffices/
OfficeofMedicalProducts
andTobacco/CDRH

FDA MedWatch
U.S. Food and Drug Administration (FDA)
Toll-Free: 800-FDA-1088
(800-332-1088)
Website: www.fda.gov/safety/
medwatch

Federal Trade Commission (FTC)
600 Pennsylvania Ave. N.W.
Washington, DC 20580
Toll-Free: 877-FTC-HELP
(877-382-4357)
Phone: 202-326-2222
Toll-Free TTY: 866-653-4261
Website: www.ftc.gov

National Breast and Cervical Cancer Early Detection Program (NBCCEDP)
Centers for Disease Control and Prevention (CDC)
Toll-Free: 800-CDC-INFO
(800-232-4636)
Toll-Free TTY: 888-232-6348
Website: www.cdc.gov/cancer/
nbccedp/index.htm

National Cancer Institute (NCI)
9609 Medical Center Dr.
BG 9609 MSC 9760
Bethesda, MD 20892-9760
Toll-Free: 800-4-CANCER
(800-422-6237)
Website: www.cancer.gov

National Eye Institute (NEI)
31 Center Dr.
MSC 2510
Bethesda, MD 20892-2510
Phone: 301-496-5248
Website: www.nei.nih.gov
E-mail: 2020@nei.nih.gov

National Institute of Diabetes and Digestive and Kidney Diseases (NIDDK)
Toll-Free: 800-860-8747
Toll-Free TTY: 866-569-1162
Website: www.niddk.nih.gov

National Institute of Mental Health (NIMH)
6001 Executive Blvd.
Rm. 6200, MSC 9663
Bethesda, MD 20892-9663
Toll-Free: 866-615-6464
Phone: 301-443-4536
TTY: 301-443-8431; Toll-Free
TTY: 866-415-8051
Fax: 301-443-4279
Website: www.nimh.nih .gov
E-mail: nimhinfo@nih.gov

National Institute of Neurological Disorders and Stroke (NINDS)
P.O. Box 5801
Bethesda, MD 20824
Toll-Free: 800-352-9424
Website: www.ninds.nih.gov

National Institute on Aging (NIA)
Bldg. 31 Rm. 5C27
31 Center Dr. MSC 2292
Bethesda, MD 20892
Toll-Free: 800-222-2225
Toll-Free TTY: 800-222-4225
Website: www.nia.nih.gov
E-mail: niaic@nia.nih.gov

National Institute on Deafness and Other Communication Disorders (NIDCD)
Office of Health Communication
and Public Liaison
31 Center Dr.
MSC 2320
Bethesda, MD 20892-2320
Toll-Free: 800-241-1044
Phone: 301-827-8183
Toll-Free TTY: 800-241-1055
Fax: 301-402-0018
Website: www.nidcd.nih.gov
E-mail: nidcdinfo@nidcd.nih.gov

Substance Abuse and Mental Health Services Administration (SAMHSA)
P.O. Box 2345
Rockville, MD 20847-2345
Toll-Free: 877-SAMHSA-7
(877-726-4727)
Toll-Free TTY: 800-487-4889
Fax: 240-221-4292
Website: www.samhsa.gov
E-mail: SAMHSAinfo@samhsa.
hhs.gov

U.S. Department of Health and Human Services (HHS)
200 Independence Ave. S.W.
Washington, DC 20201
Toll-Free: 877-696-6775
Website: www.hhs.gov

U.S. Food and Drug Administration (FDA)
10903 New Hampshire Ave.
Silver Spring, MD 20993
Toll-Free: 888-INFO-FDA
(888-463-6332)
Website: www.fda.gov

U.S. National Library of Medicine (NLM)
8600 Rockville Pike
Bethesda, MD 20894
Toll-Free: 888-FIND-NLM
(888-346-3656)
Phone: 301-594-5983
Website: www.nlm.nih.gov

U.S. Preventive Services Task Force (USPSTF)
5600 Fishers Ln.
MS 06E53A
Rockville, MD 20857
Website: www.
uspreventiveservicestaskforce.
org

Private Organizations Providing Information about Medical Tests

American Academy of Allergy, Asthma, and Immunology (AAAAI)
555 E. Wells St.
Ste. 1100
Milwaukee, WI 53202-3823
Phone: 414-272-6071
Website: www.aaaai.org

American Academy of Family Physicians (AAFP)
11400 Tomahawk Creek Pkwy
Leawood, KS 66211-2680
Toll-Free: 800-274-2237
Fax: 913-906-6075
Website: www.nf.aafp.org
E-mail: aafp@aafp.org

American Academy of Pediatrics (AAP)
345 Park Blvd.
Itasca, IL 60143
Toll-Free: 800-433-9016
Fax: 847-434-8000
Website: www.aap.org
E-mail: kidsdocs@aap.org

American Association of Neurological Surgeons (AANS)
5550 Meadowbrook Dr.
Rolling Meadows, IL 60008-3852
Toll-Free: 888-566-AANS
(888-556-2267)
Phone: 847-378-0500
Fax: 847-378-0600
Website: www.aans.org
E-mail: info@aans.org

American Cancer Society (ACS)
250 Williams St. N.W.
Atlanta, GA 30303
Toll-Free: 800-227-2345
Website: www.cancer.org

American College of Physicians (ACP)
190 N. Independence Mall W.
Philadelphia, PA 19106
Toll-Free: 800-523-1546
Phone: 215-351-2600
Website: www.acponline.org

American College of Radiology (ACR)
1891 Preston White Dr.
Reston, VA 20191
Toll-Free: 800-227-5463
Phone: 703-648-8900
Website: www.acr.org
E-mail: info@acr.org

American Diabetes Association (ADA)
2451 Crystal Dr.
Ste. 900
Arlington, VA 22202
Toll-Free: 800-DIABETES
(800-342-2383)
Website: www.diabetes.org

American Gastroenterological Association (AGA)
4930 Del Ray Ave.
Bethesda, MD 20814
Phone: 301-654-2055
Fax: 301-654-5920
Website: www.gastro.org
E-mail: member@gastro.org

American Heart Association (AHA)
National Center
7272 Greenville Ave.
Dallas, TX 75231
Toll-Free: 800-AHA-USA-1
(800-242-8721)
Phone: 214-570-5978
Website: www.heart.org

American Kidney Fund (AKF)
11921 Rockville Pike
Ste. 300
Rockville, MD 20852
Toll-Free: 800-638-8299
Website: www.kidneyfund.org
E-mail: helpline@kidneyfund.org

American Society of Echocardiography (ASE)
2530 Meridian Pkwy
Ste. 450
Durham, NC 27713
Phone: 919-861-5574
Fax: 919-882-9900
Website: asecho.org
E-mail: ase@asecho.org

American Society of Radiologic Technologists (ASRT)
15000 Central Ave. S.E.
Albuquerque, NM 87123-3909
Toll-Free: 800-444-2778
Phone: 505-298-4500
Fax: 505-298-5063
Website: www.asrt.org
E-mail: memberservices@asrt.org

American Speech-Language-Hearing Association (ASHA)
2200 Research Blvd.
Rockville, MD 20850-3289
Toll-Free: 800-638-8255
Phone: 301-296-5700
TTY: 301-296-5650
Fax: 301-296-8580
Website: www.asha.org
E-mail: actioncenter@asha.org

American Stroke Association
7272 Greenville Ave.
Dallas, TX 75231
Toll-Free: 888-4-STROKE
(888-478-7653)
Website: www.strokeassociation.
org

**Glaucoma Research
Foundation (GRF)**
251 Post St.
Ste. 600
San Francisco, CA 94108
Toll-Free: 800-826-6693
Phone: 415-986-3162
Fax: 415-986-3763
Website: www.glaucoma .org
E-mail: grf@glaucoma.org

Health Physics Society (HPS)
1313 Dolley Madison Blvd.
Ste. 402
McLean, VA 22101
Phone: 703-790-1745
Fax: 703-790-2672
Website: www.hps.org
E-mail: hps@BurkInc.com

Healthline
660 Third St.
San Francisco, CA 94107
Phone: 415-281-3100
Website: www.healthline.com

**International Foundation for
Functional Gastrointestinal
Disorders (IFFGD)**
P.O. Box 170864
Milwaukee, WI 53217
Phone: 414-964-1799
Website: www.iffgd.org

The Joint Commission
One Renaissance Blvd.
Oakbrook Terrace, IL 60181
Phone: 630-792-5000
Fax: 630-792-5005
Website: www.jointcommission.
org

**Juvenile Diabetes Research
Foundation International
(JDRF)**
26 Bdwy.
14th Fl.
New York, NY 10004
Toll-Free: 800-533-CURE
(800-533-2873)
Fax: 212-785-9595
Website: www.jdrf.org
E-mail: info@jdrf.org

March of Dimes
1275 Mamaroneck Ave.
White Plains, NY 10605
Phone: 914-997-4488
Website: www.marchofdimes.org

MedicineNet.com
Website: www.medicinenet.com

**Mental Health America
(MHA)**
500 Montgomery St.
Ste. 820
Alexandria, VA 22314
Toll-Free: 800-969-6642
Phone: 703-684-7722
Fax: 703-684-5968
Website: www.
mentalhealthamerica.net

National Kidney Foundation (NKF)
30 E. 33rd St.
New York, NY 10016
Toll-Free: 800-622-9010
Phone: 212-689-9261
Website: www.kidney.org
E-mail: info@kidney.org

National Newborn Screening and Genetics Resource Center (NNSGRC)
3907 Galacia Dr.
Austin, TX 78759
Phone: 512-921-1400
Website: genes-r-us.uthscsa.edu

National Sleep Foundation (NSF)
Website: sleepfoundation.org
E-mail: nsf@sleepfoundation.org

National Stroke Association
9707 E. Easter Ln.
Ste. B
Centennial, CO 80112
Toll-Free: 800-STROKES (800-787-6537)
Phone: 303-649-9299
Website: www.stroke.org
E-mail: info@stroke.org

The Nemours Foundation
10140 Centurion Pkwy N.
Jacksonville, FL 32256
Phone: 904-697-4100
Website: www.nemours.org

Radiological Society of North America (RSNA)
820 Jorie Blvd.
Oak Brook, IL 60523
Toll-Free: 800-381-6660
Phone: 630-571-2670
Fax: 630-571-7837
Website: www.rsna.org
E-mail: membership@rsna.org

Resolve: The National Infertility Association
7918 Jones Branch Dr.
Ste. 300
McLean, VA 22102
Phone: 703-556-7172
Fax: 703-506-3266
Website: www.resolve.org
E-mail: info@resolve.org

Susan G. Komen
5005 LBJ Fwy
Ste. 526
Dallas, TX 75244
Toll-Free: 877-GO-KOMEN (877-465-6636)
Website: ww5.komen.org
E-mail: Helpline@komen.org

University of Maryland Medical Center (UMMC)
22 S. Greene St.
Baltimore, MD 21201
Toll-Free: 800-492-5538
Phone: 410-328-8667
Website: www.umms.org

WebMD
Website: www.webmd.com

Index

Index